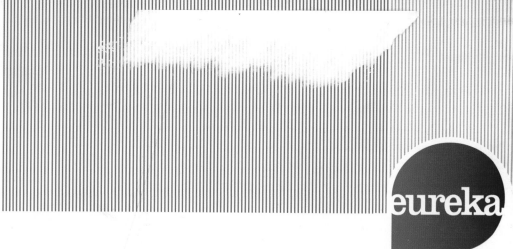

eureka

Gastrointestinal Medicine

D1418782

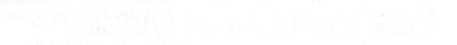

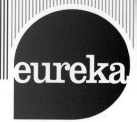

Gastrointestinal Medicine

Rachel Shakespeare MB BCh BSc
MRCP
Specialist Registrar in Gastroenterology
Wales Deanery
Cardiff, UK

Jeff Turner MB BCh MD FRCP PGCME
Consultant Gastroenterologist
Cardiff & Vale University Health Board
Cardiff, UK

John Green MB BCh MD FRCP PGCME
FAcadMEd
Consultant Gastroenterologist
Cardiff & Vale University Health Board
Clinical Senior Lecturer
Institute of Medical Education
Cardiff University
Cardiff, UK

Series Editors

Janine Henderson MRCPsych
MClinEd
MB BS Programme Director
Hull York Medical School
York, UK

David Oliveira PhD FRCP
Professor of Renal Medicine
St George's, University of London
London, UK

Stephen Parker BSc MS DipMedEd
FRCS
Consultant Breast and General
Paediatric Surgeon
St Mary's Hospital
Newport, UK

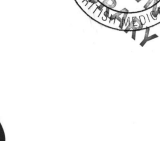
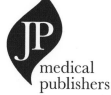
JP
medical
publishers

London • New Delhi • Panama City

© 2017 JP Medical Ltd.

Published by JP Medical Ltd, 83 Victoria Street, London, SW1H 0HW, UK

Tel: +44 (0)20 3170 8910   Fax: +44 (0)20 3008 6180

Email: info@jpmedpub.com   www.jpmedpub.com, www.eurekamedicine.com

ISBN: 978-1-909836-27-3

British Library Cataloguing in Publication Data
A catalogue record for this book is available from the British Library

Library of Congress Cataloging in Publication Data
A catalog record for this book is available from the Library of Congress

Publisher:	Richard Furn
Development Editors:	Thomas Banister-Fletcher, Paul Mayhew, Alison Whitehouse
Editorial Assistants:	Katie Pattullo, Adam Rajah
Copy Editor:	Carrie Walker
Graphic narratives:	James Pollitt
Cover design:	Forbes Design
Interior design:	Designers Collective Ltd

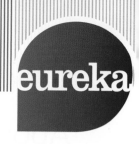

Series Editors' Foreword

Today's medical students need to know a great deal to be effective as tomorrow's doctors. This knowledge includes core science and clinical skills, from understanding biochemical pathways to communicating with patients. Modern medical school curricula integrate this teaching, thereby emphasising how learning in one area can support and reinforce another. At the same time students must acquire sound clinical reasoning skills, working with complex information to understand each individual's unique medical problems.

The *Eureka* series is designed to cover all aspects of today's medical curricula and reinforce this integrated approach. Each book can be used from first year through to qualification. Core biomedical principles are introduced but given relevant clinical context: the authors have always asked themselves, 'why does the aspiring clinician need to know this'?

Each clinical title in the series is grounded in the relevant core science, which is introduced at the start of each book. Each core science title integrates and emphasises clinical relevance throughout. Medical and surgical approaches are included to provide a complete and integrated view of the patient management options available to the clinician. Clinical insights highlight key facts and principles drawn from medical practice. Cases featuring unique graphic narratives are presented with clear explanations that show how experienced clinicians think, enabling students to develop their own clinical reasoning and decision making. Clinical SBAs help with exam revision while Starter questions are a unique learning tool designed to stimulate interest in the subject.

Having biomedical principles and clinical applications together in one book will make their connections more explicit and easier to remember. Alongside repeated exposure to patients and practice of clinical and communication skills, we hope *Eureka* will equip medical students for a lifetime of successful clinical practice.

Janine Henderson, David Oliveira, Stephen Parker

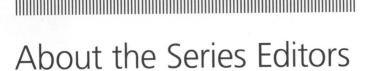

About the Series Editors

Janine Henderson is the MB BS undergraduate Programme Director at Hull York Medical School (HYMS). After medical school at the University of Oxford and clinical training in psychiatry, she combined her work as a consultant with postgraduate teaching roles, moving to the new Hull York Medical School in 2004. She has a particular interest in modern educational methods, curriculum design and clinical reasoning.

David Oliveira is Professor of Renal Medicine at St George's, University of London (SGUL), where he served as the MBBS Course Director between 2007 and 2013. Having trained at Cambridge University and the Westminster Hospital he obtained a PhD in cellular immunology and worked as a renal physician before being appointed as Foundation Chair of Renal Medicine at SGUL.

Stephen Parker is a Consultant Breast & General Paediatric Surgeon at St Mary's Hospital, Isle of Wight. He trained at St George's, University of London, and after service in the Royal Navy was appointed as Consultant Surgeon at University Hospital Coventry. He has a particular interest in e-learning and the use of multimedia platforms in medical education.

About the Authors

Rachel Shakespeare is a Specialist Registrar in Gastroenterology. She takes an active role in teaching gastroenterology and clinical skills to undergraduates, and enjoys delivering regular bedside teaching sessions.

Jeff Turner is a Consultant Gastroenterologist. He is a specialty lead for Cardiff University's C21 undergraduate curriculum and teaches clinical skills to medical students. He is also involved in writing endoscopy e-learning modules and is a Training Programme Director for postgraduate trainees in Wales.

John Green is the gastroenterology lead for the undergraduate medical course at Cardiff University. He is also the Year 3 director and is actively involved in teaching, assessment and the development of the new case-based curriculum. John is also a Consultant Gastroenterologist with an interest in endoscopy.

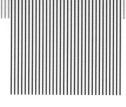

Preface

Eureka Gastrointestinal Medicine provides students with the knowledge they need to understand the digestive system and its disorders. It focuses on patients, how they present, the underlying causes of their conditions and the management strategies for treating them.

Chapter 1 outlines the normal structure and function of the gastrointestinal tract, thereby helping you to understand the scientific basis and consequences of the various disease states that affect it. Chapter 2 explains how to carry out a comprehensive patient assessment before going on to describe the range of investigations and management options available in this specialty. Subsequent chapters focus on disorders of different segments of the gastrointestinal tract, as well as the liver, biliary tree and pancreas. Clinical cases supplemented by graphic narratives provide insight into how experienced clinicians think, while full-colour artworks clarify concepts described in the text. The final chapters focus on emergency presentations and on how care of the patient is integrated between different health professionals in a variety of settings.

We have drawn from our own clinical practice and teaching experience to write *Eureka Gastrointestinal Medicine*. We hope the content, focus and learning points it contains will enable you to confidently evaluate a wide range of clinical presentations and equip you for success in exams and professional assessments in the future. Not only that, but we also hope it will stimulate your interest in this diverse, fascinating specialty.

Rachel Shakespeare, John Green, Jeff Turner
June 2017

Contents

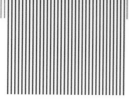

Glossary

5-ASA	5-aminosalicylic acid
5-HT	5-hydroxytryptamine
ACh	acetylcholine
AIDS	acquired immune deficiency syndrome
ALP	alkaline phosphatase
ALT	alanine transaminase
AMP	adenosine monophosphate
ANCA	anti-neutrophil cytoplasmic antibody
AST	aspartate transaminase
ATP	adenosine triphosphate
BMI	body mass index
CA	carbonic anhydrase
CCK	cholecystokinin
CRP	C-reactive protein
CT	computed tomography
CTZ	chemoreceptor trigger zone
DEXA	dual-energy X-ray absorptiometry
ECL	enterochromaffin-like
EMR	endoscopic mucosal resection
ERCP	endoscopic retrograde cholangiopancreatography
ESR	erythrocyte sedimentation rate
EUS	endoscopic ultrasound
FBC	full blood count
FODMAP diet	Fermentable oligosaccharides, disaccharides, monosaccharides and polyols diet
GGT	gamma-glutamyl transferase
GI	gastrointestinal
GORD	gastro-oesophageal reflux disease
GP	general practitioner
GTN	glyceryl trinitrate
HBA1c	haemoglobin A1c
HIDA	hydroxyl iminodiacetic acid
HIV	human immunodeficiency virus
IBD	inflammatory bowel disease

IBS	irritable bowel syndrome
IDA	iron deficiency anaemia
Ig	immunoglobulin
INR	international normalised ratio
IV	intravenous
LFTs	liver function tests
LOS	lower oesophageal sphincter
MDT	multidisciplinary team
MRCP	magnetic resonance cholangiopancreatography
MRI	magnetic resonance imaging
NAFLD	non-alcoholic fatty liver disease
NASH	non-alcoholic steato-hepatitis
NSAID	non-steroidal anti-inflammatory drug
OGD	oesophagogastroduodenoscopy
PBC	primary biliary cholangitis
PGE2	prostaglandin E2
PSC	primary sclerosing cholangitis
PET scan	positron emission tomography scan
PPI	proton pump inhibitor
PSC	primary sclerosing cholangitis
SAAG	serum–ascites albumin gradient
SBP	spontaneous bacterial peritonitis
SeHCAT	23-seleno-25-homotaurocholic acid testing
TFT	thyroid function test
TIPS	transjugular intrahepatic portosystemic shunt
TNM	tumour, node, metastases
tTG	tissue transglutaminase
ULN	upper limit of normal
US	ultrasound
VC	vomiting centre
VIP	vasoactive intestinal peptide

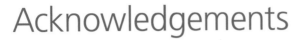

Acknowledgements

Our thanks go to Thomas Banister-Fletcher, Alison Whitehouse and Paul Mayhew from JP Medical for their expertise and patience when guiding us to write this book. We would particularly like to thank our families, colleagues and teachers who have supported us over many years.

Thanks to Meleri Morgan and Rwth Ellis-Owen for the images they supplied, and to Josh Ludlow and Helen Ludlow for the examination photos.

RS, JG, JT

The following figures are reproduced from other books published by JP Medical Ltd:

Figure 1.2 is copyright of Sam Scott-Hunter and is reproduced from Tunstall R, Shah N, *Pocket Tutor Surface Anatomy*. London: JP Medical 2012.

Figures 2.8 and 2.9 are reproduced from Cartledge P, Cartledge C, Lockey A, *Pocket Tutor Clinical Examination*. London: JP Medical Ltd, 2014.

Chapter 1
First principles

Starter questions

Answers to the following questions are on page 79.

1. Why does the GI system have its own nervous system?
2. What changes occur in the GI system as we age?
3. How might the GI system affect a person's mood and sleep pattern?
4. Why is the gut home to so many species of bacteria?

Overview of the gastrointestinal system

The gastrointestinal (GI) system comprises:

- the GI tract: a hollow tube that runs from the mouth to the anus, via the stomach and the small then the large intestine
- several secretary organs or glands: the salivary glands, liver, biliary system (gallbladder and biliary tree), spleen and pancreas

Its primary function is to provide the body with the hydration, nutrients and energy that it needs to function; these are obtained from fluids and food by the processes of digestion and absorption. The digestive process begins in the mouth and continues in the stomach, where a limited amount of absorption occurs. However, most digestion and absorption takes place in the small intestine. Fats, proteins and carbohydrates are broken down here into their smaller building blocks. These are then absorbed into the bloodstream alongside other nutrients, electrolytes and vitamins, and transported to the liver for metabolism, breakdown and storage.

Most of the water in food is absorbed in the small intestine; most of the remaining fluid is absorbed in the large intestine. Undigested material and waste products of digestion are eliminated by defaecation.

> 'Intestine' and 'bowel' are interchangeable terms, i.e. the small intestine is the same as the small bowel.

Overview of the GI tract

The GI tract is a continuous, hollow muscular tube that runs from the mouth to the anus (**Figure 1.1**). It comprises the:

- mouth
- pharynx
- oesophagus
- stomach
- small intestine (or bowel): duodenum, jejunum and ileum
- large intestine (or bowel): colon and rectum
- anus

Its regions or divisions have different functions and their structure is adapted to be as effective as possible at carrying out these functions (**Table 1.1**). Accessory organs – the salivary glands, liver, gallbladder and pancreas – facilitate the functioning of the different regions by releasing secretions into the GI tract, including enzymes which digest food.

From mouth to anus, the GI tract is approximately 9 m long in adults (**Table 1.2**).

> The small intestine is longer than the large intestine. 'Small' describes the diameter of its lumen (average 3 cm) compared with the lumen of the large intestine (average 7 cm).

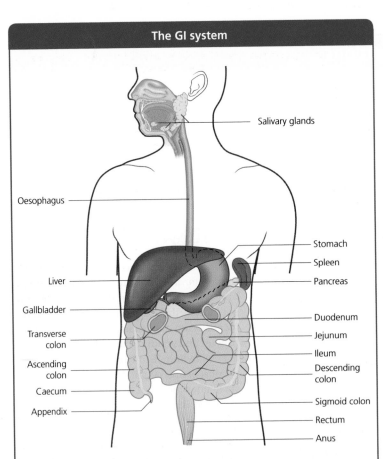

The GI system

Oesophagus

Liver

Gallbladder

Transverse colon

Ascending colon

Caecum

Appendix

Salivary glands

Stomach

Spleen

Pancreas

Duodenum

Jejunum

Ileum

Descending colon

Sigmoid colon

Rectum

Anus

Figure 1.1 The gastrointestinal system. Part of the transverse colon has been cut away here, to reveal the underlying duodenum; the spleen is shown displaced leftwards from its normal position, in which most of it lies posterior to the stomach.

Functions and adaptations of the GI system		
Region	Major function(s)*	Adaptation for GI function(s)
Mouth	Intake of food Start of mechanical digestion	Hollow cavity to receive food Teeth and tongue to help form a bolus which is moved to the pharynx then oesophagus
Salivary glands	Production of saliva for lubrication and chemical digestion through release of amylase	Millions of secretory cells
Pharynx	Common channel for swallowing and respiration	Muscular to propel food Protects airways from aspiration
Oesophagus	Transmission of food and liquids	Muscular tube with contractile waves
Stomach	Short-term storage of food (as a reservoir) Digestion – mechanical and chemical	Container that distends and contracts Produces gastric acid
Small intestine	Predominant GI site for digestion and absorption of nutrients	Surface area greatly increased by folds and finger-like villi
Liver	Filters blood travelling from intestines to IVC Produces bile, metabolises nutrients Major centre for synthesis (e.g. cholesterol, clotting factors, transporter proteins) and detoxification	Receives venous drainage from GI tract via portal vein Lobular structure puts arteries, veins, bile ducts and liver cells in close proximity
Spleen	B- and T-cell proliferation, immune response to blood-borne antigens, removal of old blood cells	No specific GI adaptations
Gallbladder	Storage and concentration of bile (a fat emulsifier)	Situated at start of small intestine and contracts when food arrives
Pancreas	Production of digestive enzymes (exocrine function) and hormones, e.g. insulin and glucagon (endocrine function)	Rich in secretory cells
Large intestine	Reabsorption of water Formation of faeces to excrete waste products	Wall and muscle layer thicken distally as contents become more solid
* Many regions also have other functions.		

Table 1.1 Major functions of the different regions of the GI system: each region is adapted to its functions. IVC, inferior vena cava

Length of regions of GI system	
Areas	Approximate length (cm)
Oesophagus	25
Stomach	25
Pancreas	15
Liver	15–20
Small intestine*	600–700
Duodenum	25
Jejunum	240
Ileum	350
Large intestine*	100–150

*The total surface areas of the small and large intestines are approximately 30 and 2 m², respectively.

Table 1.2 Normal length of regions of the GI system in adults

Anatomy

The digestive organs are contained within the abdominal cavity (**Figure 1.2**). This is bordered anteriorly and laterally by the abdominal wall, and posteriorly by the spinal column. The muscles of the diaphragm are above and the pelvic organs lie below.

Sphincters

Most regions of the GI tract are separated from the neighbouring regions by muscular thickenings called sphincters (**Table 1.3**). These sphincters open to allow the contents of the GI tract to pass from one section to the next. Ineffective sphincter function often results in symptoms, for example faecal incontinence.

Location of abdominal organs

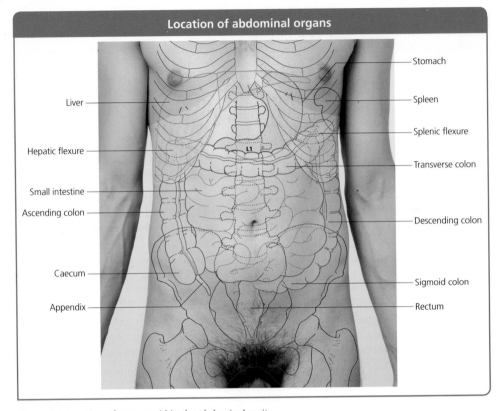

Figure 1.2 Location of organs within the abdominal cavity.

Sphincters of the GI tract	
Sphincter	**Situated between**
Upper oesophageal sphincter	Pharynx and oesophagus
Lower oesophageal sphincter	Oesophagus and stomach
Pylorus	Stomach and duodenum
Sphincter of Oddi	Common bile duct/pancreas and duodenum
Ileocaecal valve	Ileum and colon
Anal sphincter	Rectum and anus

Table 1.3 Sphincters of the GI tract

Most sphincters of the GI tract are involuntary (i.e. cannot be opened by conscious control) and are supplied by the autonomic nerves. The exception is the external anal sphincter which is voluntary and innervated by somatic nerves.

Peritoneum and peritoneal cavity

The peritoneum is a thin, transparent double-layered membrane within the abdominal cavity (**Figure 1.3**). Each layer is composed of a layer of squamous cells (mesothelium) and connective tissue. The two layers are:

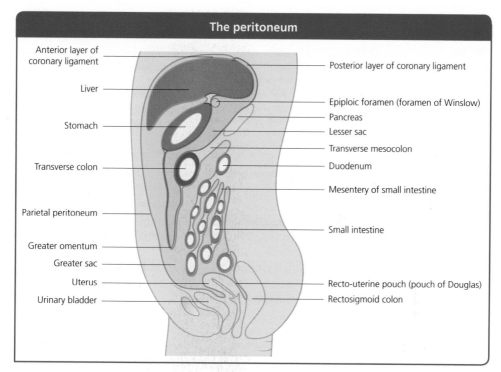

| The peritoneum |

Anterior layer of coronary ligament

Liver

Stomach

Transverse colon

Parietal peritoneum

Greater omentum

Greater sac

Uterus

Urinary bladder

Posterior layer of coronary ligament

Epiploic foramen (foramen of Winslow)

Pancreas

Lesser sac

Transverse mesocolon

Duodenum

Mesentery of small intestine

Small intestine

Recto-uterine pouch (pouch of Douglas)

Rectosigmoid colon

Figure 1.3 The peritoneum (female). The greater sac is shown in pink and the lesser sac in blue.

- **The visceral peritoneum**, which forms a continuous layer that covers the intestines and organs in the abdominal cavity
- **The parietal peritoneum**, which lines the internal surface of the abdominal and pelvic walls, as well as the undersurface of the diaphragm

The gap between the two layers of peritoneum is called the peritoneal cavity. It contains a small amount of lubricating fluid, which minimises friction.

As well as minimising friction, the peritoneum supports the abdominal organs and acts as a pathway for their blood vessels, nerves and lymphatic drainage. It also resists infection by exuding cells and fluid, and it stores fat.

A number of different structures are made out of the peritoneum:

- Greater omentum
- Lesser omentum
- Mesocolon
- Falciform ligament

- Greater sac (or general cavity)
- Lesser sac (or omental bursa)

These are described in **Table 1.4**. The greater omentum is a fatty apron composed of a fold of the visceral peritoneum. It cushions the intestines, and has a particularly important role, forming separate areas within the abdominal cavity, which help contain and prevent the spread of infection.

Peritoneal innervation and pain sensation

The two layers of the peritoneum are derived from different embryological layers of the mesoderm and therefore have different nerve supplies:

- The parietal peritoneum is derived from the 'somatic' mesoderm and has the same nerve supply as the overlying skin. It is very sensitive to pain, pressure, laceration and temperature.

Structures formed by the peritoneum		
Structure	**Location**	**Components**
Greater omentum	From greater curve of stomach and 1st part of duodenum, passing in front of small intestine and folding back on itself to enclose transverse colon, diaphragm and spleen, finally connecting to posterior abdominal wall	Gastrocolic ligament (greater curve of stomach and 1st part of duodenum to transverse colon)
		Gastrophrenic ligament (greater curve of stomach to diaphragm)
		Gastrosplenic ligament (greater curve of stomach to spleen)
Lesser omentum	From lesser curve of stomach and 1st part of duodenum to liver	Hepatogastric ligament (lesser curve of stomach to liver)
		Hepatoduodenal ligament (duodenum to liver)
Mesocolon	Attaching colon to posterior abdominal wall	Corresponds to region of colon attached (i.e. ascending, transverse, descending and sigmoid)
Mesentery	Attaching small intestine to posterior abdominal wall	Ileal and jejunal mesentery
Falciform ligament	Connecting liver to abdominal wall and diaphragm	–
Greater sac (or general cavity)	Forms majority of peritoneal cavity; connected to lesser sac via epiploic or omental foramen	–
Lesser sac (or omental bursa)	Smaller peritoneal cavity formed by lesser and greater omentum	–

Table 1.4 Structures formed by the peritoneum

■ The visceral peritoneum is derived from the 'splanchnic' mesoderm and has the same nerve supply as the organ it covers. It is sensitive only to stretch and chemical irritation. Pain from the visceral peritoneum is poorly localised. It is referred to the dermatome innervated by the same sensory ganglia and spinal cord segments as the underlying organ

> **The greater omentum is called the 'abdominal policeman' because of its role in cushioning the intestines and fighting intra abdominal infection.**

> **Referred pain is when pain is felt at a place away from the organ involved.** For instance the phrenic nerve supply to the diaphragm has the same origin as nerves supplying the skin around the shoulder tip. Injury or irritation (e.g. due to blood) to the diaphgram presents with shoulder tip pain.

Microstructure: walls of the GI tract

Along the length of the GI tract, the structure of its walls is adapted to optimise the differing functions of the different regions, so the detailed microstructure of the walls of the oesophagus and small intestine is very different for example. However, all regions have the same underlying microstructure, comprising four layers (**Figure 1.4**):

Layers of the GI wall

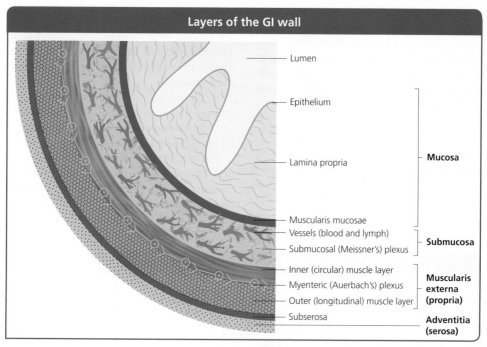

Figure 1.4 The layers of the GI wall have the same general structure throughout the length of the GI tract, with specialisations in different regions (see Figures **1.21, 1.25,** and **1.44**).

- Mucosa
- Submucosa
- Muscularis externa
- Adventitia (or serosa)

Mucosa

The mucosa is the innermost layer. It lies next to the luminal contents and has three components:

- **Epithelium** – a layer directly lining the lumen and containing glandular tissue. Its cells are regularly shed and rapidly replaced. In the mouth, oesophagus and anus this layer comprises stratified squamous cells which have a similar structure to the skin. In the rest of the intestine it is a single layer of columnar or glandular epithelium, which is best suited to digestion and absorption. The epithelium is robust and withstands the trauma of passing food or solid faeces
- **Lamina propria** – connective tissue containing capillaries that supply blood to the epithelium. This is where nutrients are absorbed into the bloodstream. The lamina propria also contains lymphoid follicles and plasma cells for immune regulation, as well as mucosal glands.
- **Muscularis mucosae** – a thin layer of muscle that facilitates local movement of the mucosa

Submucosa and submucosal plexus

The submucosa consists of connective tissue. Within it there are lymphatics, larger blood vessels, mucus-secreting glands and nerve endings, including the submucosal (Meissner's) plexus. This supplies the mucosa and submucosa.

Muscularis externa and myenteric plexus

This is made up of two layers of smooth muscle – an inner circular and an outer longitudinal layer. These are responsible for peristalsis, waves of muscle contraction that propel the contents along the GI tract (see page 19). The muscles are supplied by a network of nerves that run between the two layers – the myenteric (Auerbach's) plexus. Skeletal muscle rather than smooth muscle is present in certain areas, for example the proximal oesophagus and anus.

Adventitia (serosa)

The adventitia is the outer layer of the wall. It is composed of connective tissue and contains blood vessels, nerves and lymphatics. It is covered by visceral peritoneum.

Embryology of the GI tract

The human embryo has three layers that lie alongside the yolk sac – the ectoderm, mesoderm and endoderm. The gut is derived from the endoderm.

In the second week after fertilisation, the embryo begins to surround parts of the yolk sac. The enveloped portions form the basis of GI tract (**Figure 1.5**).

Folding of the embryo occurs between 3 and 4 weeks after fertilisation. This results in formation of the embryonic gut tube, which has three parts (**Table 1.5**):

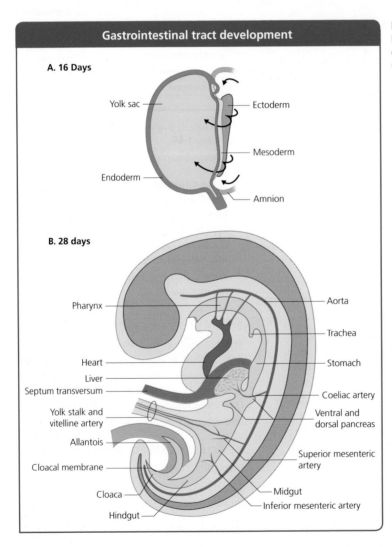

Gastrointestinal tract development

A. 16 Days

Yolk sac

Ectoderm

Mesoderm

Endoderm

Amnion

B. 28 days

Pharynx

Heart

Liver

Septum transversum

Yolk stalk and vitelline artery

Allantois

Cloacal membrane

Cloaca

Hindgut

Aorta

Trachea

Stomach

Coeliac artery

Ventral and dorsal pancreas

Superior mesenteric artery

Midgut

Inferior mesenteric artery

Figure 1.5 Embryological development of the GI tract.

Embryonic sections of the GI system		
Part	What it becomes	Blood supply
Foregut	Oesophagus, stomach, 1st and 2nd parts of duodenum, liver, gallbladder and pancreas (spleen is supplied by coeliac artery but is derived from dorsal mesentery)	Coeliac artery
Midgut	3rd and 4th parts of duodenum, jejunum, ileum, appendix, caecum and proximal ⅔ of transverse colon	Superior mesenteric artery
Hindgut	Distal ⅓ of transverse colon, descending colon, rectum and upper part of anal canal	Inferior mesenteric artery

Table 1.5 The three embryonic sections of the GI system

- foregut
- midgut
- hindgut

The boundaries of each part correlate to the artery that supplies them. Initially, the vitelline arteries, which supply and surround the yolk sac, form a plexus. This is later organised into the three main arteries that supply the abdominal GI tract:

- coeliac artery or trunk
- superior mesenteric artery
- inferior mesenteric artery

The stomach and colon develop as dilatations of the gut. Derivatives of the gut, such as the pancreas, develop as outpouchings. Further development occurs during embryonic maturation to produce the adult GI tract, as described in later subsections of this chapter.

In the GI tract the embryological origins of each part's neurovascular supply underpins many clinical characteristics, for example the locations of metastases from GI tumours.

Foregut

This extends from the buccopharyngeal (oral) membrane to the septum transversum (a mass of mesenchyme, i.e. embryonic connective tissue, that later develops into the thoracic diaphragm and ventral mesentery of the foregut). The foregut is divided into three parts:

- The first part becomes the pharynx
- The second (or thoracic) part gives rise to the respiratory bud and oesophagus

- The third (or abdominal) part passes through the septum transversum and gives rise to the intra-abdominal oesophagus, stomach and first half of the duodenum. This part is supplied by the coeliac artery, which runs in the embryonic septum transversum

Midgut

This is connected with the yolk sac, which provides nourishment via the vitelline duct. It is supplied by the superior mesenteric artery. It forms the second half of the duodenum (from the ampulla of Vater), jejunum, ileum, caecum, ascending colon and proximal two thirds of the transverse colon.

In Meckel's diverticulum the vitelline duct persists and forms a diverticulum from the small bowel. This is usually asymptomatic but rarely can cause bleeding; it is present in around 2% of the population.

Hindgut

This communicates with the allantoic diverticulum, which is the remnant of the allantois, the area where new blood vessels form outside the embryo and induce formation of the placenta. The hindgut extends to the cloacal membrane. It is supplied by the inferior mesenteric artery. This forms the distal third of the transverse colon, descending colon, sigmoid colon, rectum and upper part of the anal canal.

Blood and lymphatic vessels

Arterial supply

Three major arteries supply the GI system and accessory organs with oxygenated blood from the heart. These are the coeliac artery, superior mesenteric artery and inferior mesenteric artery, corresponding to the embryological foregut, midgut and hindgut, respectively (**Figure 1.6**, **Table 1.6**). They arise from the anterior surface of the abdominal aorta, which runs from the diaphragm to where it bifurcates into the common iliac arteries.

The three major arteries give rise to the vasa recta, which are smaller vessels that encircle the muscle layers of the intestinal wall and penetrate them to form an arterial plexus in the submucosa. Small arterial branches from the larger arteries also form an anastomosis (connection) on the mesenteric borders of the intestine to provide a collateral blood supply between the three major vessels. The mouth, pharynx, oesophagus and lower anal canal have a different arterial supply (see pages 25, 28, 32 and 77).

> The coeliac artery is only 1 cm long, hence the synonym 'coeliac trunk'. Almost immediately after branching from the aorta it divides into the left gastric, splenic and common hepatic arteries.

Venous drainage

The venous drainage from the GI system broadly follows the arterial supply (**Figure 1.7**):

- **The splenic vein,** which runs along the length of the pancreas underneath its posterior surface. It drains the spleen, stomach and part of the pancreas

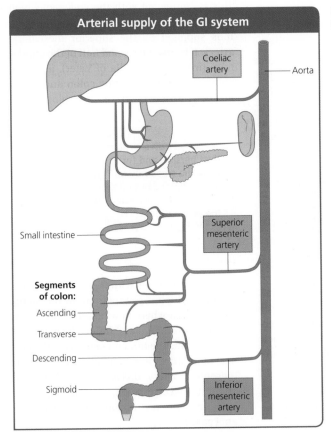

Arterial supply of the GI system

Coeliac artery

Aorta

Small intestine

Segments of colon:

Ascending

Transverse

Descending

Sigmoid

Superior mesenteric artery

Inferior mesenteric artery

Figure 1.6 Arterial supply of the GI system. See also **Figure 1.53**.

Arterial supply of the GI system

	Coeliac artery	Superior mesenteric artery	Inferior mesenteric artery
Region supplied	Foregut	Midgut	Hindgut
Extent	From abdominal oesophagus to midway down 2nd part of duodenum, at the ampulla of Vater (also includes pancreas, liver, biliary tree and spleen)	From midway down 2nd part of duodenum, at major papilla, to ⅔ of way across transverse colon	From ⅔ of way across transverse colon to halfway down anal canal
Vertebral level of origin from abdominal aorta	Upper L1	Lower L1	Lower L3
Major branches	Common hepatic (branches into hepatic, right gastric and gastroduodenal arteries) Left gastric Splenic	Ileal and jejunal Ileocolic Right colic Middle colic	Left colic Sigmoid Superior rectal

Table 1.6 Arterial supply of the GI system

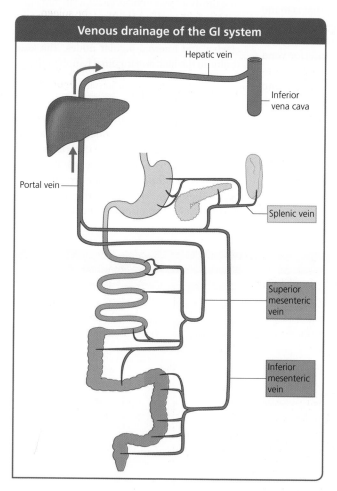

Venous drainage of the GI system

Hepatic vein

Inferior vena cava

Portal vein

Splenic vein

Superior mesenteric vein

Inferior mesenteric vein

Figure 1.7 Venous drainage of the GI system. See also **Figure 1.54**.

- **The superior mesenteric vein (SMV),** which drains the small intestine, caecum, ascending colon, proximal two thirds of the transverse colon and part of the pancreas
- **The inferior mesenteric vein (IMV),** joins the splenic vein. The IMV drains the distal third of the transverse colon, descending colon, and sigmoid colon to half way down the anal canal

The splenic vein and superior mesenteric vein combine to form the portal vein (or hepatic portal vein), the final common pathway for blood leaving the GI system. The portal vein also has veins which join it directly, draining parts of the stomach and pancreas. Blood that is deoxygenated, but carrying the nutrients absorbed from the GI tract, enters the liver via the portal vein (**Table 1.7**). There is a vascular bed within the liver that is made up of a network of microscopic vessels called sinusoids. These drain into the left and right hepatic veins which enter the inferior vena cava just before it passes through the diaphragm into the thorax and ultimately into the right atrium of the heart (see **Figure 1.32**).

Lymphatic drainage

Lymph is a fluid derived from plasma that contains nutrients, oxygen and carries lymphocytes and antibodies from lymph nodes to blood to help with fighting infection. In the intestinal lymphatic vessels, lymph is milky in colour (chyle) due to high levels of absorbed fatty acids.

Small-calibre lymphatic vessels (lacteals) within the intestinal wall take the lymph from the mucosa and submucosa, and drain through the muscularis externa. They then drain into larger channels that run alongside the arteries and veins. These channels enter local mesenteric lymph nodes, where lymphocytes and monocytes join the lymph from venules (small veins). These cells have a role in the immune function. The lymph drains via further lymphatics into larger para-aortic lymph nodes, and cisterna chyli (**Figure 1.8**). This becomes the thoracic duct which runs alongside the aorta into the thorax. Here, the duct empties into the junction of the left subclavian and internal jugular veins.

Lymphatic drainage of the oesophagus is into the thoracic, cervical, subclavian and internal jugular lymph nodes. The lymphatics of the mouth and thorax drain into the cervical, subclavian and internal jugular nodes. The anus drains to the iliac and inguinal lymph nodes.

Nerve supply

The GI tract has its own enteric nervous system, which does not need any external innervation to function. The enteric nervous system contains approximately 100 million neurones, a similar number to the spinal cord. These are located in the submucosa and between the circular and longitudinal

	Venous drainage of the GI system			
	Portal vein	Splenic vein	Superior mesenteric vein	Inferior mesenteric vein
Drainage	All GI tract below the gastro-oesophageal junction	Spleen, gastric fundus and part of pancreas	Stomach, pancreas Small intestine, caecum, ascending colon and proximal ⅔ of transverse colon	Distal ⅓ of transverse colon to halfway down anal canal
Venous tributaries	Splenic Superior mesenteric Gastric Cystic	Inferior mesenteric Short gastric Left gastroepiploic Small pancreatic	Right gastroepiploic Inferior pancreaticoduodenal Ileal and jejunal Ileocolic Right colic Middle colic	Left colic Sigmoid Superior rectal Rectosigmoid

Table 1.7 Venous drainage of the GI system

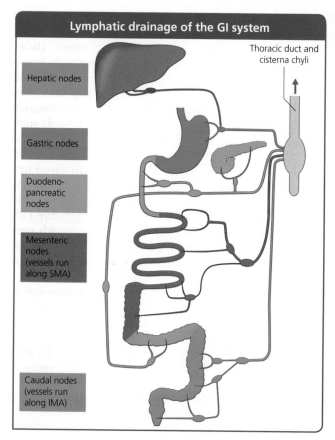

Lymphatic drainage of the GI system

Hepatic nodes

Gastric nodes

Duodeno-pancreatic nodes

Mesenteric nodes (vessels run along SMA)

Caudal nodes (vessels run along IMA)

Thoracic duct and cisterna chyli

Figure 1.8 Lymphatic drainage of the GI system. SMA, superior mesenteric artery; IMA, inferior mesenteric artery.

muscle layers of the muscularis externa (see **Figure 1.4**), making up the submucosal and myenteric plexuses:

■ **The submucosal plexus** aids secretion, e.g. of mucus, from nearby glands by providing a nerve stimulus. It also aids contraction of the muscularis mucosae which induces movement of the mucosa to expel contents from glands and increase the contact between the epithelium and luminal contents.
■ **The myenteric plexus** is responsible for peristalsis as impulses generated from here cause the nearby muscularis externa to contract.

As well as functioning as an independent nervous system, these plexuses receive input from the sympathetic and parasympathetic nervous systems, forming the 'gut–brain' axis, i.e. the signalling system between the GI tract and brain (**Figure 1.9**):

■ **Sympathetic supply** is from the thoracolumbar system. Sympathetic stimulation decreases smooth muscle activity, inhibiting peristalsis, resulting in sphincter contraction and reducing blood flow to the GI tract.
■ **Parasympathetic supply** is from the vagus (Xth cranial) nerve, which supplies the GI tract down to the distal two thirds of the transverse colon. The rest of the colon, the rectum and the anus are supplied by the sacral plexus from the S2–S4 spinal roots. Parasympathetic nerves in the GI tract stimulate motility and sphincter activity as well as increasing blood flow

The vagus (Xth cranial) nerve also supplies the GI tract with:

■ Motor nerves to the pharynx, larynx and soft palate
■ Sensory innervation of the viscera
■ Taste sensation at the root of the tongue

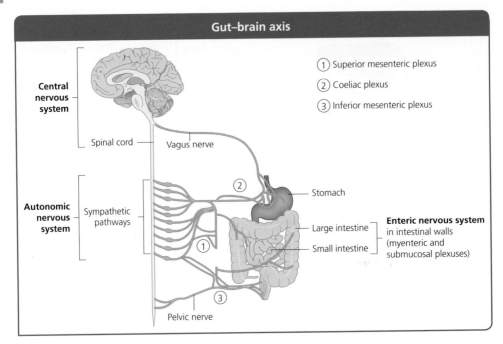

Figure 1.9 The gut–brain axis.

It also supplies the heart and airways.

All the preganglionic fibres of the autonomic nervous system (both sympathetic and parasympathetic divisions) release acetylcholine, as do parasympathetic postganglionic fibres. Postganglionic sympathetic fibres release noradrenaline (norepinephrine). Other neurotransmitters used in the enteric nervous system include serotonin, nitric oxide, somatostatin and vasoactive intestinal peptide (VIP).

> Over 90% of the body's serotonin (5-hydroxytryptamine or 5-HT) is present in the GI tract where it is produced by the enteric nervous system; only a small amount is in the brain.

Function

The main functions of the GI system are digestion and absorption. These are supported by movement of the tract (i.e. its motility) and are regulated by hormones and the enteric nervous system. Faecal matter is excreted as a by-product of these processes. Key terms relating to gastrointestinal function are outlined in **Table 1.8**.

Key terms in GI function	
Term	Meaning
Ingestion	Intake of food and fluids through mouth
Mastication	Chewing of food
Deglutition	Swallowing
Peristalsis	Coordinated movements in the GI tract
Digestion	Breaking down food into smaller components – a mechanical (chewing, mixing) and chemical (via enzymes) process
Absorption	Transport of nutrients, electrolytes and water from GI lumen into the bloodstream
Defaecation	Passage of waste products (faeces) from the body

Table 1.8 Key terms in GI function

Digestion

The human diet is mostly composed of macromolecules that have to be broken down into smaller components, i.e. digested, to be absorbable. Digestion is both a mechanical and chemical process:

- Digestion begins with food being chewed and mixed with saliva in the mouth before being swallowed.
- Further mechanical breakdown mainly takes place in the stomach but does continue in the small intestine
- Many enzymatic and non-enzymatic secretions are involved (**Table 1.9**), and one result is a significant variation in pH along the GI tract (**Table 1.10**).
- Most enzymatic digestion takes place in the small intestine, where the three major food groups are absorbed – carbohydrates, proteins and fats – along with nucleic acids.

Overview of digestion in the stomach and small intestine

Once food has reached the stomach, gastric acid is secreted by cells of the stomach wall

pH in the GI tract	
Area	Average pH
Mouth	6.5–7.5
Stomach – fundus	4.0–6.5
Stomach – antrum	1.5–4.0
Duodenum	6.0–6.5
Jejunum	6.0–6.5
Ileum	6.5–7.5
Colon	6.5–7.5

Table 1.10 Normal pH in the GI tract: pH falls significantly in the stomach due to secretion of gastric acid, then rises along the length of the rest of the GI tract

Digestive secretion in the GI system			
Region	Non-enzymatic secretion	Enzyme secretion	Food digested
Mouth	Saliva: salt, water and mucus	Amylase	Complex carbohydrates
		Lipase	Fats
Oesophagus	Mucus	None	None
Stomach	Gastric acid: hydrochloric acid and mucus	Pepsin	Proteins
		Lipase	Fats
Small intestine	Salt, water and mucus	Peptidases	Proteins
Pancreas	Pancreatic fluid*: bicarbonate	Amylase	Carbohydrates
		Lipase	Fats
		Trypsinogen, chymotrypsinogen and elastase†	Proteins
		Nucleases	Nucleic acids
Liver	Bile*: bile salts, salt and water, waste products	None	Fats
Large intestine	Mucus	None	Bacteria ferment undigested carbohydrates

*Secreted into the small intestine to aid digestion.

†Secreted at the same time.

Table 1.9 Digestive secretion in the different regions of the GI system

and added to the food to produce a mixture called chyme. The acid kills bacteria, denatures proteins (aiding subsequent digestion) and activates pepsinogen to become pepsin, a protein-digesting enzyme. The stomach performs mechanical digestion by contracting the muscle layers in its walls to mix and crush the food. It also acts as a store for the food, and delivers it in a slow and measured way into the duodenum through the pylorus.

The entry of acidic chyme into the duodenum reduces its pH. The fall in pH stimulates production of the hormone secretin by the duodenum and jejunum, which increases pancreatic bicarbonate production and secretion into the duodenum. As a result the pH level rises in the proximal small intestine. On the mucosal lining of the small intestine this optimises the environment for enzymes that break down the food into its constituents (see page 66). These enzymes are predominantly produced in the pancreas (see page 57) and transported to the duodenum in pancreatic juice (e.g. pancreatic amylase, lipase and trypsinogen), but some are produced in the small intestine itself (see page 66).

Entry of food into the duodenum also stimulates it to produce cholecystokinin; this makes the gallbladder contract to deliver bile, which assists in digestion of fats.

The further the food moves along the small intestine, the less digestion takes place. Once it reaches the colon there is no further significant enzymatic digestion, but some of the indigestible carbohydrate such as soluble fibre is fermented here by bacteria.

> **pH variation along the length of the GI tract is taken into account when developing drugs.** Examples include drugs to treat peptic ulcers, which raise the pH of the stomach, and drugs that are enterically coated to survive the acidic environment of the stomach and then dissolve in the small intestine.

Control of digestion

There are three phases that regulate digestion:

- Cephalic: control by the central nervous system

- Gastric: control by the stomach
- Intestinal phase: control by the small intestines

Different stimuli and inhibitors promote and inhibit these phases, as summarised in **Figure 1.10**.

The luminal contents exert chemical effects (e.g. concentration of digestive products, pH and osmolarity) and mechanical effects (e.g. stretch due to the volume of food in the lumen), promoting secretion of gastric acid and enzymes and fluid from the small intestine and pancreas.

Local control is exerted by the enteric nervous system and by hormones (**Table 1.13**). These hormones perform several functions, such as activation of acid secretion in response to food in the stomach, contraction of the gallbladder, transport of pancreatic secretions into the duodenum, release of enzymes and stimulation of gut motility.

External control of digestion is exerted by the central nervous system, via the 'gut–brain' axis. External sensory stimuli such as smell induce the cephalic phase of digestion, leading to processes such as salivation, gastric acid production and stimulation of motility via nerves that communicate between the brain and the mouth and intestine (**Figure 1.10**).

Absorption

A summary of water and electrolyte movements in the intestine is given in **Table 1.11**. Most of this activity occurs in the small intestine (see pages 67-69), with a lesser amount of water absorption occurring in the colon.

> **If a high concentration of unabsorbed solutes remains in the lumen of the small intestine, water cannot be reabsorbed; this leads to 'osmotic' diarrhoea.** Examples include diarrhoea due to a high lactose concentration in lactase deficiency and diarrhoea deliberately induced magnesium hydroxide, prescribed as a laxative.

Fluid fluxes through the intestine are summarised in **Figure 1.11**. Water moves passively along osmotic gradients predominantly

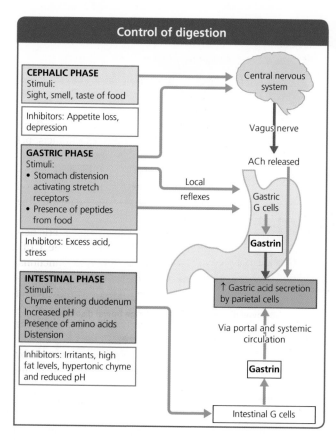

Figure 1.10 Digestion is controlled by three phases. In addition to the effects on gastric acid secretion, the cephalic phase stimulates saliva production and promotes intestinal motility via the vagus nerve. During the intestinal phase, distension of the duodenum and the presence of chyme stimulate local hormone production and neural factors to promote intestinal motility, gallbladder contraction and the release of pancreatic and small intestinal secretions that contain digestive enzymes.

Daily fluxes of water and electrolytes				
	Water (mL)	Sodium (mmol)	Chloride (mmol)	Potassium (mmol)
Input				
Diet	2000	150	150	80
Secretions	8000	1000	750	40
Total	10,000	1150	900	120
Absorption				
Small intestine	8500	950	800	115
Colon	1400	195	97	−4
Stool output	100	5	3	9

Table 1.11 Typical daily fluxes of water and electrolytes in the GI tract

through a paracellular route, i.e. through the 'tight' junctions that are present between enterocytes. These gradients are created by active absorption of osmotic electrolytes, particularly sodium and glucose for example in the small intestine. Most water is absorbed in the jejunum and less in the ileum.

Water absorption from the large intestine can increase threefold to compensate for abnormalities of the small intestine, for example

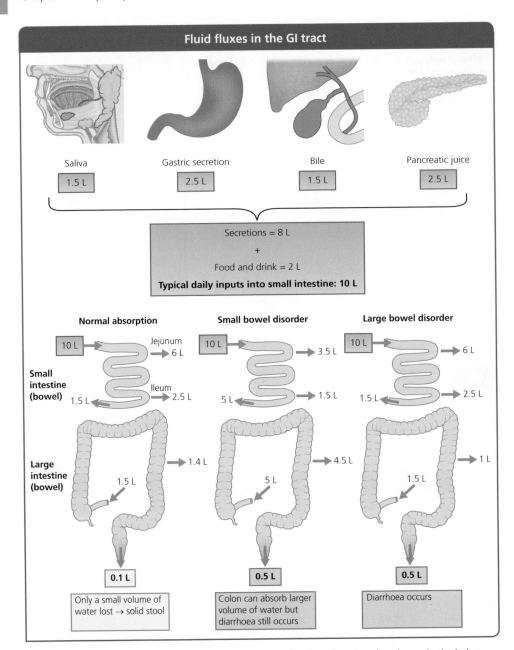

Figure 1.11 Fluid fluxes through the GI tract. Diarrhoea results when there is a disturbance in the balance between the volume of water entering the small intestine and the volume absorbed through the walls of the small and large intestine.

abnormalities of the ileum in Crohn's disease or after surgical resection of part of the small intestine. Whether a person develops diarrhoea largely depends on how efficiently his or her colon absorbs water. Even modest disturbances in colonic function increase stool (faecal) volume because of failure to absorb water, and this leads to diarrhoea (for example as occurs when there is inflammation of the large intestine due to ulcerative colitis).

Absorption by the GI tract is very efficient, with only very small amounts of water and electrolytes being excreted in the faecal matter. The rest is absorbed for use by the body.

Motility

This term describes physical movement in the walls of the GI tract to propel food and liquid along the tract and facilitate mixing. Motility is essential for effective functioning of the GI tract, and it has a distinct pattern in each region.

Motility starts in the mouth with chewing and mixing, and continues in the pharynx as swallowing. From the oesophagus downwards it is largely the result of peristalsis, which is a process of automatic synchronised contrac-

tion that carries food as a bolus down the oesophagus and later on propels semi-digested food (chyme) through the stomach and small intestine, and then moves liquid faeces and then solid faeces along the large intestine (**Figure 1.12a**). Movement called 'segmentation' occurs along the length of the small intestine. Segmental rings of contraction move food forwards and backwards in a way that chops and mixes it (**Figure 1.12b**); this produces a net movement towards the large intestine.

During peristalsis, the inner circular muscle layer relaxes in front of the food to allow it to be moved and contracts behind it to prevent reflux; the outer longitudinal layer contracts to to propel the food forwards (**Figure 1.12a**). This is controlled by the myenteric nerve plexus, which runs between the circular and longitudinal muscle layers of the muscularis externa (see **Figure 1.4**). Intrinsic activity of these muscles is constant and is initiated by the

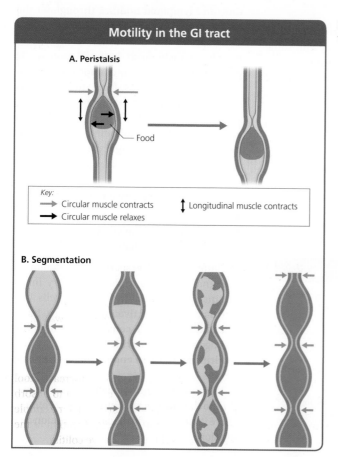

Figure 1.12 Motility in the GI tract.

interstitial cells of Cajal ('pacemaker' cells), situated in both the submucosal and myenteric nerve plexuses. However, there is also modulation of the rate of firing of these cells, and hence the rate of peristalsis, by the autonomic nervous system, the enteric nervous system and hormones such as cholecystokinin, secretin and motilin produced locally by intestinal cells.

There are three GI reflexes:

- Enterogastric reflex – the passage of acidic chyme from the stomach into the duodenum inhibits the release of gastrin from the stomach cells
- Gastroileal reflex – as the stomach empties, chyme is moved through the ileocaecal valve
- Gastrocolic reflex – peristaltic waves of contraction in the large intestine are stimulated by stomach distension due to the presence of food, and this forward movement helps create space for incoming food

Mass movements and the gastrocolic reflex happen three or four times a day and some will ultimately end with defaecation.

The time it takes for the contents to travel the whole length of the GI tract varies between individuals; normal transit times are given in **Table 1.12**. It is also influenced by the amount of food, type of diet, medication, co-morbidity, previous GI surgery and ageing. Colonic transit time is on average slower in women.

Hormones

Enteroendocrine cells in the stomach, small intestine and pancreas produce many peptide hormones. These hormones, their site of production, stimulus and effect are summarised in **Table 1.13**. Most are carried in the blood to nearby parts of the GI tract or other parts of the body. They are also released into intestinal fluid – as are histamine and somatostatin, for example – where they bind to nearby cells; this is called paracrine signalling. Some of the hormones involved in GI function are also neurotransmitters that play a role in the central and peripheral nervous systems, e.g. substance P and secretin.

Immunology

The GI tract contains a significant number of immune cells, including lymphocytes and macrophages. These are diffusely present in the mucosal epithelium and lamina propria. They are also present in lymphoid tissue, such as Peyer's patches in the small intestine, and lymphoid nodules throughout the GI tract.

Lymphoid tissue in or close to the gut is able to distinguish between potentially pathogenic organisms and innocuous (harmless) antigens such as food, host proteins and commensal (non-pathogenic) bacteria. Tolerance to harmless antigens in normal conditions is from antibodies (humoral immunity) as well as phagocytes, cytotoxic T-lymphocytes and cytokines (cell-mediated immunity).

Protection from pathogens is provided by:

- a physical barrier: the intestinal mucosa
- a number of pathways involving inflammatory mediators

The latter include the secretion of chemotactic signals, such as proinflammatory interleukins, which attract effector B cells (i.e. plasma cells) and activated T cells (i.e. helper T and cytotoxic T cells) to the site of the pathogen. Together with macrophages and dendritic cells, these engulf and degrade the toxins.

The antibody immunoglobulin A is secreted onto the mucosa and into the bowel lumen, where it interferes with bacterial adhesion and invasion.

Normal gut transit times	
Region	Approximate transit (total emptying) time*
Oesophagus	<10 seconds
Stomach	4–5 hours
Small intestine	2–4.5 hours
Large intestine	20–45 hours

*These times often vary significantly between individuals and at different times.

Table 1.12 Normal gut transit times

Hormones of the gastrointestinal system			
Name	**Major site of production**	**Stimulus for production**	**Main GI actions**
Gastrin	Stomach and duodenum	Food entering stomach	Stimulates: secretion of gastric acid, pepsinogen and intrinsic factor; intestinal mucosal growth; gastric and intestinal motility (including large intestine)
Somatostatin	Stomach, duodenum and pancreas	Acidic pH Sympathetic nervous system	Inhibits release of gastrin in stomach, secretin and cholecystokinin in duodenum, and glucagon in pancreas
Cholecystokinin	Duodenum	Food entering duodenum (especially fatty meals)	Inhibits gastric emptying Contraction of gallbladder and relaxation of sphincter of Oddi to release bile into duodenum Stimulates pancreatic secretion of enzymes, insulin and glucagon Via vagal neurones provides sensation of satiety to medulla oblongata in brain
Secretin	Duodenum and jejunum	Gastric acid	Stimulates pancreatic production of bicarbonate, enzymes and insulin Reduces gastric and duodenal motility Inhibits gastrin and gastric acid secretion
Vasoactive intestinal polypeptide	Enteric nerves	Food entering small intestine	Relaxes smooth muscle in wall of GI tract Increases water and electrolyte secretion in pancreas and gut Inhibits gastric acid production
Gastric inhibitory peptide	Duodenum	Food entering duodenum (particularly if rich in fats and glucose)	Stimulates release of insulin Inhibits gastric secretion and motility
Ghrelin	Stomach and liver	Fasting	Acts on hypothalamus to stimulate hunger Increases gastric emptying
Motilin	Duodenum	Fasting	Increases gastric emptying and small intestine motility

Table 1.13 Hormones produced by the GI system

> **The GI tract contains more immune cells than any other region of the body.**

Gut flora

The intestinal gut flora (gut microbiota) is predominantly composed of bacteria but does include some fungi adapted to life in the GI tract. The fetal gut is sterile but microbial colonisation occurs during or immediately after birth. It is later affected by hygiene levels, medication and diet (breastfeeding or bottle feeding and its contents).

Distribution

A healthy adult has trillions of commensal microorganisms (up to 1000 different species) in his or her GI tract. This is more than 10 times the total number of cells present in the organs and tissues of the body. The microorganisms weigh up to 2 kg in total. Bacteria contribute over half of the faecal mass.

The number and species of bacteria vary along the gut (**Table 1.14**). Aerobic species predominate in the upper GI tract, and anaerobic species from the middle of the small intestine downwards. Approximately one third of the gut microbiota is common to all people; two thirds is specific to the individual.

> **Gastric acid, bile and pancreatic secretions keep the stomach and proximal small intestine virtually sterile.** Bacterial colonisation then increases through the small intestine and into the large intestine.

Function

The most important role of commensal (resident) organisms is to protect their host from infection with other, potentially harmful, bacteria. Commensal bacteria resist colonisation with pathogens by competing for nutrients and preventing their attachment to the epithelium. They also stimulate the activity of the immune cells in the intestinal mucosa.

In addition, the commensal bacteria synthesise vitamins and aid digestion by producing enzymes, e.g. those to break down polysaccharides (starches). Other functions are described on pages 71 and 76.

> **Germ-free animals have an impaired mucosal immune system and reduced integrity (i.e. a compromised mucosal barrier) so they are more susceptible to infection.**

Bacterial flora of the GI tract		
Region	Viable bacteria per gram of intestinal content	Predominant species
Mouth	10^6–10^{10}	Streptococci, lactobacilli and staphylococci
Stomach	0–10^3	*Lactobacillus* and *Helicobacter pylori*
Jejunum	0–10^4	*Lactobacillus* and *Enterococcus faecalis* Few Gram-positive organisms
Ileum	10^5–10^8	As for jejunum, plus coliforms (e.g. *Escherichia coli*) and *Bacteroides*
Colon	10^{10}–10^{12}	*Bacteroides* and *Bifidobacterium* predominate Also coliforms, enterococci, lactobacilli and clostridia

Table 1.14 Bacterial flora of the GI tract

Mouth

Starter questions

Answers to the following questions are on page 79.

5. How does saliva help prevent tooth decay?
6. How does the mouth prepare food for digestion?

The mouth is the start of the GI tract and is responsible for intake of food and initiation of digestion. The food bolus created in the mouth reaches the pharynx via swallowing.

The mouth is also part of the respiratory tract and helps to produce speech.

Anatomy

The mouth includes the lips, gingivae (gums), teeth, hard and soft palates, tongue, cheeks and floor of the mouth (**Figure 1.13**).

Teeth (dentition)

Humans have two sets of teeth. Milk (baby or deciduous) teeth start to appear at approximately 6 months of age. By about 2½ years of age, all 20 milk teeth have appeared. These are replaced from the age of 6 until the late teens to give a full set of up to 32 adult (permanent) teeth (**Figure 1.14** and **Table 1.15**).

The general structure of a tooth is shown in **Figure 1.15**. Teeth are shaped for different functions:

- Incisors are thin and blade-like to cut food
- Canines are pointed to pierce and tear food
- Molars and premolars have a wide surface with pointed cusps to grind food

Tongue

This lies on the floor of the mouth. It is a strong, mobile, muscular organ composed

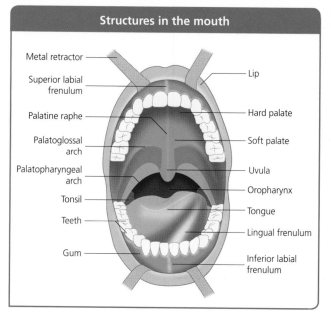

Figure 1.13 Structures in the mouth.

Structures in the mouth

- Metal retractor
- Superior labial frenulum
- Palatine raphe
- Palatoglossal arch
- Palatopharyngeal arch
- Tonsil
- Teeth
- Gum
- Lip
- Hard palate
- Soft palate
- Uvula
- Oropharynx
- Tongue
- Lingual frenulum
- Inferior labial frenulum

Adult dentition

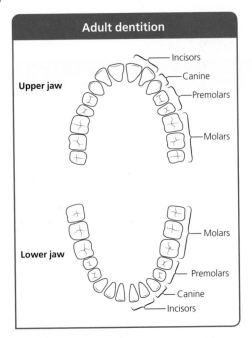

Upper jaw — Incisors, Canine, Premolars, Molars

Lower jaw — Molars, Premolars, Canine, Incisors

Figure 1.14 Adult dentition. In complete adult dentition there are 32 teeth. The third (posterior) molars or wisdom teeth erupt into the jaw several years after the other 28 teeth and do not always develop.

Number of teeth

Type of tooth	Milk (baby) teeth in children	Adult (permanent) teeth
Incisors	8	8
Canines	4	4
Premolars	0	8
Molars	8	12*
Total	20	32

*Includes four 'wisdom' (third molar) teeth. These do not always all erupt.

Table 1.15 Number of teeth

of interlacing bundles of skeletal muscle (see **Figure 1.18**) that run in the vertical, longitudinal and transverse planes. These muscles control its shape for speech and swallowing. Gross (large) movements are produced by external muscles that originate on the skull bones and hyoid – the genioglossus, hyoglossus and styloglossus muscles.

The tongue has a rough surface as it is covered with tiny projections or papillae that contain the taste buds.

Figure 1.15 Tooth structure. A molar tooth is shown in longitudinal section.

Tooth structure

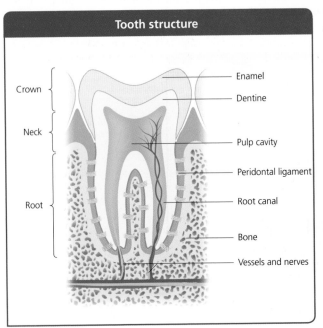

Crown
Neck
Root

Enamel
Dentine
Pulp cavity
Peridontal ligament
Root canal
Bone
Vessels and nerves

Microstructure

The mouth is lined by moist mucous membranes composed of protective, stratified squamous mucosa. The tongue, hard palate and gums are keratinised to resist noxious stimuli such as abrasion, heat and chemical irritation.

Salivary glands

Three pairs of major salivary glands open into the mouth: the parotid, sublingual and submandibular glands (**Figure 1.16**). There are also up to 1000 minor salivary glands in the mouth. The glands are composed of numerous acini lined by secretory epithelium (**Figure 1.17**). Their exocrine function is production and secretion of saliva, which enters the mouth via ducts. Saliva is a serous (pale yellow and watery) fluid containing mucin, which acts as a lubricant. It also contains the enzymes amylase and lipase which aid digestion of food as well as immunoglobulin A, lysozyme and defensins which are all antimicrobial agents.

Various stimuli, including the taste, smell and the sight of food, activate the autonomic nervous system to produce saliva.

Blood vessels and lymphatics

The blood supply to the mouth is via three branches of the external carotid artery. Venous drainage is into the internal jugular vein.

The lymphatics go directly into the deep cervical lymph nodes or via the submandibular or submental nodes. Lymph then enters the thoracic trunk on the left side of the neck,

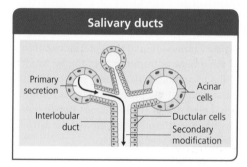

Figure 1.17 Salivary ducts. Acinar cells line the hemispherical lobules (i.e. acini) and produce the primary salivary secretion. These drain into interlobular ducts that unite to form interlobar ducts; ductular cells line both.

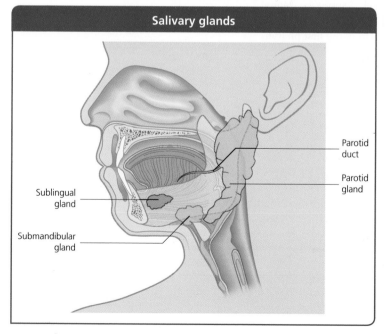

Figure 1.16 Salivary glands.

and the internal jugular vein or brachioce-phalic vein on the right.

Nerve supply

Sensation of the lips, cheeks, gums, teeth, hard palate and floor of the mouth is pro-vided by the second (maxillary) and third (mandibular) divisions of the trigeminal (Vth cranial) nerve.

The motor function supply of the four muscles of mastication is via the mandibular branch of the trigeminal (Vth cranial) nerve.

The tongue receives motor innervation from the hypoglossal (XIIth cranial) nerve. Sensory innervation of the anterior two thirds of the tongue is from the mandibular branch of the trigeminal (Vth cranial) nerve. Sensory innervation of the posterior third is from the glossopharyngeal (IXth cranial) nerve. Some innervation at the root of the tongue is from the vagus (Xth cranial) nerve.

Function

The teeth facilitate the mechanical break-down of food by tearing and grinding (mas-tication). This forms smaller pieces that are then easily swallowed.

Mastication is powered by four different muscles – the masseter, temporalis, lateral pterygoid and medial pterygoid. These are de-rived from the mesoderm of the first pharyn-geal arch. They are supplied by the mandibu-lar nerve, which is a branch of the trigeminal (Vth cranial) nerve.

The tongue has several functions:

- It moves food around the mouth during chewing
- It mixes food and saliva together
- It contains taste buds and receptors for touch and temperature
- It starts the process of swallowing by pushing the food bolus towards the pharynx
- It is involved in forming some sounds during speech

The taste buds on the tongue distinguish between sweet, salty, bitter, sour and savoury. Together with the sense of smell, this allows us to recognise and appreciate different flavours.

The lubricant action of saliva helps in chew-ing and swallowing. Saliva also contains enzymes that start digestion, for example salivary amylase, which contributes to breakdown of complex carbohydrates (see page 66). Saliva helps clean the mouth after eating and also helps to kill bacteria, fungi and viruses.

Pharynx

Starter questions

Answers to the following questions are on pages 79–80.

7. What processes are triggered by the smell of food?
8. How is aspiration of food and fluids into the airways prevented during swallowing?

The pharynx is a muscular tube that connects the nasal cavity and mouth to the larynx and oesophagus. It extends from the base of the skull to the lower border of the cricoid cartilage (vertebral level C6).

Anatomy

The pharynx has three regions: naso-, oro- and hypopharynx (**Figure 1.18**).

Nasopharynx

This is continuous with the posterior nasal cavity and lies between the base of the skull and the soft palate. It is functionally part of the respiratory system and is lined by respiratory epithelium containing goblet cells that produce mucus. In it is located a collection of lymphoid tissue (the nasopharyngeal tonsils or adenoids). In addition, there are the openings of the auditory (Eustachian or pharyngotympanic) tubes, which connect the nasopharynx to the tympanic cavities of the ears.

Oropharynx

This extends from the soft palate to the superior part of the epiglottis. It contains the

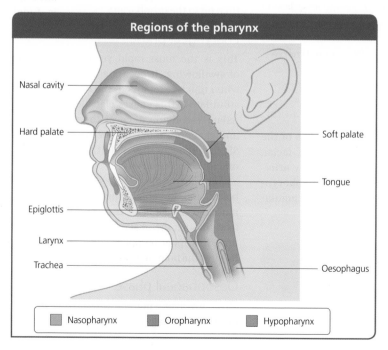

Figure 1.18 Regions of the pharynx.

Regions of the pharynx

- Nasal cavity
- Hard palate
- Epiglottis
- Larynx
- Trachea
- Soft palate
- Tongue
- Oesophagus

☐ Nasopharynx   ☐ Oropharynx   ☐ Hypopharynx

posterior part of the tongue together with the palatine, lingual and tubal tonsils.

Hypopharynx

This stretches from the superior border of the epiglottis to the inferior border of the cricoid cartilage, where it becomes the oesophagus.

Microstructure

The pharynx is lined by a stratified squamous epithelium and contains skeletal muscle. The three circular constrictor muscles (superior, middle and inferior pharyngeal constrictors) contract in sequence from the top to the middle of the pharynx. The inferior ones then propel the food bolus into the oesophagus. The circular muscles are innervated by the vagus (Xth cranial) nerve.

The longitudinal muscles shorten and widen the pharynx and elevate the larynx during swallowing. They are innervated by the vagus (Xth cranial) and glossopharyngeal (IXth cranial) nerves.

The sensory innervation of the pharynx differs between the three regions:

- Nasopharynx – mandibular (i.e. second) branch of the trigeminal (Vth cranial) nerve
- Oropharynx – glossopharyngeal (IXth cranial) nerve
- Hypopharynx – vagus (Xth cranial) nerve

Blood vessels and lymphatics

The arterial supply is from branches of the external carotid artery (the lingual, facial, ascending pharyngeal and maxillary arteries). The venous drainage is via the pharyngeal venous plexus into the internal jugular vein.

> The 'throat' incorporates the pharynx and larynx (or voice box).

Function

The mouth and pharynx act as a common passageway for food and air during the processes of swallowing and respiration.

Swallowing

The swallowing of food and liquids must occur in a coordinated manner for two reasons:

- to deliver the food into the rest of the digestive GI tract, and
- to prevent entry into the trachea, which would lead to choking and pulmonary aspiration (food entering the lower respiratory tract)

The swallowing reflex causes temporary closure of the airway by the epiglottis, which ensures that food is deviated laterally to the sides of the hypopharynx, so it is in the correct alignment to enter the oesophagus. There are three phases of swallowing: oral, pharyngeal and oesophageal. The oropharyngeal phases are shown in **Figure 1.19**.

Oral phase

This phase is entirely voluntary. First a bolus of food is formed in the mouth. The tongue then pushes it against the hard palate and then on to the oropharynx.

Pharyngeal phase

This is the most rapid yet complex phase of swallowing. It occurs as a reflex activity when touch receptors in the oropharynx are stimulated. This causes elevation of the soft palate and uvula to cover the nasopharynx and therefore block off the nasal passages. Simultaneously, the epiglottis moves posteriorly to cover the larynx.

The pharynx then elevates to receive the food bolus, and the three pharyngeal constrictor muscles contract in succession. This forces the food through the pharynx. At almost the same time, the upper oesophageal sphincter relaxes to allow the bolus to pass into the oesophagus.

Oesophageal phase

This involves peristaltic waves and is described on page 33.

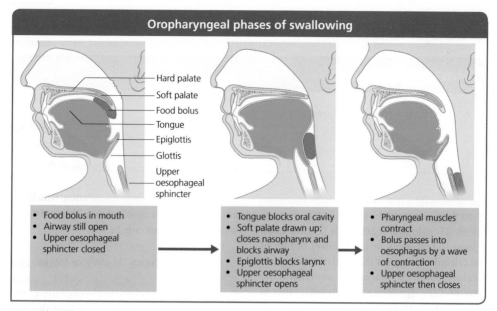

Figure 1.19 Oropharyngeal phases of swallowing.

Oesophagus

Starter questions

Answer to the following question is on page 80.

9. How is peristalisis in the oesophagus similar to the movement of an earthworm?

The oesophagus is a muscular tube that connects the pharynx to the stomach. It is approximately 25 cm long and 2 cm wide (**Figure 1.20**). It joins the pharynx near the lower border of the cricoid cartilage at the level of C6 (6th cervical vertebra), and reaches the stomach at the level of T11 (11th thoracic vertebra). Most of the oesophagus is in the thorax but, as it penetrates the diaphragm, the lower approximately 2 cm is in the abdominal cavity.

Its function is to transport food, drink and saliva to the stomach. The contents are propelled not just by gravity, but also by peristalsis. It is therefore possible to swallow when lying flat and or even when upside down. The peristaltic waves cannot generally be felt.

Oesophagus means 'to carry to eat' in Greek.

Anatomy

The oesophagus is subdivided into three parts based on location, blood supply, venous drainage and lymphatic drainage:

Figure 1.20 Oesophagus.

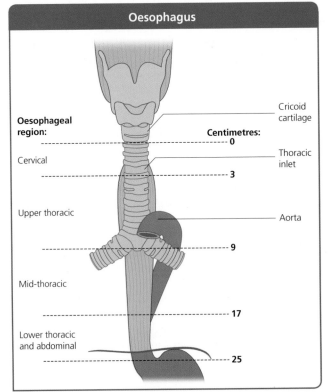

- **Cervical oesophagus** – from the cricopharyngeus muscle in the pharynx to the suprasternal notch, i.e. in the neck
- **Thoracic oesophagus** – from the suprasternal notch to the diaphragm, i.e. in the chest
- **Abdominal oesophagus** – from the diaphragm to the cardia region of the stomach, i.e. in the abdominal cavity

The cervical oesophagus

This is located posterior to the trachea and anterior to the prevertebral muscles and fascia that cover the C6–C8 vertebral bodies. The common carotid and left carotid arteries, internal jugular vein and vagus (Xth cranial) nerve run laterally up each side of the oesophagus within in a carotid sheath, a layer of fibrous connective tissue. The thoracic duct runs along the left side at the level of the C6 vertebral body.

The thoracic oesophagus

This begins where the oesophagus enters the superior mediastinum. It passes behind the aortic arch and enters the posterior mediastinum at the level of the T4–T5 intervertebral disc.

The oesophagus passes through the thorax behind the trachea, right pulmonary artery, left main bronchus, left atrium and diaphragm. It is located anterior to the vertebral column, right posterior intercostal arteries, thoracic duct, thoracic aorta and diaphragm. On its left is the thoracic duct, aorta and left subclavian artery. To the right is the azygos vein.

The abdominal oesophagus

This starts where the oesophagus passes through the right crus of the diaphragm at the level of the tenth thoracic vertebra (T10). Here the oesophagus is covered by peritoneum – the greater sac anteriorly and to its left, and the lesser sac on the right – and it lies in the oesophageal groove on the posterior surface of the left lobe of the liver.

The abdominal oesophagus ends at the cardia of the stomach, where its right side is continuous with the lesser curve of the stomach. Its left side is separated from the gastric fundus by the cardiac notch.

Oesophageal sphincters

There are ring-shaped muscles at both ends of the oesophagus: the upper and lower oesophageal sphincters. Unlike other sphincters in the GI tract, they do not show distinct thickenings. The sphincters open and close to allow the contents to pass onwards, but they prevent the reflux of stomach contents into the oesophagus, the pharynx and therefore the airways.

The two sphincters differ in composition and neurological control:

- **The upper oesophageal (cricopharyngeal) sphincter** consists of skeletal muscle, primarily the cricopharyngeus part of the inferior constrictor muscle. This is not under direct conscious control but is triggered to open by several actions. Some of these – eating and drinking, breathing, vomiting and belching – can be deliberately performed.
- **The lower oesophageal (gastro-oesophageal) sphincter** is smooth muscle that surrounds the junction between the oesophagus and stomach. This relaxes along with peristalsis to allow food from the oesophagus into the stomach and prevents reflux of gastric contents. It is not under conscious control.

Microstructure

The wall of the oesophagus consists of four layers (**Figure 1.21**):

- **Mucosa** – the oesophagus is lined by layers of tough, non-keratinising stratified squamous epithelial cells in continuity with the mucosa of the pharynx. This covers all except the lower 2 cm of the oesophagus, which is lined by columnar epithelium
- **Submucosa** – this contains glands which secrete mucus. This has a lubricating effect and creates a protective barrier. Lymphoid aggregates, blood vessels and a plexus of nerves are also located within it

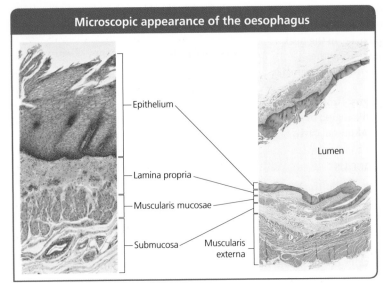

Microscopic appearance of the oesophagus

Epithelium

Lumen

Lamina propria

Muscularis mucosae

Submucosa   Muscularis externa

Figure 1.21
Microscopic appearance of the oesophagus. Compared with the general appearance of the GI tract in **Figure 1.4**, the epithelium is very much thickened: it is lined with stratified squamous cells (i.e. similar to the skin). Like the rest of the GI tract, the oesophagus has a further layer external to the muscularis externa: the adventitia (serosa); however, this is not shown in these sections.

- **Muscularis externa** – the inner circular and outer longitudinal muscle layers of the upper third of the oesophagus are striated. There is smooth muscle in the lower third, and mixed striated and smooth muscle in the middle third. The inner circular muscle is continuous with the cricopharyngeal part of the pharyngeal inferior constrictor muscle and the oblique muscle fibres in the stomach. The muscle in the oesophagus is strong in order to fulfil its function as a transporting region for ingested, often solid, food
- **Adventitia** – this outer layer is formed by connective tissue containing many elastic fibres. The abdominal oesophagus and the more distal GI tract are covered in peritoneum.

Embryology

The oesophagus develops in different stages. In chronological order these are:

1. Elongation occurs in the second month of gestation, and the lumen is partly occluded by proliferating epithelium
2. In the second month of gestation, induction of muscle formation in the splanchnic mesoderm occurs in response to signals from the splanchnic endoderm.

This leads to the formation of smooth muscle. In the upper two thirds of the oesophagus, skeletal muscle is derived from the branchial arches
3. Re-canalisation happens during the third month by vacuolation of the multi-layered columnar epithelium
4. Differentiation of stratified squamous epithelium occurs in the fourth month

Blood vessels and lymphatics

Arterial supply and venous drainage

The cervical oesophagus and upper oesophageal sphincter are supplied by the inferior thyroid artery. Venous drainage is into the inferior thyroid vein, which in turn drains into the superior vena cava.

The thoracic oesophagus is supplied by the bronchial and oesophageal branches of the thoracic aorta, and venous blood drains into the azygos, hemiazygos, bronchial and intercostal veins (branches of the superior vena cava).

The intra-abdominal oesophagus is supplied by the left gastric and left phrenic arteries. Venous drainage is into the left costal vein, a tributary of the portal vein.

Lymphatic drainage

The oesophagus has a continuous submucosal lymphatic system that runs along its whole length. As a result, the drainage of the three different areas of the oesophagus is interconnected. The cervical oesophagus drains mainly to the deep cervical lymph nodes in the neck (i.e. the same nodes as the pharynx). The lymph drainage from the thoracic oesophagus is to the superior and mediastinal nodes in the chest. The abdominal oesophagus drains into the coeliac nodes and the nodes around the left gastric blood vessels.

> Knowledge of the pattern of lymph drainage of the whole GI tract, including the oesophagus, is necessary to be able to plan investigations that seek metastases in patients with GI cancer.

Nerve supply

Motor supply to the skeletal muscle in the proximal oesophagus and the upper sphincter is provided by the recurrent laryngeal nerves, branches of the vagus (Xth cranial) nerve. These also supply parasympathetic fibres to innervate the smooth muscle of the distal oesophagus and lower oesophageal sphincter. The parasympathetic nerves synapse with the ganglia of the enteric nerve plexuses and then supply the muscle and glands in the oesophageal wall.

The oesophagus receives a sympathetic nerve supply from T4–T6 (from the spinal cord at the level of the fourth to sixth thoracic vertebrae). These are vasomotor (innervate its blood vessels).

Afferent fibres run through sympathetic fibres to the T1–T4 segments of the spinal cord and transmit visceral pain. Gross sensation is carried by the vagus (Xth cranial) nerve.

Function

Swallowing

Food and liquid enter the oesophagus when the upper oesophageal sphincter relaxes (**Figure 1.22**). Rhythmic contractile peristaltic waves propel food downwards during the oesophageal phase of swallowing (see **Figure 1.12**). They start when food is in the mouth and continues when it is in the oesophagus. Contraction begins in the skeletal muscle proximally, followed by contraction of the smooth muscle of the distal oesophagus. The movements are involuntary. They are initiated by the enteric plexus and by motor impulses from the vagus (Xth cranial) nerve.

The lower oesophageal sphincter (**Figure 1.23**) temporarily relaxes as the peristaltic waves reach the distal end to allow the contents to enter the stomach. The sphincter then contracts, helping to reduce gastric reflux.

Primary peristaltic waves occur automatically during swallowing. Secondary waves help to clear residual food in the oesophagus and are a reflex action that involves oesophageal afferent nerves. Tertiary contractions describe peristalsis that occurs without a precipitant.

> The oesophagus does not have a direct role in digestion or absorption. It exists to carry contents from the pharynx to the stomach.

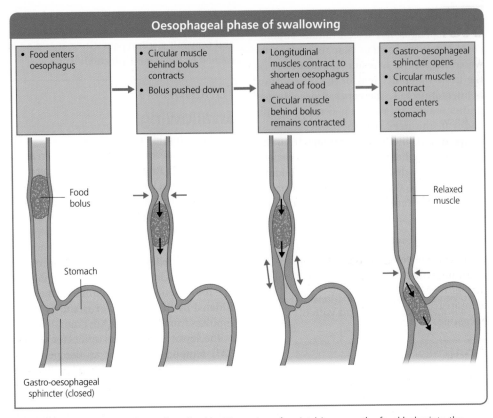

Figure 1.22 Oesophageal phase of swallowing. The action of peristalsis moves the food bolus into the stomach.

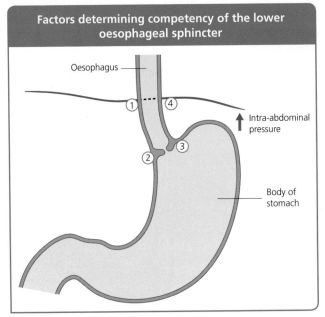

Figure 1.23 The balance of pressures either side of the lower oesophageal sphincter (LOS) determines its competency. Factors involved are: ① the LOS itself; ② an acute angle where the oesophagus meets the stomach; ③ flaps of the gastric mucosa covering this entrance; ④ diaphragmatic contraction. The LOS pressure increases with a rise in intrathoracic and intra-abdominal pressure.

Stomach

Starter questions

Answers to the following questions are on page 80.

10. How is the stomach protected from the effects of gastric acid?
11. How does the stomach expand from the size of a fist to a size that will accommodate a large meal?
12. What causes the noise of a 'rumbling stomach'?

The stomach is a sac-like structure that forms the GI tract between the oesophagus and the small intestine. It acts as a reservoir where further digestion takes place before its contents are passed into the duodenum in smaller volumes as chyme.

Anatomy

The stomach is located in the left upper quadrant of the abdomen. It is a J-shaped organ that is divided into four main regions (**Figure 1.24**):

- Fundus, positioned below the left diaphragm
- Cardia
- Body
- Pylorus (includes the antrum)

The lower and upper curvatures of the stomach are called the greater and lesser curves (**Figure 1.24**). Respectively, the greater and lesser omentum (see pages 5–6) are attached to these.

The volume of the stomach increases from approximately 45 mL when empty to hold

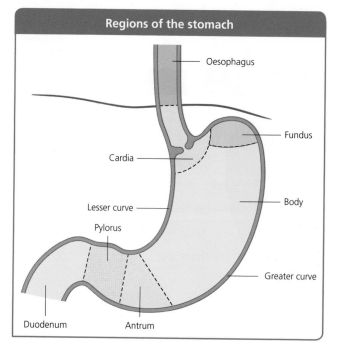

Regions of the stomach

- Oesophagus
- Fundus
- Cardia
- Body
- Lesser curve
- Pylorus
- Greater curve
- Duodenum
- Antrum

Figure 1.24 Regions and curves of the stomach.

between 1 and 2 litres of food and fluid when fully expanded. The lining of the stomach is made up of longitudinal folds called rugae, which increase the surface area for storage and digestion. These flatten as the stomach fills.

The junction of the gastric body and pylorus is marked by the incisura angularis, an angulation in the lesser curve.

The pyloric region includes the antrum, which narrows to form the pyloric canal and orifice. The orifice is surrounded by the pyloric sphincter, which controls the passage of stomach contents into the duodenum. The stomach wall is thicker at this point because of thickening of the smooth muscle layer (muscularis externa). This muscle relaxes in response to stimulation by the vagus (Xth cranial) nerve and contracts in response to feedback from duodenal hormones.

> On an erect (upright) chest X-ray, the gastric fundus is usually visible under the left diaphragm because it contains a bubble of gas that is present from swallowing air.

Microstructure

The wall of the stomach contains the same four layers as the rest of the GI tract (see page 7). However, the stomach's muscularis

externa differs in composition in that it contains an inner oblique muscle layer that is not present in the rest of the GI tract. Thus the muscularis externa contains three layers of muscle: outer longitudinal, middle circular and inner oblique (**Figure 1.25**). These contract to mechanically break up the gastric contents.

The stomach wall is lined with mucus-secreting columnar epithelial cells that provide protection against gastric acid, digestive enzymes and microorganisms. This gastric mucosa has multiple gastric pits that form the entrances to the gastric glands (**Figure 1.26**). The glands are lined with several different specialised cells that secrete components of the gastric juice, as described in **Table 1.16**. The predominant cells are the parietal cells that produce hydrochloric acid and the chief (zymogenic) cells that form pepsinogen. The glands are emptied by contraction of the muscularis mucosae.

Primitive and multipotent stem cells in the gastric gland produce new specialised cell types. These migrate up or down the glands depending upon what type of cell they are destined to become.

Embryology

In the fourth week of gestation, the stomach starts to develop as a dilatation of the foregut

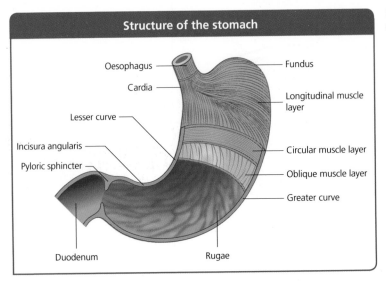

Figure 1.25 Structure of the stomach.

Structure of the stomach

Oesophagus — Fundus

Cardia — Longitudinal muscle layer

Lesser curve —

Incisura angularis — Circular muscle layer

Pyloric sphincter — Oblique muscle layer

Greater curve

Duodenum   Rugae

A gastric pit and gastric gland

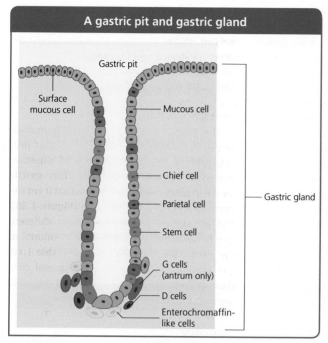

Gastric pit

Surface mucous cell

Mucous cell

Chief cell

Parietal cell

Stem cell

G cells (antrum only)

D cells

Enterochromaffin-like cells

Gastric gland

Figure 1.26 A gastric pit and gastric gland. The gastric pit is the opening in the gastric mucosa, through which pass the secretions of the gastric glands. Stem cells proliferate in the middle regions of the pits and migrate upwards as they divide to become mucous cells, or downwards to become specialised secretory cells. The gastric glands contain gastric parietal cells (produce gastric acid), chief cells (produce pepsinogen) and enteroendocrine cells (the hormone-secreting cells of the GI tract, e.g. G-cells, D-cells and enterochromaffin-like cells).

Cells of the gastric mucosa

Cell type	Principal location	Secretion	Stimulus for release
Parietal (oxyntic) cell	Gastric body Fundus	Hydrochloric acid Intrinsic factor	Acetylcholine Gastrin Histamine
Mucous cell	Cardia Pylorus	Mucus Bicarbonate	Acetylcholine Gastrin Histamine
Chief cell	Gastric body Fundus	Pepsinogens Gastric lipase	Acetylcholine Gastric acid Secretin
G cell	Antrum	Gastrin	Acetylcholine Peptides and amino acids Gastric distension
D (delta) cell	Antrum	Somatostatin	Gastric acid
Enterochromaffin-like (ECL) cell	Gastric body Fundus	Histamine	Acetylcholine Gastrin
P/D1 cell	Fundus	Ghrelin	Fasting state

Table 1.16 Cells of the gastric mucosa

(see **Figure 1.5**). The dorsal (back) aspect of the tube grows more rapidly, to form the greater curve; the shorter, more slowly growing ventral (front) aspect forms the lesser curve (**Figure 1.27**). During week 5, the stomach gradually rotates 90° in a clockwise direction around its longitudinal axis.

The stomach is attached to the body walls by the ventral and dorsal mesenteries (or mesogastrium). The ventral mesentery attaches to the superior aspect of the stomach and later forms the lesser omentum, which attaches to the liver. It also forms the falciform ligament, which connects the liver to the anterior abdominal wall. The dorsal mesentery attaches to the inferior aspect of the stomach and later forms the greater omentum.

During the eighth week of gestation, a combination of rotations moves the duodenum into a C shape. Hormone-containing cells develop between 8 and 11 weeks.

Blood vessels and lymphatics

Arterial supply and venous drainage

Branches of the coeliac artery, which originates from the aorta, supply the stomach with blood (**Figure 1.28**). The lesser curve is supplied by branches of the right and left gastric arteries. The short gastric arteries and right and left gastroepiploic (gastro-omental) arteries run along and supply the greater curve.

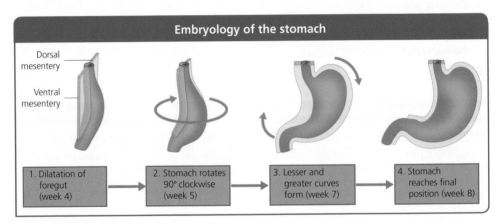

Embryology of the stomach

Dorsal mesentery

Ventral mesentery

| 1. Dilatation of foregut (week 4) | 2. Stomach rotates 90° clockwise (week 5) | 3. Lesser and greater curves form (week 7) | 4. Stomach reaches final position (week 8) |

Figure 1.27 Embryology of the stomach.

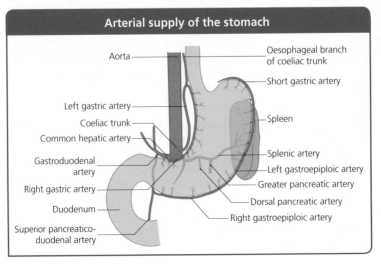

Arterial supply of the stomach

Aorta

Oesophageal branch of coeliac trunk

Short gastric artery

Left gastric artery

Coeliac trunk

Common hepatic artery

Spleen

Gastroduodenal artery

Splenic artery

Right gastric artery

Left gastroepiploic artery

Greater pancreatic artery

Duodenum

Dorsal pancreatic artery

Superior pancreatico-duodenal artery

Right gastroepiploic artery

Figure 1.28 Arterial supply of the stomach.

The gastric veins follow the same path as the arteries and have corresponding names, e.g. right gastric vein. They ultimately drain into the portal vein.

Lymphatic drainage

Lymph vessels follow the arteries along the lesser and greater curves of the stomach. They initially drain into local gastric nodes and then to the coeliac lymph nodes. Lymph from these drains into the cisterna chyli.

Nerve supply

The stomach is supplied by autonomic nerves which join the submucosal and myenteric nerves plexuses:

- The sympathetic nerve supply is from the coeliac plexus
- The parasympathetic nerve supply is from the vagus (Xth cranial) nerve

The anterior vagal trunk [a branch of the left vagus (Xth cranial) nerve] enters the abdominal cavity on the anterior wall of the oesophagus and runs towards the lesser curve of the stomach. It supplies the pylorus and forms the anterior gastric branches. The posterior vagal truck [a branch of the right vagus (Xth cranial) nerve] enters the posterior oesophageal wall and follows the lesser curve to supply the coeliac plexus.

Function

The stomach has several functions, predominantly aiding digestion:

- Mechanical breakdown of food
- Secretion of digestive fluid
- Storage of undigested food
- Movement of material into the small intestine
- Limited absorption of nutrients
- Production of intrinsic factor which helps to absorb vitamin B_{12} in the distal ileum

Motility

Coordinated contractions of the stomach churn the food to break it down into smaller particles prior to pushing it onwards into the duodenum.

Interstitial cells of Cajal (pacemaker cells) are present in the stomach wall. They create slow-wave potentials which lead to contraction of smooth muscle and peristaltic waves. These waves start in the proximal gastric body and move towards the pylorus to move the stomach content downwards. There are around three contractions per minute. Release of acetylcholine by parasympathetic nerve fibres and other neurotransmitters (e.g. substance P) open calcium channels during maximal electrical potentials, with movement of calcium into the smooth muscle cells increasing the rate and force of contraction.

Contractions occurring in the antrum help to move liquid and small food particles of less than 2 mm in diameter through the pylorus. Larger food particles are pushed in a retrograde direction towards the gastric body, in a grinding and mixing action (**Figure 1.29**).

As the contents of the stomach empty into the duodenum, the hormone cholecystokinin, which is produced in the small intestine, causes relaxation of the gastric reservoir and the first part of the duodenum (the bulb).

> Around 5 mL of chyme are emptied from the stomach into the duodenum at a time.

Gastric secretions

Secretions from a number of specialised cells in the gastric mucosa form the gastric juice that helps chemically break food down and digest it. They also form a protective layer over the mucosa, preventing autodigestion.

The hormones involved in regulating gastric function are listed in **Table 1.17**.

Gastric acid

Parietal cells located in the gastric glands of the body and fundus secrete hydrochloric acid into the gastric lumen to maintain an acidic pH in the stomach (**Figure 1.30**). However, these cells are absent from the pyloric region. The acid pH:

- begins the hydrolysis of macromolecules
- helps the functioning of enzymes such as pepsin and gastric lipase

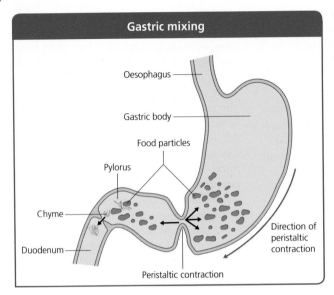

Gastric mixing

Oesophagus

Gastric body

Food particles

Pylorus

Chyme

Duodenum

Peristaltic contraction

Direction of peristaltic contraction

Figure 1.29 Gastric mixing. 'Churning' waves of contraction pass down the stomach, grinding and mixing its contents.

Principal regulators of gastric function

Endocrine	Paracrine	Neurocrine (work as neurotransmitters)
Gastrin	Prostaglandin	Cholecystokinin
Motilin	Histamine	Somatostatin
Secretin	Somatostatin	Acetylcholine
Cholecystokinin		Vasoactive intestinal peptide
		Nitric oxide

Table 1.17 Principal hormones regulating gastric function

■ forms a hostile environment for ingested microorganisms

Gastric acid is secreted at a basal rate of 1–8 mmol/h. The rate rises and falls in response to a number of stimulatory and inhibitory substances acting at the surfaces of parietal cells (**Figure 1.31**), rising to 6–40 mmol/h in response to the presence of gastrin. Secretion is stimulated by:

■ **Gastrin,** a polypeptide hormone produced by G cells in response to two factors: gastrin-releasing peptide neurotransmitter released by fibres of the vagus nerve that innervate the G-cells (**Figure 1.10**), and the presence of dietary oligopeptides in the gastric lumen. Gastrin binds to receptors on the parietal cells to stimulate acid secretion, and binds to enterochromaffin-like (ECL) cells to release histamine. It also stimulates growth of the mucosa of the stomach, small intestine and large intestine. An increase in acidity in the gastric antrum inhibits gastrin secretion through negative feedback

■ **Histamine,** produced by gastric endocrine (ECL) cells to stimulate acid secretion from the parietal cells by binding to H_2 histamine receptors

■ **Acetylcholine,** released into the fundus by enteric nerve endings of vagal nerve fibres, to stimulate the parietal and chief cells; the former secrete acid and the latter secrete pepsinogen, the proenzyme of pepsin

> In conditions such as peptic ulcer disease, proton pump inhibitors and H_2 receptor antagonists are used to suppress excessive gastric acid secretion.

Secretion of acid by the parietal cells is inhibited by:

■ **Somatostatin,** which inhibits release of histamine and gastrin by ECL and G cells, respectively

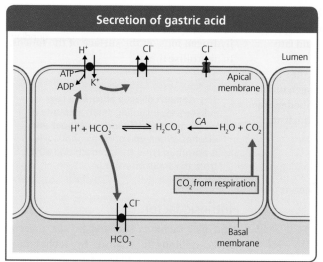

Secretion of gastric acid

Figure 1.30 Secretion of gastric acid. Parietal cells secrete hydrochloric acid (HCl) into the gastric lumen. Carbonic anhydrase (CA) acts on water to generate H^+ ions that are secreted into the lumen via the K^+/H^+ ATPase antiporter. HCO_3^- leaves via basolateral exchange for Cl^-, which passes through apical channels to the lumen.

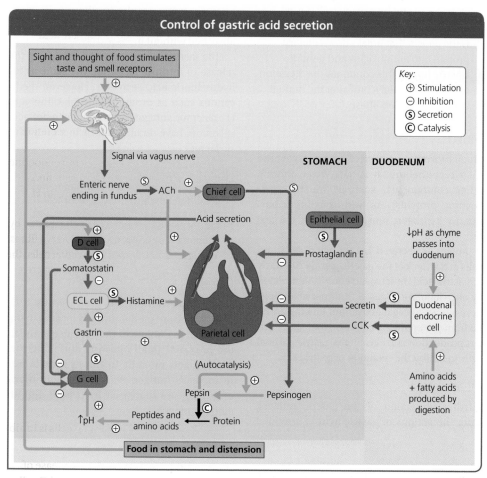

Figure 1.31 Control of gastric acid secretion. ACh, acetylcholine; CCK, cholecystokinin; ECL, enterochromaffin-like

- **Cholecystokinin** (CCK), which is released from duodenal endocrine cells in response to the presence of amino acids and fatty acids
- **Secretin**, which is released from the duodenal cells when acid (hydrogen ions) from the stomach pass into the duodenum
- **Prostaglandin E**, receptors for which are present on the parietal cells

Enzymes

The chief cells of the stomach secrete two digestive enzymes:

- **Pepsinogen:** this is released in response to gastrin and to the acetylcholine released when the vagal nerve is stimulated (see above). It is converted to pepsin by gastric acid and by pepsin itself (i.e. by autocatalysis) in the stomach lumen; it is the pepsin that breaks down dietary protein into amino acids and peptides
- **Gastric lipase:** this continues the digestion of dietary triacylglycerol after the limited actions of salivary lipase

Mucus

Mucus forms a protective coating over the gastric epithelium. It is 95% water and 5% other components, such as mucins (gel-forming proteins). As well as being a barrier to hydrogen ions, it provides surface lubrication.

Mucus is secreted by epithelial cells and cells at the neck of the gastric glands. Similarly to gastric acid, mucus secretion is stimulated by acetylcholine released from nerve endings in response to vagal activation. Prostaglandin E2 from the epithelial cells also increases mucus production and acts on the gastric parietal cells to inhibit the secretion of gastric acid.

Bicarbonate

Further protection of the gastric mucosa from the actions of gastric acid is provided by bicarbonate ions secreted by the surface epithelial cells. The bicarbonate ions bind to hydrogen ions on the surface of the mucosa to neutralise them.

> **The stomach directly absorbs a few substances, including small amounts of water, trace metals such as copper and alcohol.** When you drink alcohol, 20% is absorbed from the stomach and 80% from the small intestine.

Intrinsic factor

Intrinsic factor is secreted by the parietal cells. It binds to vitamin B_{12} (cobalamin) to form a complex that is later absorbed in the terminal ileum. Reduced production of intrinsic factor results in vitamin B_{12} deficiency because the vitamin is not readily absorbed without it.

The factors stimulating and inhibiting the release of intrinsic factor are the same as for hydrochloric acid secretion. However, medications such as proton pump inhibitors and H2 receptor antagonists, which decrease acid secretion, have no inhibitory effect on intrinsic factor.

> **Pernicious anaemia is an autoimmune condition in which there is destruction of the parietal cells** leading to reduced production of intrinsic factor and then vitamin B_{12} deficiency.

Ghrelin

This peptide hormone is produced by P/D_1 cells, which are predominantly located in the fundus of the stomach. They are also found in the proximal small intestine and pancreas. Ghrelin acts on cells in the hypothalamus to increase hunger. Plasma concentrations of ghrelin are increased by fasting and an empty stomach.

Liver

Starter questions

Answers to the following questions are on pages 80–81.

13. How does the liver repair itself?
14. What is the liver's role in nutrition?
15. What is the portal circulation system and why is it important?
16. What gives bile its colour?

The liver is the largest solid organ in the body and one of the heaviest, weighing around 1.5 kg. Most of it lies in the right side of the abdomen beneath the diaphragm and extends into the epigastrium. It has several vital roles, including protein, carbohydrate and lipid metabolism, storage, and bile and protein synthesis. It is also responsible for the breakdown of toxins and drugs.

Anatomy

Occupying most of the right hypochondrium (see **Figure 1.2**), the liver is attached to the

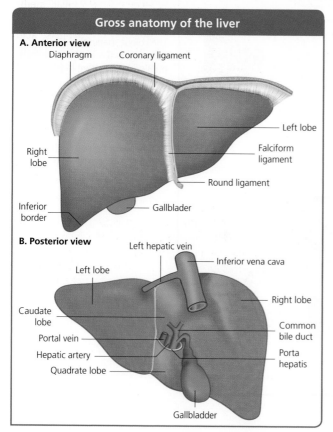

Gross anatomy of the liver

A. Anterior view

Diaphragm · Coronary ligament · Left lobe · Falciform ligament · Round ligament · Right lobe · Inferior border · Gallblader

B. Posterior view

Left hepatic vein · Inferior vena cava · Left lobe · Right lobe · Caudate lobe · Common bile duct · Portal vein · Hepatic artery · Porta hepatis · Quadrate lobe · Gallbladder

Figure 1.32 Gross anatomy of the liver. There is also a right hepatic vein, which runs in the right hepatic fissure but is not visible from this angle.

diaphragm above it by the falciform ligament. This also acts to divide the liver into two lobes, the right and left (**Figure 1.32**). The right lobe is larger and is made up of the caudate and quadrate lobes. The liver is further divided into eight smaller segments on the basis of their blood supply (see **Figure 1.35**).

The liver is surrounded by a capsule of strong connective tissue called Glisson's capsule which helps keep it in position. The porta hepatis lies on the posterior–inferior surface of the liver. This is the region where the portal vein and hepatic artery enter the liver. The porta hepatis also contains the common hepatic duct and hepatic lymph nodes.

The tissue of the liver is described in two ways (**Figure 1.33**):

- **structurally**, according to its division into lobules
- **functionally**, by its division into units named **acini**

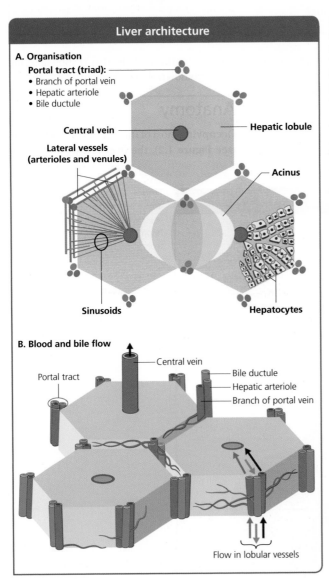

Liver architecture

A. Organisation

Portal tract (triad):
- Branch of portal vein
- Hepatic arteriole
- Bile ductule

Central vein

Lateral vessels (arterioles and venules)

Hepatic lobule

Acinus

Sinusoids

Hepatocytes

B. Blood and bile flow

Central vein

Portal tract

Bile ductule
Hepatic arteriole
Branch of portal vein

Flow in lobular vessels

Figure 1.33 Liver architecture. (A) The liver is organised structurally as lobules and functionally as acini. Each lobule has a central vein (forms the hepatic vein) and peripheral portal tracts (triads). As shown in the lower left lobule, these course through the centre of the acinus and specialised capillaries branch from them to connect with the central vein. These capillaries are called sinusoids and run between the columns of hepatocytes shown in the lower right lobule. The colour shading on the acinus indicates its three zones (see text). (B) Blood flows from hepatic arterioles and branches of the portal vein into lateral vessels and then via sinusoids to the central vein, and bile secreted by hepatocytes flows in the opposite direction. For simplicity, the sinusoids are not drawn here.

Lobules

- In transverse section, lobules are approximately hexagonal structures about 1 mm in diameter. In the middle of each is a central vein, a tributary of the hepatic vein. At each corner is a portal tract that contains branches of the portal vein, hepatic artery, bile duct (or canaliculus), lymphatic vessels and vagus (Xth cranial) nerve.

> The portal tract is also called the 'portal triad', even though it contains five structures (vein, artery, bile duct, lymphatics and nerve).

Acini

Each acinus is an elliptical unit with a terminal branch of a hepatic arteriole and venule at its centre (**Figure 1.33**). Blood flows into each acinus from the portal tract via lateral branches of the portal vein and hepatic artery. It flows outwards along sinusoids (see below), into the central vein (terminal hepatic venule) at the pole of the acinus.

Bile flows in the opposite direction, from the periphery of the acinus into the interlobular bile ducts in the portal tracts.

The hepatocytes in each acinus are arranged into three zones depending on their position in relation to the portal tract:

- Zone 1 (periportal zone) – these cells are in the centre of the acinus closest to the portal tract and are the most metabolically active. Their position means not only do they receive the most oxygenated and nutrient-rich blood, but are also the most exposed to toxins
- Zone 2 (midzone) – these have an intermediate level of metabolic activity and exposure to toxins
- Zone 3 (centrilobular zone) – these cells are furthest from the portal tract and are less metabolically active. They receive less oxygenated blood, which makes them more susceptible to ischaemic injury

Microstructure

The liver is composed of a number of different cell types, as summarised in **Table 1.18** and **Figure 1.34** and discussed below.

Hepatocytes

These specialised epithelial cells make up around 80% of all liver cells. They are the main functional and metabolic cells of the liver and are responsible for many of the liver's secretory functions. One of their functions is to produce bile, which drains into the biliary system (see page 54).

Sinusoids

Networks of specialised, highly permeable capillaries called sinusoids run between the columns of hepatocytes. These deliver blood to the hepatocytes from the portal vein and hepatic artery and drain into the central hepatic vein. The sinusoids are lined by endothelial cells. These differ from the endothelial cells of other capillary beds as they have no basement membrane. This allows easy movement of solutes from the blood to the hepatocytes.

Stellate cells

Individual hepatocytes are separated from the leaky endothelial lining of the sinusoids by the space of Disse. This contains non-parenchymal cells called stellate cells, which secrete collagen to provide a supporting mesh. They are also able to store 80% of the body's vitamin A. It is these cells which contribute to fibrosis in liver damage as they secrete collagen to form scar tissue.

Kupffer cells

Kupffer cells are macrophage-like cells located within the sinusoids. They phagocytose (ingest) bacteria as part of the immune response.

Embryology

The liver develops from the liver bud. In the middle of the third week of gestation, this appears as an outgrowth of the endodermal

Cells of the liver	
Cell type	**Role**
Hepatocyte	Main functional liver cell
	Metabolism (protein, carbohydrate, fat, drugs), storage (e.g. glycogen and fat), bile production
Endothelial cell	Line sinusoids
	Scavenger cells for pathogens and denatured collagen
Stellate (Perisinusoidal) cells	Replace damaged hepatocytes
	Secrete collagen
Kupffer cell	Immune cells, phagocytosis
Haemopoietic cell	Haemopoiesis in fetus

Table 1.18 Cells of the liver

epithelium at the distal end of the primitive foregut. Between the 6th and 11th weeks of development, the stomach, liver and spleen rotate, reaching their final positions.

The hepatic sinusoids are formed by epithelial liver cords (linear arrangement of epithelial cells) which join to the umbilical and vitelline veins. These liver cords also differentiate into hepatocytes, bile canaliculi and hepatic ducts. The hepatocytes begin to produce bile at around week 12.

The mesoderm of the nearby septum transversum gives rise to the haemopoietic cells, Kupffer cells and connective tissue cells. Haemopoiesis (the formation of blood cells) begins in the liver by the 4th week of gestation.

Blood vessels and lymphatics

The blood supply to the liver is unique in that it is part arterial and part venous:

- 30% is supplied by the hepatic artery, which enters through the porta hepatis to provide oxygenated blood (**Figure 1.35**).
- 70% is supplied by the portal vein, which drains nutrient-rich deoxygenated blood from the gut to the liver; this is called the portal circulation (**Figure 1.36**).

Arterial supply

The hepatic artery is a branch of the coeliac artery and divides into right and left branches to supply the right and left lobes of the liver, respectively. An accessory left hepatic artery sometimes arises from the left gastric artery. In total, the liver receives 25–30% of the cardiac output.

Venous drainage and the portal circulation

The portal vein receives venous drainage from all regions of the GI tract, from the lower part of the oesophagus down to the upper part of the rectum. It enters the liver via the porta hepatis alongside the hepatic artery, and passes through liver tissue (**Figure 1.33**) before draining into the inferior vena cava via the hepatic veins. This is called the portal circulation (**Figure 1.36**). It allows substances to be metabolised by the

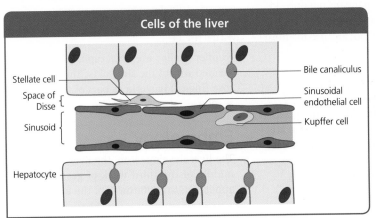

Cells of the liver

Stellate cell
Space of Disse
Sinusoid
Hepatocyte

Bile canaliculus
Sinusoidal endothelial cell
Kupffer cell

Figure 1.34 Cells of the liver. Hepatocytes are arranged in plates between sinusoids, lined by fenestrated endothelial cells. The area between these endothelial cells and the hepatocytes is known as the space of Disse and contains stellate cells. Kupffer cells lie in the sinusoids.

Segments of the liver

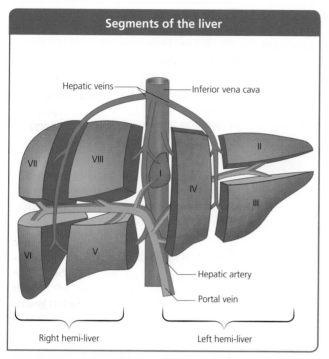

Hepatic veins

Inferior vena cava

VII

VIII

II

I

IV

III

VI

V

Hepatic artery

Portal vein

Right hemi-liver

Left hemi-liver

Figure 1.35 Segments of the liver; each segment has its own arterial and portal venous supply and its own venous drainage. Segments are used to describe the location of lesions, e.g. liver metastases.

Portal circulation

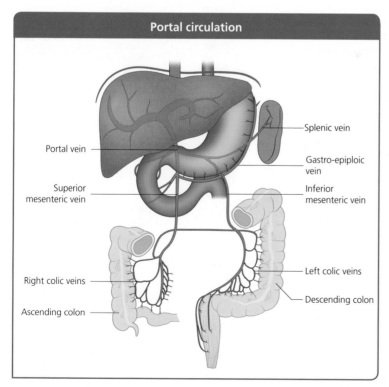

Splenic vein

Portal vein

Gastro-epiploic vein

Superior mesenteric vein

Inferior mesenteric vein

Right colic veins

Left colic veins

Descending colon

Ascending colon

Figure 1.36 The portal venous circulation. Venous blood from almost the entire GI tract (from the lower oesophagus to upper rectum) drains via the portal vein and through the liver before entering the systemic circulation.

liver before passing into the systemic circulation. The blood in the portal vein is only 60–70% oxygenated and it is at low pressure, only 7 mmHg.

> **Pressure in the portal vein often increases in liver disease, i.e. there is portal hypertension.** Sequelae include ascites, splenomegaly and the development of collateral blood vessels called varices.

The central veins of each lobule drain into the hepatic veins and then the inferior vena cava.

Lymphatic drainage

Lymphatic drainage is into deep and superficial vessels. The deep vessels join at the porta hepatis and end at the hepatic lymph nodes, which are scattered along the hepatic artery and portal vein. These drain into the coeliac lymph nodes and from there into the thoracic duct.

The superficial lymph vessels follow a similar drainage pattern, although they sometimes also drain to the mediastinal nodes.

Nerve supply

Innervation is via the hepatic plexus, which enters the liver at the porta hepatis.

The sympathetic supply arises from sympathetic ganglia from T7–T10 spinal segments, which synapse in the coeliac plexus. The parasympathetic supply is from the vagus (Xth cranial) nerve. The right phrenic nerve from the C3–C5 spinal levels provides sensory innervation to the liver capsule.

Biliary tree

The bile produced by hepatocytes is transported from the liver to the small intestine and the gallbladder via the biliary tree. This is a series of ducts: ductules drain from hepatic lobules into intrahepatic bile ducts, which drain into extra-hepatic ducts and then into the duodenum via the common bile duct and into the gallbladder via the cystic duct (see **Figure 1.37**; see also page 54).

Function

The liver has many vital roles (**Table 1.19**):

- Metabolism
- Synthesis
- Breakdown (catabolism) and excretion
- Storage
- Immune and haematological functions

It has a central role in the metabolism of carbohydrate, protein and lipids and in coordinating their availability to other tissues. This is tightly regulated by different hormones that interact to synchronise liver metabolism with the body's needs.

Carbohydrate metabolism

Storage of glucose

After a meal, the rise in blood glucose concentrations stimulates the release of insulin

Liver functions	
Function	Description
Metabolism and synthesis of:	
Protein	Makes plasma proteins, including albumin and clotting factors
Carbohydrate	Makes glycogen from excess glucose; gluconeogenesis
Fat	Makes cholesterol, lipoproteins and fatty acids
Bile	Produces bile acids; bilirubin metabolism
Breakdown	Amino acids
	Ammonia into urea
	Metabolism of steroid hormones
	Detoxification and breakdown of drugs and toxins
Bone metabolism	Vitamin D hydroxylation
Storage	Glycogen
	Fat-soluble vitamins, vitamin B12, folate, iron
Immune	Removal of bacteria by Kupffer cells (phagocytosis)
Haematological	Production of blood cells in fetus (before the bone marrow takes over)

Table 1.19 Functions of the liver

from the pancreas. Glucose diffuses into the hepatocytes where it is converted by insulin into glycogen. This process is called glycogenesis. Glycogen is stored in the liver to be used later when it is needed.

> **The liver contains around 80 g of glycogen.** This is enough to maintain a normal blood glucose level for around 24 hours.

Mobilisation of glucose

The liver maintains the blood glucose level in one of two ways:

- Glycogenolysis – in which glycogen stored in the liver is broken down into glucose
- Gluconeogenesis – the manufacture of new glucose from non-sugar substrates such as lactate and pyruvate

Lipid metabolism

Most of the fat in the diet is in the form of triacylglycerols. As lipids are insoluble in water, they are combined with protein to form complexes known as lipoproteins which are then transported in the blood to body tissues. This process takes place in the liver. Lipoproteins are also stored in the liver and broken down during fasting to be used as an energy source.

As well as being a dietary component, cholesterol is synthesised in the liver. It is required to make steroid hormones and bile acids.

Protein metabolism

The liver synthesises the majority of plasma proteins; these are listed in **Table 1.20**. It also has a key role in the excretion of nitrogenous waste.

Amino acids from the breakdown of dietary proteins are used by hepatocytes for endogenous protein synthesis and to produce plasma proteins, including albumin. Albumin is the predominant plasma protein and has two main roles:

- Binding and transporting small molecules in the blood, e.g. hormones, drugs, lipid-based molecules such as bilirubin, and ions such as calcium

Plasma proteins	
Protein	Role
Albumin	Maintains oncotic pressure
	Transports insoluble molecules, e.g. bilirubin and hormones
Globulins	Antibody functions
	Transport lipids, iron or copper in blood
Fibrinogen	Blood clotting/coagulation cascade
Clotting factors (prothrombin, factors V, VII, IX, X, XII)	
Complement	Immune and inflammatory roles
Lipoprotein	Transports lipids
α1-Antitrypsin	Inhibitor of enzyme trypsin
Alpha-fetoprotein	Produced by embryonic liver cells
	Increased level in adulthood is a marker of primary liver cancer
Caeruloplasmin	Transports copper
Transferrin	Transports iron

Table 1.20 Plasma proteins

- Maintaining oncotic pressure, i.e. the force that retains water in the blood vessels

> **The blood level of albumin falls in liver disease but because its half-life is long (approximately 20 days) it is usually normal in acute liver injury.**

Urea metabolism

The liver is also the major site for protein breakdown. Some amino acids are used for the production of new proteins whilst others are broken down forming ammonia. The ammonia joins with carbon dioxide in the urea cycle to form urea, which is less toxic and more easily excreted in the urine.

Clotting factors

Most of the proteins responsible for blood clotting – clotting factors – are produced by the liver; consequently bleeding occurs in liver disease. These clotting factors have a short half-life. The prothrombin time is therefore a very useful marker of the severity of acute liver damage: it becomes prolonged in the hours soon after the damage has occurred.

> Vitamin K is a fat-soluble co-factor in the synthesis of clotting factors II, VII, IX and X. The synthesis of these clotting factors is therefore impaired in vitamin K deficiency, e.g. caused by biliary obstruction where a malabsorption of fat would occur.

Vitamin metabolism and storage

Hepatocytes are the main storage site for fat-soluble vitamins (A, D, E, K) after they are absorbed from the small intestine and for vitamin B$_{12}$ absorbed from the terminal ileum. These stores are usually large enough to last 2–3 years. Folate, iron and copper are also stored in the liver.

The liver metabolises vitamins, for example vitamin D is converted into calcidiol which then travels in the bloodstream to the kidneys where it becomes calcitriol, the biologically active form of vitamin D.

Bile production

Bile is a greenish yellow liquid produced by the liver. It contains bile salts, cholesterol, phospholipid, bilirubin (from the breakdown of haemoglobin – see pages 51–52), electrolytes, drugs and their metabolites, proteins and water. Its role is to:

- Supply bile salts to emulsify fats (make them soluble in water) in the small intestine, promoting their digestion and absorption
- Excrete bilirubin and excess cholesterol synthesised in the liver

> In clinical practice the terms 'bile acids' and 'bile salts' are often used interchangeably.

The hepatocytes synthesise the primary bile acids cholic acid and deoxycholic acid from cholesterol. Bile acids are conjugated with glycine and taurine in the liver to form bile salts. These have both hydrophilic and hydrophobic properties, which aids solubility to transport lipids and the emulsification of fats, respectively.

Bile salts are released into the intestine in response to cholecystokinin which is released from the duodenum in the presence of a meal, particularly a fatty one. Bile salts are involved in the absorption of lipids and fat-soluble vitamins (A, D, E and K). The majority (95%) of bile salts are absorbed in the terminal ileum and recycled to the liver via the enterohepatic circulation and reused (**Figure 1.37**). The remaining unabsorbed bile salts enter the large intestine where they are modified by intestinal bacteria to form secondary bile acids which are excreted in the faeces.

Bile production is driven by the secretion of bile salts, electrolytes and cholesterol from the hepatocytes into the bile canaliculi. This creates an osmotic gradient for water movement. The bile duct cells secrete bicarbonate in response to the hormone secretin. The bicarbonate makes the fluid alkaline which, together with pancreatic juice, neutralises gastric acid and activates digestive enzymes in the duodenum and small intestine. Bile travels from the bile canaliculi, via the bile ducts in the liver and then into either the gallbladder for storage or directly into the duodenum.

> Bile salt malabsorption may occur after surgical resection of the terminal ileum or if the terminal ileum is damaged by diseases such as Crohn's disease or treatments including radiotherapy. This causes symptoms of diarrhoea, which is worse after meals.

Bilirubin metabolism

Because the body has a high turnover of red blood cells (erythrocytes) there is a high rate of release of breakdown products from the cells. These include haemoglobin and

Enterohepatic circulation

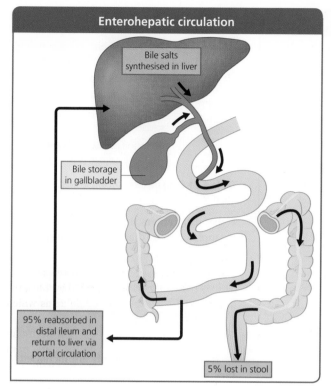

Bile salts synthesised in liver

Bile storage in gallbladder

95% reabsorbed in distal ileum and return to liver via portal circulation

5% lost in stool

Figure 1.37 Enterohepatic circulation. This is the route through which bile salts are reabsorbed from the terminal ileum to return them via the portal vein to the liver to be reutilized again.

haem-containing proteins, which are converted to the insoluble substance bilirubin in many tissues but principally in the liver and spleen. It is released into the circulation bound to albumin to render it water soluble. This circulating bilirubin is described as being unconjugated. It is taken up by hepatocytes, which conjugate it (i.e. combine it) with glucuronic acid; this makes it water soluble and allows it to be excreted in the bile (**Figure 1.38**).

Failure of bilirubin excretion results in its build up in the circulation and the yellow colour of bilirubin becomes visible leading to jaundice. Causes include blockage in the biliary tree or failure of conjugation by the liver.

Once the bile has reached the large intestine, bacteria break down the conjugated bilirubin into urobilinogen. The majority is excreted in

the stool as stercobilinogen, which contributes to its brown colour. If the flow of bile is blocked, there is less stercobilinogen in the stools and they often look pale. The rest is reabsorbed into the bloodstream and either excreted via the kidneys or recirculated to the liver, where it is metabolised, to be excreted in the urine as urobilinogen and urobilin. These give urine its typical yellow colour.

Defence and immune regulation

Because all venous blood from the GI tract drains to the vena cava via the portal circulation, it is processed by the liver. Toxins and bacteria are removed and destroyed within the liver, before the blood is returned to the systemic circulation. Kupffer cells in the sinusoids facilitate this by phagocytosis. This processing protects the body from harmful substances that have breached the gut's defence mechanisms.

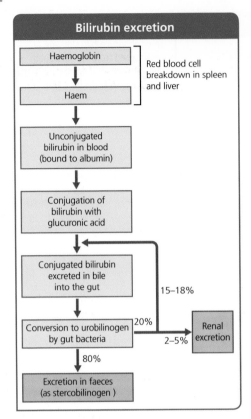

Figure 1.38 Bilirubin excretion.

Detoxification phase	Metabolic process
1	Hydroxylation and oxidation reaction Cytochrome P450 activation
2	Conjugation to make substance water soluble
3	Elimination of conjugated substance by excretion in urine or stool

Table 1.21 Drug metabolism in the liver

active drug enters the systemic circulation; examples include diazepam and morphine.

> **Medications metabolised by the liver may need to be avoided or reduced in dose in liver diseases (e.g. cirrhosis) to avoid toxic side-effects.**

The systemic drug levels are increased if they are given by another route, e.g. intravenously or in cirrhosis, which leads to greater toxicity and side effects.

Drug detoxification occurs in three phases, as summarised in **Table 1.21**.

Processing drugs and hormones

Another major role of the liver is detoxification. It converts active compounds, such as drugs or hormones, into inactive substances that are excreted in the urine or stool. When given orally, some drugs are metabolised almost completely by the liver and little

Haemopoiesis

During embryonic development, the liver is the main site of haemopoiesis – the formation of blood cells. As development progresses, this role is taken over by the bone marrow. Sometimes, for example in bone marrow failure, the adult liver resumes this role. This is referred to as extramedullary haemopoiesis.

Spleen

The spleen is the largest secondary lymphoid organ (organs where lymphocytes are activated, including lymph nodes and tissue in the GI tract). It plays a major role in the immune system.

Although the spleen is not actually part of the gastrointestinal tract it is frequently enlarged in chronic liver disease and shares blood vessels with the nearby digestive system (unlike the kidneys, for example).

Anatomy

The spleen sits in the left upper quadrant of the abdomen, behind the stomach. It is 7–14 cm long (see **Figure 1.2**) and mainly consists of two types of tissue:

- **Red pulp** – this is composed of sinuses lined by connective tissue. These are connected to branches of the splenic artery. Large numbers of macrophages and dendritic cells line the sinuses and filter the blood that flows through them removing old erythrocytes, white blood cells and platelets from the circulation.
- **White pulp** – this has a structure similar to lymphoid follicles and contains predominantly T cells. Its main role is in active immune responses via humoral (antibody) and cell-mediated pathways.

In embryonic development, the spleen develops as a mesodermal proliferation of the primitive gut during the fifth week of gestation. Its arterial blood supply is from the splenic artery. Its venous drainage is via the splenic veins, which join with the superior mesenteric vein to form the portal vein (see **Figure 1.36**).

Function

The spleen filters and takes up old blood cells from the circulation, and is a major site of the immune response against blood-borne antigens. It is also the site where B and T cells (types of white blood cell) proliferate and antibodies are produced.

The spleen also functions as a blood reservoir; it contains up to a third of the body's platelets. If the spleen becomes enlarged (e.g. due to portal hypertension), it filters more cells from the circulation, either pooling them or destroying them. This therefore reduces the number of cells in the circulation.

Biliary system

Starter questions

Answers to the following questions are on page 81.

19. What kind of diet prevents gallstones?
20. What controls bile release into the small intestine?

The biliary system (also called biliary tract or tree) stores and concentrates bile, and transports bile salts to the gut, where they help with digestion.

Anatomy

The biliary system comprises the gallbladder and the bile ducts (**Figure 1.39**).

Gallbladder

The gallbladder is a hollow, pear-shaped sac in the right upper quadrant of abdomen, just beneath the right lobe of the liver. The gallbladder has three regions: the fundus, body and neck. When fully distended, it measures around 8 cm in length and 4 cm in diameter. It holds around 100 mL of bile.

The presence of food in the duodenum stimulates the gallbladder to release bile into the cystic duct, which is continuous with the tapered neck of the gallbladder. The cystic duct is 2–4 cm long. It joins the common hepatic duct to form the common bile duct (see **Figure 1.39**).

Biliary tree

The extrahepatic biliary tree starts from the right and left hepatic bile ducts, which drain the right and left lobes of the liver, respectively. These two bile ducts join at the porta hepatis to form the common hepatic duct. After about 4 cm, the common hepatic duct joins the cystic duct to form the common bile duct. This descends behind the superior part of the duodenum and head of the pancreas. It

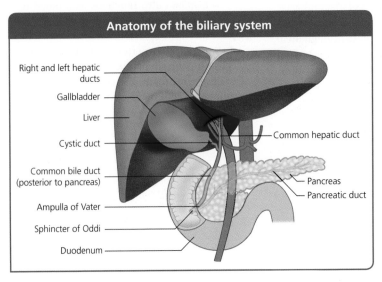

Anatomy of the biliary system

Right and left hepatic ducts
Gallbladder
Liver
Cystic duct
Common bile duct (posterior to pancreas)
Ampulla of Vater
Sphincter of Oddi
Duodenum
Common hepatic duct
Pancreas
Pancreatic duct

Figure 1.39 Anatomy of the biliary system.

is around 7.5 cm long and less than 7 mm in diameter.

The common bile duct joins the pancreatic duct to form the ampulla of Vater (hepatopancreatic ampulla) which opens into the second part of the duodenum. The sphincter of Oddi, an area of smooth muscle at this opening, contracts and relaxes to control the secretion of the mixture of bile and pancreatic juice into the duodenum when food is present (see pages 50 and 55).

Microstructure

The gallbladder mucosa is lined with columnar epithelial cells that have a border of microvilli on their apical surface. In the gallbladder, the muscularis externa is not organised into distinct layers but is interspersed with longitudinal, transverse and oblique fibres.

The extrahepatic bile ducts are lined with columnar epithelial cells.

Embryology

As the liver bud develops from the foregut (duodenum), the connection between them narrows to form the bile duct. A small ventral outgrowth from the bile duct gives rise to the gallbladder and cystic duct.

Blood vessels and lymphatics

Arterial supply of the biliary system is from the cystic artery, a branch of the right hepatic artery. Venous drainage is via the cystic veins. Lymph drains into the cystic nodes, which are located near the neck of the gallbladder, and from there into the hepatic and coeliac nodes.

Nerve supply

The biliary system is supplied via the vagus (Xth cranial) nerve (parasympathetic), coeliac plexus (sympathetic), right phrenic nerve (sensory) and hepatic plexus (this is formed by nerve fibres from all three sources).

Function

The biliary system has three main roles:

- Bile storage (in the gallbladder)
- Concentration of bile (in the gallbladder)
- Transport of bile (via the bile ducts)

Storage and concentration

Bile secreted by the liver is stored by the gallbladder. Half of the bile secreted during fasting is collected in the gallbladder. The remaining bile passes into the duodenum.

The epithelial cells of the gallbladder are highly specialised for absorption – up to 90% of the water in the bile is absorbed, raising its concentration. The water passively follows the active transport of sodium from the gallbladder epithelium into the lateral intracellular spaces.

Bile release

Contraction of the gallbladder to release bile is brought about in two ways:

- The smell and taste of food stimulates the vagus (Xth cranial) nerve, which acts on the muscle wall of the gallbladder
- Fat in food within the gut is detected by the I cells of the duodenum. These then release cholecystokinin, which causes the gallbladder to contract and the sphincter of Oddi to relax

After removal of the gallbladder, there is a constant slow release of bile from the liver into the bile ducts and duodenum. This means that fats are still digested. However patients occasionally have diarrhoea, particularly after large fatty meals, because there is not the volume of bile that would have been released by gallbladder contraction.

Pancreas

Starter questions

Answers to the following questions are on page 81.

21. How does the pancreas not digest itself?
22. Can you live without a pancreas?

The pancreas is a digestive gland that lies behind the stomach and towards the back of the abdomen. It has two modes of action:

- Exocrine – secretion of fluid into a duct
- Endocrine – release of hormones directly into the bloodstream

Anatomy

The pancreas is located in the epigastric region and is mostly retroperitoneal bar its tail, meaning that it lies behind the visceral peritoneum. It extends transversely across the posterior abdominal wall from the curve of the duodenum to the spleen. It lies posterior to the stomach and anterior to the aorta, inferior vena cava and L1–L3 vertebral bodies (see **Figure 1.39**). The pancreas is 12–15 cm long and weighs about 80 g.

The pancreas is divided into four main parts: head, neck, body and tail (**Figure 1.40**). The head lies in the C-shaped curve of the duodenum, anterior to the inferior vena cava and left renal vein. The common bile duct lies in a groove on the posterior surface of the head. The uncinate process is a small portion of the head that extends superiorly around the superior mesenteric vessels - uncinate means 'hooked'. The pancreatic duct courses through the pancreas from tail to head, where it joins the common bile duct to enter the ampulla of Vater. The sphincter (sphincter of Oddi) of the pancreatic duct controls the flow of pancreatic secretions into the duodenum via this ampulla. An accessory duct is sometimes also present which drains into the duodenum separately.

Microstructure

The pancreas comprises of both exocrine and endocrine cells.

Exocrine cells

Most of the exocrine cells are pyramidal epithelial cells that are grouped to form pancreatic acini (**Figure 1.41**). They produce hydrolytic enzymes that digest proteins, lipids and carbohydrates (see **Table 1.22**). Each cell contains many secretory (zymogen) granules, which empty into the lumen of the pancreatic acinus.

A bicarbonate-rich fluid, which neutralises the gastric acid and helps enzymes to function more effectively, is produced by the epithelial cells of the pancreatic duct and is added to the acinar cell secretion.

These secretions then drain into a series of ducts and eventually into the main pancreatic duct, which enters the duodenum at the sphincter of Oddi.

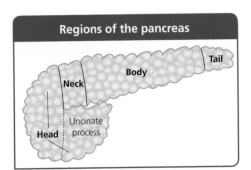

Regions of the pancreas

Tail
Body
Neck
Uncinate process
Head

Figure 1.40 The four regions of the pancreas (the uncinate process is a portion of the head of the pancreas)

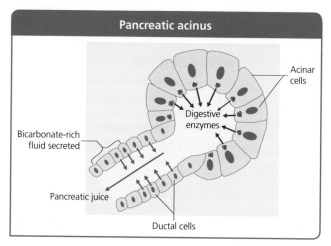

Pancreatic acinus

Acinar cells

Digestive enzymes

Bicarbonate-rich fluid secreted

Pancreatic juice

Ductal cells

Figure 1.41 A pancreatic acinus.

Pancreatic exocrine secretions		
Pancreatic cell type	Secretion	Role
Acinar cells	Amylase	Breakdown of starch and glycogen
	Lipase, cholesterol esterase and phospholipase	Fat digestion
	Proteolytic enzymes:	Digestion of proteins
	Trypsinogen	
	Proelastase	
	Chymotrypsinogen	
	Procarboxypeptidase	
	Elastase	
	Ribonuclease	RNA breakdown
	Deoxyribonuclease	DNA breakdown
Ductal epithelial cells	Water and electrolytes	Fluid volume
		Membrane gradients and transport
	Bicarbonate	Neutralises gastric acid

Table 1.22 Pancreatic exocrine secretions

Endocrine cells

The endocrine cells of the pancreas are arranged in clusters called islets of Langerhans. They are present throughout the gland but are more prevalent in the tail. They consist of:

- Alpha cells, which produce insulin
- Beta cells, which produce glucagon
- Delta cells, which secrete somatostatin
- PP cells, which secrete pancreatic polypeptide

The islets are highly vascular and have a rich capillary bed which facilitates the release of hormones into the systemic circulation.

> The islets of Langerhans make up only 1–2% of the overall mass of the pancreas.

Embryology

The pancreas develops from the endodermal layer of the caudal foregut during the fourth to sixth week of gestation.

A dorsal and a ventral bud develop one on each side of the foregut (see **Figure 1.5**), each with its own duct. The dorsal bud forms the head, body and tail of the pancreas, and the ventral bud forms the uncinate process. The two buds fuse at around week 7. The two developing ducts fuse to form the pancreatic duct.

The islets of Langerhans cells develop from pancreatic parenchymal tissue in the third month of gestation and are scattered throughout the gland. Insulin secretion begins at around 20 weeks.

Blood vessels and lymphatics

Arterial supply

The pancreas has a rich blood supply (**Figure 1.42**). The head of the pancreas and uncinate process are supplied by two arteries:

- Superior pancreaticoduodenal artery, a branch of the common hepatic artery from the coeliac artery
- Inferior pancreaticoduodenal artery, a branch of the inferior mesenteric artery

The body and tail of the pancreas are supplied by branches of the splenic artery. The inferior border is supplied by the pancreatic artery.

Venous drainage

Venous drainage is to the superior and inferior pancreaticoduodenal veins. The superior pancreaticoduodenal vein drains into the portal vein, and the inferior pancreaticoduodenal veins into the superior mesenteric vein. The body and tail drain into the splenic vein.

Lymphatic drainage

Lymph drains to the pancreaticosplenic or suprapancreatic nodes, which run alongside the splenic artery, and to the preaortic nodes around the superior mesenteric and coeliac vessels.

Nerve supply

Sympathetic innervation of the pancreas arises from the splanchnic and coeliac plexuses which have a nerve supply from the T6 to T10 levels of the spinal cord. The parasympathetic supply is from the coeliac branch of the vagus (Xth cranial) nerve.

Function

Exocrine role

The main role of the exocrine pancreas is to secrete pancreatic juice (**Table 1.22**), approximately 1–1.5 L of clear fluid each day. As well as enzymes this contains water, bicarbonate

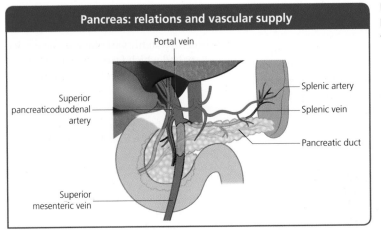

Pancreas: relations and vascular supply

Portal vein

Superior pancreaticoduodenal artery

Superior mesenteric vein

Splenic artery

Splenic vein

Pancreatic duct

Figure 1.42 The pancreas: relations and vascular supply.

and electrolytes that help to neutralise the acidic chyme and halt the digestive enzymes already active in the chyme.

Alkaline secretion

Fluid rich in sodium and bicarbonate is secreted by the small duct cells, neutralising the gastric acid as it enters the duodenum. This raises the pH to 6 or 7 and produces an optimum pH for pancreatic enzyme activity.

Within the duct cells bicarbonate for excretion is produced by two mechanisms:

- carbonic anhydrase catalyses the conversion of carbon dioxide and water to hydrogen and bicarbonate
- a sodium/bicarbonate co-transporter in the membrane of duct cells actively transports sodium into the cells from the surrounding interstitial fluid. This is followed by the active transport of bicarbonate into the duct lumen in exchange for chloride.

Pancreatic bicarbonate secretion is stimulated by secretin, which is produced by endocrine cells in the duodenal mucosa.

Exocrine enzyme secretion (**Table 1.22**)

Pancreatic enzymes are synthesised by the rough endoplasmic reticulum of the acinar cells. The enzymes are stored in either an active or a precursor (proenzyme) state in secretory granules within the cells.

Enzymes for protein metabolism

The presence of food and gastric acid in the duodenum stimulates the release of enterokinase (enteropeptidase) from cells in the small intestine, by cholecystokinin. This in turn converts trypsinogen produced by the pancreas into trypsin in the small intestine. This acts as a proenzyme, i.e. trypsin activates other enzymes in the small intestine, for example converting pancreatic chymotrypsinogen into chymotrypsin.

> **Pancreatic enzymes involved in digestion of protein are released in their proenzymatic (inactive) form** to avoid self-digestion of the pancreas.

Enzymes for carbohydrate metabolism

Pancreatic amylase hydrolyses polysaccharides in the gut to form disaccharides. These are then cleaved to glucose by enzymes in the small intestine.

Enzymes for lipid metabolism

Pancreatic lipase is the principal enzyme involved in the digestion of fat. It converts triacylglycerols into glycerol and free fatty acids, which can then be absorbed from the gut lumen. The pancreas also secretes cholesterol esterase, which catalyses the breakdown of cholesterol esters, and phospholipase, which breaks down phospholipids.

> **In patients with pancreatic insufficiency there is reduced lipase secretion.** Fats are not broken down and therefore cannot be easily absorbed by the gut. Instead they pass through into the stools, causing fatty, greasy motions that are difficult to flush away. This condition is called steatorrhea.

Control of secretion of pancreatic juice

Pancreatic exocrine secretion is regulated by a combination of neural and hormonal signals in response to eating. The following occur:

- Acinar cell secretion is stimulated by distension of the stomach with food
- Cholecystokinin is released into the bloodstream from the duodenal I cells in response to fatty acids and peptides within the lumen of the duodenum. It acts via receptors on vagal afferent fibres to increase pancreatic acinar cell secretion
- Cholecystokinin also acts on the gallbladder causing it to contract, and relaxes the sphincter of Oddi allowing bile and pancreatic juice to enter the duodenum
- Secretin is released from duodenal S cells in response to a falling pH within the duodenum. It acts directly on the ductal cells of the pancreas to increase bicarbonate secretion

Endocrine role

The pancreas secretes several hormones (**Table 1.23**). Its main endocrine function is blood glucose control, through the release of the hormones insulin and glucagon which have opposing actions:

- **Insulin** is secreted in greater amounts as blood glucose increases, and promotes the uptake of glucose into the cells to reduce blood sugar. It is also involved in protein and fat synthesis.
- **Glucagon** stimulates the production of glucose from glycogen stores in the liver (glycogenolysis) and stimulates gluconeogenesis (see page 49) to increase blood sugar. It also promotes the breakdown of lipids to provide a source of energy.

> **Blood glucose must be tightly controlled:** a high level has metabolic consequences such as diabetic ketoacidosis and in the long term causes damage to blood vessels and nerve endings, leading to blindness, ischaemic heart disease and peripheral neuropathies. Low blood glucose leads to confusion and fits.

Role of pancreatic hormones			
Hormone	Source	Stimulus for production	Action
Insulin	β (B) cells	High blood glucose	Increases cellular uptake of glucose from the blood
Glucagon	α (A) cells	Low blood glucose	Increases gluconeogenesis and glycogenolysis to increase blood sugar
Somatostatin	δ (D) cells	Food	Inhibits release of insulin and glucagon
			Inhibits release of secretin, cholecystokinin, motilin and gastrin (gut peptides)
Pancreatic polypeptide	PP (F) cells	Ingestion of food	Reduces pancreatic exocrine activity, gastric motility and gallbladder activity

Table 1.23 Role of pancreatic hormones

Small intestine

Starter questions

Answers to the following questions are on page pages 81–82.

23. How is the small intestine adapted to aid nutrient absorption?
24. How is gastric acid neutralised in the small intestine?

The small intestine is a tubular structure connecting the stomach and large intestine. With an average length of 7 m in adults, it is the longest part of the GI tract.

Anatomy

The small intestine is divided into three segments:

- Duodenum
- Jejunum
- Ileum

The large surface area facilitates efficient absorption of nutrients. The area is increased by circular folds and villi:

- **Circular folds** ('plicae circulares' or 'valvulae conniventes') are composed of mucosa and submucosa (**Figure 1.43a**). They slow the movement of food through the intestine but, unlike gastric rugae, do not disappear when the lumen distends. They are smaller and less prominent towards the distal end of the small intestine
- **Villi** are mucosal folds that form finger-like projections of up to 1.5 mm in height (**Figures 1.43b** and **1.44**). Along the length of the small intestine they vary in shape and size (**Figure 1.45**): short, broad and leaf shaped in the duodenum; long and thin in the jejunum; and short in the ileum

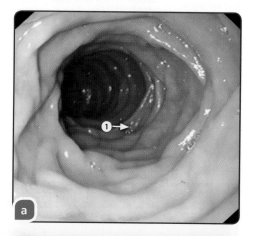

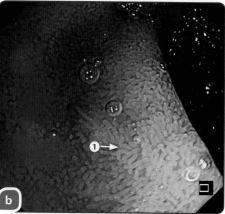

Figure 1.43 Endoscopic appearance of the small intestine: (a) circular folds ① (valvulae conniventes); (b) villi ①, finger-like projections that line the walls.

Duodenum

This is C-shaped and starts at the pylorus, where it envelops the head of the pancreas. It is the shortest section of the small intestine.

The duodenum is divided into four parts (**Figure 1.46**); all except the first are retroperitoneal. The combined pancreatic and

Structure of the small intestine

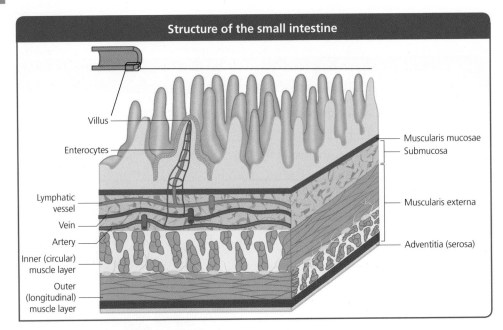

Figure 1.44 Microstructure of the small intestine.

Segments of the small intestine

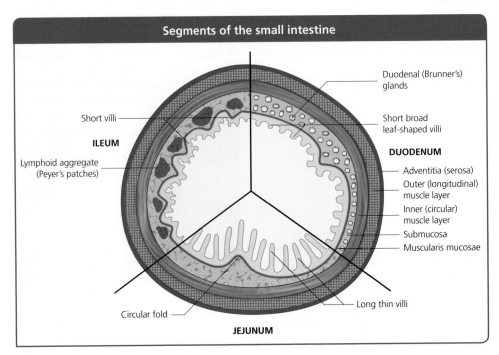

Figure 1.45 Characteristics of different segments of the small intestine.

common bile ducts open into the second part of the duodenum at the ampulla of Vater.

> The name duodenum derives from the Latin word for 12 – duodecimi – because it is 12 fingerbreadths (25 cm) long.

Jejunum

The duodenum becomes the jejunum at the ligament of Treitz (also called the suspensory 'muscle' of the duodenum). The lower portion of this ligament extends from connective tissue surrounding the coeliac artery and superior mesenteric artery to the duodenojejunal flexure.

The jejunum is approximately 2.4 m long.

Ileum

The ileum is the longest segment of the small intestine – approximately 3.5 m. It joins the large intestine at the ileocaecal valve. Along with the jejunum, it is attached to the posterior abdominal wall by a fan-shaped mesentery.

> There is no external point of demarcation between the jejunum and the ileum but there are some microscopic differences.

Microstructure

Like the rest of the GI tract, the wall of the small intestine has four layers (**Figure 1.4**). The columnar epithelial cells (enterocytes) that line the finger-like villi, have many, very small projections on their surface. They are called microvilli and form the 'brush border' of the wall. The enterocytes have intracellular, apical and basolateral membrane receptors for various nutrients that are involved in regulating intestinal absorption and secretion.

The small intestine has two types of gland:

- **Brunner's glands**: these are tubular submucosal glands that are mainly located in the duodenum above the ampulla of Vater
- **Crypts of Lieberkühn**: these small tubular glands lie between the villi and extend inwards to the muscularis mucosae, and contain a variety of cells, as listed in **Table 1.24**

Embryology

The intestinal loop starts to lengthen at 4 weeks of gestation (**Figure 1.47**). It grows so rapidly that there is not enough room for it so it herniates from the abdominal cavity, through the navel opening into the umbilical cord. At 39 days, the developing intestine undergoes a 90° clockwise rotation, and the configuration starts to be recognisable as the small and large intestine. The intestine continues to lengthen and rotate.

During the 10th week of gestation, the intestinal loops undergo a further 180° clockwise rotation around the axis of the superior mesenteric artery. They then return to the abdominal cavity where there is now enough room to accommodate them. First the proxi-

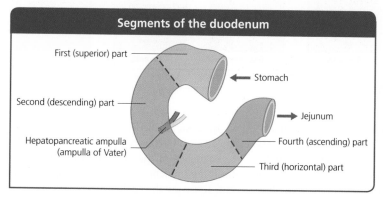

Segments of the duodenum

First (superior) part

Stomach

Second (descending) part

Jejunum

Hepatopancreatic ampulla (ampulla of Vater)

Fourth (ascending) part

Third (horizontal) part

Figure 1.46 Four parts or segments of the duodenum. These are often used in clinical practice to describe the location of an abnormality or how far an oesophagogastroduodendoscope has reached.

Cells of the crypts of Lieberkühn		
Cell type	**Function**	**Products**
Enterocyte	Absorb water and electrolytes Contain digestive enzymes	See Table 1.25
Goblet cell	Secrete mucus, which protects against gastric acid and digestive enzymes	Mucus
Enteroendocrine cells (e.g. I cell, S cell)	Secrete hormones	Secretin Somatostatin Enteroglucagon Serotonin Motilin
Paneth cell	Secrete antimicrobial peptides	Defensins Lysozyme Tumour necrosis factor alpha
Stem cell	Replicating cells	Replace all cell types

Table 1.24 Cells of the crypts of Lieberkühn in the small intestine

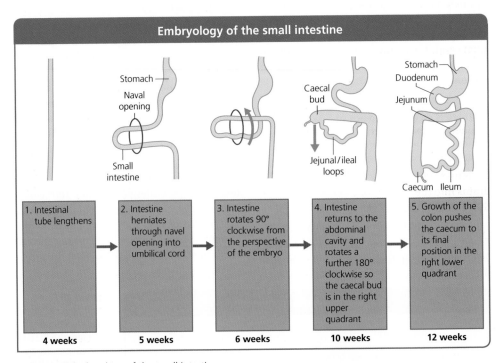

Figure 1.47 Embryology of the small intestine.

mal jejunum re-enters the left side of abdominal cavity. The next loop then moves to the right side. The caecal bud is initially located in the right upper quadrant but later descends to its final position in the right iliac fossa.

By week 13, the neural crest cells have migrated to and colonised the developing intestine.

Branches of the vitelline arteries fuse to form the branches of the aorta supplying the gut. These are the coeliac artery and superior and inferior mesenteric arteries.

Errors of embryological development of the small intestine lead to congenital abnormalities such as intestinal malrotation, Meckel's diverticulum and Hirschsprung's disease.

Blood vessels and lymphatics

Arterial supply

The proximal sections of the duodenum down to the level of the ampulla are supplied by the superior pancreaticoduodenal artery, which originates from the coeliac artery (see **Figure 1.28**). This anastomoses with the inferior pancreaticoduodenal artery, which arises from the superior mesenteric artery and supplies the distal sections of the duodenum. Jejunal and ileal arteries are formed from the superior mesenteric artery (see **Figure 1.53**). Branches from all these arteries run through layers of the mesentery to form arterial arcades.

Venous drainage

Duodenal veins follow the arteries and drain into the portal vein either directly or indirectly via the superior mesenteric or splenic veins first. Blood from the jejunum and ileum drains into the superior mesenteric vein and then into the portal vein.

Lymphatic drainage

The submucosa contain lacteals that empty lymphatic fluid into the lymph vessels:

- Lymph from the duodenum drains into the pancreaticoduodenal, pyloric and superior mesenteric lymph nodes
- Lymph from the jejunum and ileum passes to vessels located between the layers of the mesentery and into the superior mesenteric lymph nodes

Lymph drained from all regions of the small intestine ultimately drains into the cisterna chyli.

Nerve supply

The duodenum is supplied by the parasympathetic (vagus – Xth cranial) and sympathetic nerves through plexuses lying on the pancreaticoduodenal arteries.

The jejunum and ileum are supplied by the vagus (Xth cranial) and splanchnic (sympathetic) nerves.

Function

The functions of the small intestine are:

- Digestion of chyme produced by the stomach
- Absorption of nutrients and bile salts
- Movement of the bowel contents into the large intestine
- Provision of a barrier against pathogenic organisms and toxins, and immune functions to protect against infection (e.g. *E. coli*)

Digestion

Digestion takes place in the small intestine, where carbohydrates, proteins, fats and nucleic acids are absorbed. Within the small intestine, it is the duodenum that has the principal role in regulating digestion:

- **Brunner's glands** secrete urogastrone and pepsinogen, which inhibit secretions from the chief and parietal cells in the stomach
- **Enteroendocrine cells** secrete cholecystokinin (from I cells) and secretin (from S cells), which stimulate gallbladder contraction and secretion of pancreatic enzymes into the duodenum. Secretin increases the secretion of bicarbonate from the pancreas and biliary tree as well as inhibiting gastric emptying to optimise digestion before further food arrives.

Brunner's glands also secrete an alkaline mucus (pH 9) that lines the mucosa and helps to neutralise the acidic chyme. Alkaline mucus is also secreted by Goblet cells.

Digestion of carbohydrates

Large carbohydrate molecules are not absorbable across the wall of the small intestine and must be broken down into smaller components first. This is accomplished by the digestive enzymes amylase, lactase, maltase and sucrase (see **Table 1.25**).

Polysaccharides

These are large carbohydrate molecules consisting of long chains of linked monosaccharides. Their breakdown begins in the mouth with salivary amylase but predominantly occurs in the small intestine where bonds between monosaccharides are cleaved by enzymes to form smaller oligosaccharide and disaccharide components. Some polysaccharides, for example cellulose, are not digestible.

Disaccharides

These are sugars composed of two bonded monosaccharides. They are broken down by enzymes on the brush border of the small intestinal mucosa, allowing the constituent simple sugars to be absorbed.

Monosaccharides

These simple sugars (e.g. glucose, galactose, fructose) are ingested in food or produced by enzymatic digestion and are freely absorbed.

Digestion of proteins

Pepsin in the stomach begins the breakdown of proteins (proteolysis) into large polypeptides. Pancreatic enzymes in the lumen of the small intestine continue the process by breaking the large polypeptides into smaller polypeptides and peptides (see **Table 1.25**).

Over 20 peptidases on the brush border break down peptides into amino acids, dipeptides and tripeptides.

Digestion of fats

Most dietary fat is in the form of triacylglycerols (glycerol molecules plus a fatty acid chain). There is a very small amount of lipase present in saliva and gastric secretions which has a minor effect on the breakdown of fat. However, pancreatic lipase is responsible for the majority of fat breakdown, which occurs in the small intestine. Lipases work optimally on fat that has been emulsified by the detergent action of bile salts produced by the liver. Their action produces monoglycerides and fatty acids.

Digestion of major food groups				
Food Group	Enzymes	Site of enzyme production	Substrate	Product
Carbohydrate	Amylase*	Mouth Pancreas	Polysaccharides	Disaccharides, e.g. lactose, maltose, sucrose
	Lactase	Small intestine	Lactose	Glucose and galactose
	Maltase	Small intestine	Maltose	Two glucose molecules
	Sucrase	Small intestine	Sucrose	Glucose and fructose
Proteins	Pepsin	Stomach	Proteins	Polypeptides
	Trypsin Chymotrypsin Elastase	Pancreas	Polypeptides	Smaller polypeptides, peptides
	Carboxypeptidase Aminopeptidase Dipeptidase	Brush border of small intestinal mucosa	Smaller polypeptides and peptides	Amino acids
Fats	Lipase	Pancreas	Triacylglycerols	Monoglycerides and fatty acids

*Amylase is also secreted in saliva.

Table 1.25 Digestion of major food groups.

Digestion of nucleic acids (i.e. DNA and RNA)

These are hydrolysed to nucleotide monomers by pancreatic nucleases released into the small intestine.

Absorption

Absorption of nutrients and water from the lumen of the small intestine is optimised by the increased surface area provided by the circular folds, villi and microvilli. The jejunum is responsible for most of the nutrient absorption, with long thin villi maximising its absorptive area.

Cellular and molecular mechanisms of absorption

There are two routes for absorption from the lumen of the intestine: transcellular and paracellular (**Figure 1.48**). In transcellular absorption, the first stage is absorption through the apical cell membrane of the enterocyte. The nutrient then passes through the cell's basolateral membrane into the adjacent venules and from there into the superior mesenteric vein and then to the liver via the portal vein. Some absorbed fats (i.e. chylomicrons) enter the small lymph channels (lacteals) and then the lymphatic system (see **Figure 1.8**).

Absorption also occurs via tight (occluding) junctions between the enterocytes (paracellular movement).

Molecules are transported into and from the enterocytes by several different mechanisms (**Figure 1.49**):

- Diffusion
- Active transport
- Endocytosis and exocytosis

> Tight junctions, are protein complexes that hold adjacent cells closely together. They have a barrier function as they limit the regulation of molecules and ions. Tight junctions are also found in other parts of the body, e.g. the distal convoluting tubule of the kidney.

Diffusion

Simple diffusion occurs by osmosis, which is the spontaneous movement of molecules across a semi-permeable membrane from an area of low solute concentration to an area of high solute concentration. In this way, the solute concentrations are equalised. Small molecules such as water and alcohol diffuse through pores in the membrane or via the paracellular route, i.e. through the 'tight junctions' between the cells. As a result, around 80% of the water is absorbed before the gut contents reach the large intestine.

Gases diffuse passively across pores or tight junctions. Fats are able to diffuse through the lipid-based epithelium.

In facilitated diffusion the process of diffusion is facilitated by transport proteins, as

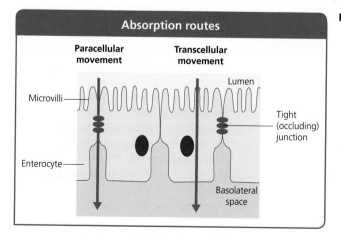

Figure 1.48 Absorption routes.

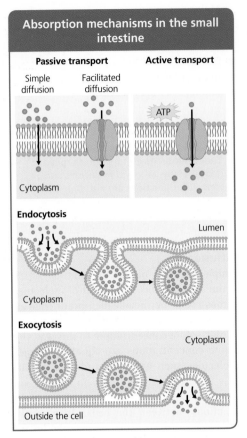

Absorption mechanisms in the small intestine

Passive transport   **Active transport**

Simple diffusion   Facilitated diffusion

ATP

Cytoplasm

Endocytosis

Lumen

Cytoplasm

Exocytosis

Cytoplasm

Outside the cell

Figure 1.49 Mechanisms of absorption in the small intestine.

is the case in transport of glucose and some amino acids for example.

Active transport

This allows nutrients to move against a concentration gradient, using adenosine triphosphate (ATP) as the energy source for the process. An example is the sodium/potassium pump, present in all intestinal cells, which imports glucose and amino acids into the cells. There are several different transport proteins to accommodate the large number of different amino acids to be absorbed.

Endocytosis and exocytosis

Larger molecules that cannot cross the membrane by diffusion or active transport are transported by these processes:

■ In endocytosis larger molecules are surrounded and engulfed into the cell, as

is the case for antibodies, which are intact large proteins
■ In exocytosis, the reverse happens: large molecules such as chylomicrons are released from the enterocytes into the lacteals

Absorption mechanisms for major food groups and nutrients

Mechanisms of absorption of the major food groups and nutrients are summarised in **Tables 1.26–1.28**. Under normal conditions, most nutrient absorption and nutrient-stimulated electrolyte absorption takes place in the jejunum. The ileum is responsible for the absorption of any residual nutrients. It also absorbs sodium against a concentration gradient and reabsorbs bile salts.

Figure 1.50 shows the major sites of absorption in the GI tract. In the duodenum, the osmotic pressure of the contents is variable. By the jejunum, however, it is almost equal to that of the plasma which means that transport of nutrients across the gut wall requires a more active mechanism.

> **80–90% of protein absorption takes place in the jejunum.**

Water

Water moves out of the lumen of the small intestine and into the enterocytes and then the bloodstream as the result of different osmotic drives:

■ The breakdown of macromolecules into monosaccharides (e.g. galactose, glucose), which makes the lumen hyperosmolar compared with the enterocytes. This causes water to move into the lumen along the osmotic gradient
■ Transport of chloride from the enterocytes into the lumen through cyclic-adenosine monophosphate (cAMP)-dependent chloride channels. Water follows by osmosis
■ These movements of osmotically active molecules are more than counterbalanced by the absorption and transport of

Absorption of the major food groups			
Food group	Substrate	Mechanism of absorption from lumen into enterocyte	Transfer from enterocyte into capillary
Carbohydrate	Glucose and galactose	Active absorption – co-transport with Na^+	Facilitated diffusion
	Fructose	Facilitated diffusion	Facilitated diffusion
Protein	Amino acids	Active absorption – co-transport with Na^+	Facilitated diffusion
	Dipeptides and tripeptides	Active absorption – co-transport with H^+, hydrolysed to amino acids in enterocytes	Facilitated diffusion
Fats	Cholesterol Monoglycerides and fatty acids	Diffusion through apical cell membrane, followed by formation of lipoproteins (chylomicrons) in enterocytes	Exocytosis (of chylomicrons into lacteals) and diffusion (of short-chain fatty acids into capillaries)

Table 1.26 Absorption of the major food groups

Mucosal absorption of major ions and nutrients	
Nutrient	Method of absorption
Sodium	Principal mechanism: active co-transport with amino acids and glucose
	Also transported via primary sodium channels and Na^+/H^+ exchanges. Quickly exported via active sodium pumps into the circulation
Potassium	Active via potassium conductance channels
	K^+/Cl^- co-transporters
Chloride	Passive diffusion
Calcium	Active: via vitamin-D dependent transporter route
Iron	Haem and Fe^{2+} are actively transported into the enterocyte
	Fe^{2+} is released from the cell into the circulation were it binds with transferrin
Fat-soluble vitamins (A, D, E, K)	Combined into chylomicrons (same pathway as fats)

Table 1.27 Mucosal absorption of the major ions and nutrients: this mostly takes place in the jejunum

osmotically active molecules from the lumen and into the bloodstream, for example glucose, amino acids, and electrolytes. Water follows along this osmotic gradient

The result is net absorption of water from the lumen.

Motility

The motility of the small intestine propels chyme from the duodenum to the colon and helps to prevent bacterial overgrowth, which lead to malabsorption and diarrhoea by interfering with normal mucosal function. Movement of the intestinal contents is mainly antegrade (i.e. from mouth to anus), but also occurs in a retrograde direction to allow mixing which increases the opportunities for absorption and digestion.

The intestinal wall has three layers of smooth muscle:

- The muscularis mucosae layer is involved in movement of the villi. It also aids secretion from the cells in the crypts of Lieberkühn (**Table 1.24**)
- The circular and longitudinal smooth muscle fibres of the muscularis externa cause peristalsis of the intestinal wall and are stimulated by nerves in the myenteric plexus

The interstitial ('pacemaker') cells of Cajal in the plexus produce bioelectrical waves at

Water-soluble vitamins			
Vitamin	Name	Absorption mechanism	Deficiency disease
B_1	Thiamine	Sodium-dependent active transport	Wernicke's syndrome Korsakoff's psychosis Beriberi
B_2	Riboflavin	Sodium-independent active transport	Ariboflavinosis Glossitis
B_3	Niacin	Sodium-dependent facilitated diffusion and passive diffusion	Pellagra
B_5	Pantothenic acid	Sodium-dependent multivitamin transporter	Paraesthesia
B_6	Pyridoxine	Simple diffusion	Peripheral neuropathy Anaemia
B_7	Biotin	Uncertain	Dermatitis
B_9	Folic acid	Sodium-dependent active transport or facilitated diffusion	Neural tube defects Megaloblastic anaemia
B_{12}	Cyanocobalamin	Intrinsic factor–vitamin B12 complex attaches to receptors on epithelial cells in the terminal ileum and is endocytosed	Anaemia Peripheral neuropathy
C	Ascorbic acid	Sodium-dependent active transport in the ileum	Scurvy

Table 1.28 Water-soluble vitamins: mechanisms of absorption and conditions caused by deficiency

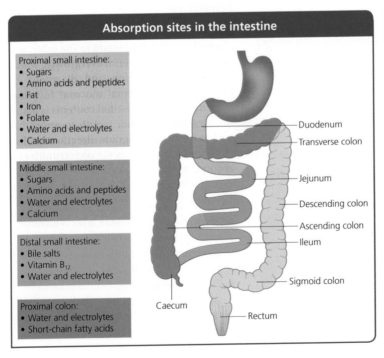

Absorption sites in the intestine

Proximal small intestine:
- Sugars
- Amino acids and peptides
- Fat
- Iron
- Folate
- Water and electrolytes
- Calcium

Middle small intestine:
- Sugars
- Amino acids and peptides
- Water and electrolytes
- Calcium

Distal small intestine:
- Bile salts
- Vitamin B_{12}
- Water and electrolytes

Proximal colon:
- Water and electrolytes
- Short-chain fatty acids

Duodenum
Transverse colon
Jejunum
Descending colon
Ascending colon
Ileum
Sigmoid colon
Caecum
Rectum

Figure 1.50 Absorption sites in the GI tract.

a rate of 12 per minute in the duodenum and 7 per minute in the ileum; leading to different rates of movement. Some of these waves result in intestinal contractions that increase the intraluminal pressure.

Motility is under the control of the enteric and autonomic nervous systems. Contraction is stimulated by luminal distension, pH changes and hyperosmolar contents. The presence of unabsorbed nutrients slows intestinal transit by reducing the frequency of intestinal contractions. Motility is also affected by several hormones, the most important are:

- Motilin – secreted by M cells in the crypts of the proximal small intestine. This promotes motility
- Gastrin – produced in the stomach increases the motility of the small intestine
- Vasoactive intestinal peptide (VIP) – produced by enteric nerves. This causes relaxation of the smooth muscle in the small intestine, thereby reducing motility. It also stimulates the secretion of water and electrolytes and inhibits gastric acid production

Neuroendocrine tumours (e.g. VIPomas) cause an excess production of gut hormones. This results in significant GI symptoms such as severe watery diarrhoea, which causes electrolyte disturbance.

Immune function

Lymphoid tissue is present throughout the GI tract and is referred to as gut-associated lymphoid tissue. For example, Peyer's patches are lymphoid aggregates in the lamina propria and submucosa of the distal small intestine; they are most numerous in the ileum (see **Figure 1.45**). They contain B cells and T cells, which differentiate commensal from foreign bacteria. B cells produce antibodies and T cells produce cytokines to neutralise gut toxins and infective agents.

Microbiota of the small intestine

The small intestine contains numerous commensal organisms (see **Table 1.14**). Their roles include:

- Carbohydrate digestion and absorption: bacterial enzymes help the breakdown of some polysaccharides, e.g. cellulose and pectin
- Production of short-chain fatty acids, e.g. acetic, butyric, propionic and succinic acid. These are formed by the fermentation of carbohydrates or proteins
- Synthesis of vitamins (folic acid, thiamine, B12 and K) by enteric and lactic acid bacteria; the vitamins are then absorbed by passive diffusion
- Metabolism of bile salts and sterols: primary bile salts are converted to secondary bile salts by dehydroxylation and these are reabsorbed via the enterohepatic circulation.
- Suppression of pathogenic microbial growth, e.g. *Clostridium difficile*
- Gut immune defences

Many of these actions are also carried out by bacteria in the large intestine, which are present in larger numbers (see page 76).

Some species of gut bacteria have not been identified and cannot be cultured as there are no suitable laboratory growth media.

Large intestine

Starter questions

Answers to the following questions are on page 82.

25. How do bacteria in the large intestine contribute to digestion?
26. How does the large intestine respond to dehydration?

The large intestine is a tubular structure that connects the small intestine to the anus. It is around 1.5 m long in its natural position.

Anatomy

The small intestine connects to the large intestine at the ileocaecal valve. The large intestine has a similar structure to the rest of the GI tract but, unlike the small intestine, does not contain villi or plicae circulares. It is divided into six segments (**Figure 1.51**):

- Caecum – lies in the right iliac fossa. Its diameter is greater than that of the left colon
- Ascending colon

- Transverse colon – the longest and most mobile part of the large intestine
- Descending colon
- Sigmoid colon – an S-shaped segment of intestine
- Rectum – around 15 cm in length. The anatomical relations of the rectum are outlined in **Table 1.29**

In addition to these segments is the appendix. This is a narrow blind-ending tube that is approximately 8 cm long. It connects to the end of the caecum, below the level of the ileocaecal valve (**Figure 1.51**).

The ascending and descending colon are retroperitoneal structures (the peritoneum covers the anterior surface only). The caecum,

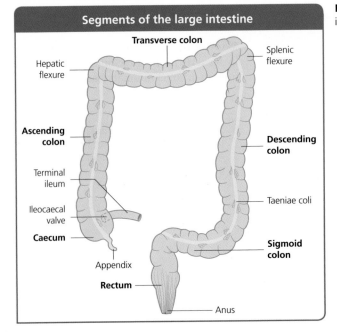

Segments of the large intestine

- Transverse colon
- Hepatic flexure
- Splenic flexure
- Ascending colon
- Descending colon
- Terminal ileum
- Taeniae coli
- Ileocaecal valve
- Caecum
- Sigmoid colon
- Appendix
- Rectum
- Anus

Figure 1.51 Segments of the large intestine (labelled in bold).

transverse colon, sigmoid colon and upper third of the rectum are peritoneal structures (completely covered by the peritoneum and suspended by the mesenteries). The lower third of the rectum is infraperitoneal (i.e. lies below the level of the peritoneum in the pelvis with other organs such as the bladder, distal ureters, uterus and prostate).

Three bands of longitudinal smooth muscle called the taeniae coli run from the rectosigmoid junction along the outside of the colon (**Figure 1.52**) and converge at the base of the appendix. They are located at 120° intervals around the large intestine. The taeniae coli contract to form haustra, which are pouches along the length of the large intestine and aid mixing of contents.

> The wall of the ascending colon and caecum is approximately 1.5 mm thick, compared with 3 mm in the descending and sigmoid colon.

Microstructure

The layers of the colon are similar to the rest of the GI tract (see **Figure 1.4**). Epithelial cells of the large intestine are called colonocytes. Within the epithelial lining of the intestinal wall there are crypts of Lieberkühn which extend to the muscularis mucosae. It also

Anatomical relations of the rectum			
		Anterior wall	Posterior wall
Male		Prostate	Sacral vertebrae
		Bladder fundus	Coccyx
		Section of the ureters	Blood vessels and nerves
		Vas deferens	
		Seminal vesicles	
Female		Vagina	Sacral vertebrae
		Cervix	Coccyx
			Blood vessels and nerves

Table 1.29 Anatomical relations of the rectum

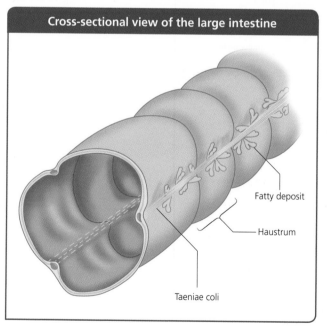

Cross-sectional view of the large intestine

Fatty deposit

Haustrum

Taeniae coli

Figure 1.52 Cross-sectional view of the large intestine.

contains a large number of goblet cells, which produce mucus to lubricate the movement of stool through the large intestine.

Embryology

The large intestine forms from the gut tube along with the small intestine, as described on page 63.

The caecum, appendix, ascending colon and proximal two thirds of the transverse colon are formed from the midgut. After the caecal bud re-enters the abdominal cavity, it moves from the right upper quadrant to the iliac fossa. This moves the ascending colon and hepatic flexure to the right side of the abdominal cavity.

The distal third of the transverse colon down to the upper part of the anal canal is formed from the hindgut.

Blood vessels and lymphatics

Arterial supply

The large intestine is supplied by the superior and inferior mesenteric arteries, which are branches of the aorta (**Figure 1.53**; see also **Figure 1.6**).

Figure 1.53 Arterial supply of the large intestine.

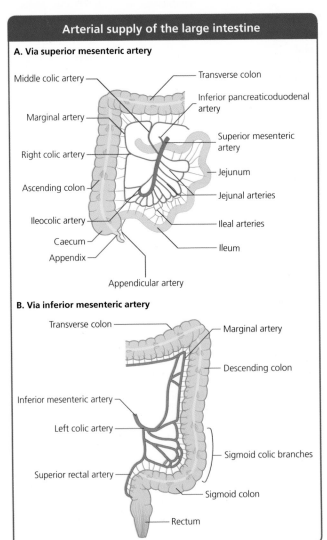

Arterial supply of the large intestine

A. Via superior mesenteric artery

- Middle colic artery
- Transverse colon
- Inferior pancreaticoduodenal artery
- Marginal artery
- Superior mesenteric artery
- Right colic artery
- Jejunum
- Ascending colon
- Jejunal arteries
- Ileocolic artery
- Ileal arteries
- Caecum
- Ileum
- Appendix
- Appendicular artery

B. Via inferior mesenteric artery

- Transverse colon
- Marginal artery
- Descending colon
- Inferior mesenteric artery
- Left colic artery
- Sigmoid colic branches
- Superior rectal artery
- Sigmoid colon
- Rectum

Venous drainage

Venous drainage of the region from the caecum down to the upper rectum is to the superior and inferior mesenteric veins. These join the splenic vein to form the portal vein (**Figure 1.54**; see also **Figure 1.7**). The lower part of the rectum drains into the systemic venous system rather than joining the portal circulation.

Lymphatic drainage

Lymphatic drainage of the large intestine is outlined in **Table 1.30**.

Nerve supply

The nerve supply is as follows:

- The coeliac and superior mesenteric ganglia supply the caecum, appendix and ascending colon
- The transverse colon is innervated by the superior and inferior mesenteric ganglia
- The descending and sigmoid colon are supplied by the superior hypogastric plexus (sympathetic) and pelvic splanchnic (parasympathetic) nerves

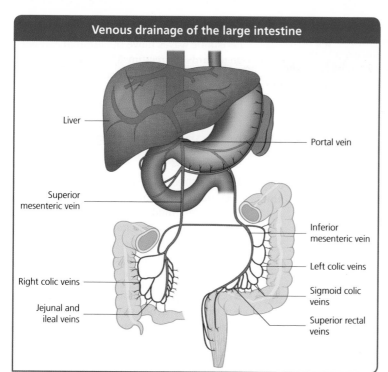

Venous drainage of the large intestine

Liver —
Portal vein
Superior mesenteric vein
Inferior mesenteric vein
Left colic veins
Right colic veins —
Sigmoid colic veins
Jejunal and ileal veins
Superior rectal veins

Figure 1.54 Venous drainage of the large intestine.

Lymphatic drainage of the large intestine

Segment	Lymphatic drainage	
Caecum and appendix	Ileocolic nodes	Superior mesenteric lymph nodes
Ascending colon	Paracolic and epicolic nodes	Superior mesenteric lymph nodes
Transverse colon	Middle colic nodes	Superior mesenteric lymph nodes
Descending colon	Intermediate colic nodes	Inferior mesenteric lymph nodes
Sigmoid colon	Intermediate colic nodes	Inferior mesenteric lymph nodes
Rectum	Superior half – pararectal nodes	
	Inferior half	Internal iliac lymph nodes

Table 1.30 Lymphatic drainage of the large intestine

■ The rectum is innervated by the inferior hypogastric plexus (sympathetic) and pelvic splanchnic (parasympathetic) nerves

Function

The main functions of the large intestine are to:

■ Absorb water from the chyme to form a more solid faecal material
■ Move faeces through the large intestine for evacuation from the body

> Water absorption is slower in the colon than the small intestine because the tight junctions connecting the epithelial cells are not as 'leaky'.

Peristaltic waves in the ileum push the chyme through the ileocaecal valve into the caecum. At all other times this valve is closed to prevent reflux of contents of the large intestine, including bacterial flora, into the terminal ileum.

Absorption

Around 1.5 L of chyme enters the large intestine each day. Most of the absorption from this occurs in the proximal (ascending and transverse) colon (see **Figures 1.11** and **1.50**). The lower part of the colon (descending and sigmoid colon, rectum) is a storage reservoir for the stools prior to their evacuation.

Sodium is actively transported into the epithelial cells through a sodium channel, and chloride is exchanged for bicarbonate (see page 68). Water is absorbed from the lumen by diffusion to equalise osmotic pressure between the plasma and the intestinal contents. Short-chain fatty acid absorption occurs as well as the completion of fluid and electrolyte absorption by active transport.

Around 90% of the fluid is absorbed, leaving behind semi-solid faecal matter containing water, undigested fibre, bacteria, fat, inorganic matter and protein.

Motility

The activity of the interstitial cells of Cajal leads to contraction of the circular and longitudinal smooth muscle in the walls of the large intestine. This has two main actions: mixing and propulsion.

Mixing

Contraction of both the circular muscle layer and the taeniae coli causes the large intestine to bulge into segments (haustrae). The faeces are moved back and forth within these haustra.

Propulsion

Peristaltic waves move the luminal contents on towards the rectum. Mass action contraction (mass movements) occurs when there is a contraction of long sections of the smooth muscle, starting in the right colon.

Microbiota of the large intestine

The large intestine contains in excess of 500 bacterial species including anaerobes (e.g. *Bacteroides*, bifidobacteria, clostridia) and aerobes (e.g. *Escherichia coli*, staphylococci) (see **Table 1.14**). The bacteria of the large intestine have similar functions to the bacteria of the small intestine:

■ Conversion of bilirubin to urobilinogen
■ Conversion of bile salts to secondary bile acids by bacterial dehydroxylases
■ Breakdown of fibre by glycosidase enzymes
■ Production of vitamins B and K
■ Prevention of growth of pathogenic bacteria

Fermentation by bacterial enzymes also results in the production of gas, which is expelled via the anus as flatus.

> **Broad-spectrum antibiotics (e.g. cephalosporins) alter the flora in the large intestine,** resulting in an overgrowth of bacteria; this causes disease, for example *Clostridium difficile* diarrhoea.

Anus

Starter questions

Answers to the following questions are on page 82.

27. How is defaecation controlled?
28. Why does the anus have two separate blood supplies?

The anal canal is approximately 4 cm long and controls the passage of faeces (defaecation) from the rectum where they are stored. It ends at the anus, which is the external opening of the GI tract.

Anatomy

The anal canal continues down from the rectum. The transition between its upper two thirds and lower third is marked by the dentate (or 'pectinate') line, at which there is a change in arterial supply and lymphatic drainage (see below). The anus has two sphincter muscles (**Figure 1.55**):

- Internal anal sphincter – the muscularis mucosae layer is thickened to form this sphincter, which extends from the rectum and surrounds the anal canal. Its action is involuntary
- External anal sphincter – this is formed from the striated sphincter ani externus muscle, with fibres connecting to the levator ani muscle

The puborectalis muscle forms a U-shaped sling around the anorectal junction, which is attached to either side of the pubic symphysis joint.

Microstructure

Inferior to the dentate line, the columnar epithelial lining of the rectum and upper anal canal is replaced by squamous epithelium.

Embryology

The dentate line forms the junction between the superior anal canal, which arises from the embryonic hindgut (endoderm), and the inferior anal canal, derived from the proctodeum (ectoderm). This explains their different innervation, vascular and lymphatic supply.

Blood vessels and lymphatics

Arterial supply and venous drainage

Superior to the dentate line, blood is supplied by the superior rectal artery, which originates

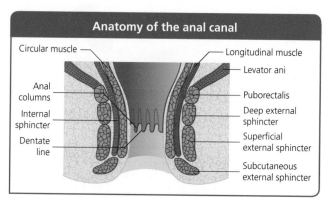

Anatomy of the anal canal

Circular muscle — Longitudinal muscle
— Levator ani
Anal columns
Internal sphincter — Puborectalis
Deep external sphincter
Dentate line — Superficial external sphincter
Subcutaneous external sphincter

Figure 1.55 Anatomy of the anal canal.

from the inferior mesenteric artery. Venous drainage is via the internal rectal plexus, which leads to the superior rectal vein. This empties into the inferior mesenteric vein.

Inferior to the dentate line, the arterial supply is from the inferior rectal arteries. Venous blood drains into the inferior rectal plexus, which empties into the inferior rectal veins.

Lymphatic drainage

Superior to the dentate line, drainage is to the internal iliac lymph nodes. The superficial inguinal lymph nodes drain the area inferior to the dentate line.

Nerve supply

The inferior hypogastric plexus (sympathetic) and pelvic splanchnic nerves (parasympathetic) innervate areas superior to the dentate line. Inferior areas are supplied by the inferior rectal nerves, which are branches of the pudendal nerves.

> The upper part of the anal canal is sensitive only to stretch; the lower part is sensitive to touch, pain and temperature. This relates to the different developmental derivation of these areas.

Function

The principal function of the anus is to control the evacuation of faeces from the large intestine.

Defaecation

The internal anal sphincter is usually contracted, but stimulation of the parasympathetic nerve fibres inhibits this contraction. This action is involuntary and occurs in response to distension of the rectum. The external anal sphincter is also maintained in a state of contraction, but it is under voluntary control.

When the pressure in the rectum starts to rise, there is an urge to defaecate. Once this reaches a certain point, both the internal and external anal sphincter muscles relax, resulting in reflex emptying of the rectal contents.

Voluntary defecation occurs on straining. It results from a combination of relaxation of the external sphincter, increased intra-abdominal pressure and relaxation of the puborectalis muscle (Figure 1.56). This makes the angle between the anus and rectum almost straight which allows the faeces to pass. Peristalsis in the rectosigmoid colon moves the faeces downwards until they are expelled through the anus.

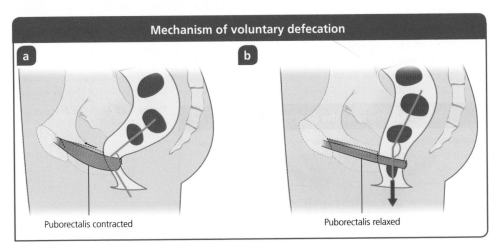

Mechanism of voluntary defecation

a

b

Puborectalis contracted

Puborectalis relaxed

Figure 1.56 Mechanism of voluntary defecation. Puborectalis is a sling-like part of the levator ani muscle, attached to the pubis on either side of the pubic symphysis and looping around the anorectal canal. When it is contracting (a), stool is retained in the rectum because of the acute angle between the rectum and anus. When it relaxes this angle increases (b), permitting defecation if the external sphincter also relaxes.

Answers to starter questions

1. The enteric nervous system of the GI tract can operate independently of the central nervous system (CNS). Its myenteric plexus, in the muscularis propria, controls peristalsis and its submucosal plexus controls epithelial function such as secretion, absorption, local blood flow and muscle movements. It responds to the presence of food in the intestinal lumen without external influence. It is also part of the autonomic nervous system: it receives a paraysmpathetic supply from the vagus nerve and a sympathetic supply from the paravertebral ganglia, so the CNS does have an influence on GI function, for example the 'cephalic' phase of digestion in which stimuli such as the smell of food or emotional factors stimulate saliva and gastric acid secretion.

2. Ageing has less effect on the GI tract than on other systems, such as the central nervous and musculoskeletal systems. However, the same reductions in muscle tone, sensation and compliance of tissue take place. As a result constipation, diverticulosis and gastro-oesophageal reflux are more common with older age. Changes to diet, physical activity, increased co-morbidity and increased medications all effect GI function and therefore cause symptoms. GI malignancies including oesophageal, gastric, pancreatic and colorectal cancer become more common.

3. There is a two-way relationship between symptoms and conditions of the GI tract and the central nervous system (CNS). The two systems are interconnected by the 'gut–brain axis' which links the CNS to nerves in the intestinal wall (the enteric nervous system) via the autonomic nervous system. Psychiatric and mood disorders commonly cause or exacerbate GI symptoms such as irritable bowel syndrome. Abdominal discomfort or diarrhoea often occurs during times of psychological stress, for example before an exam. Conversely, GI conditions such as inflammatory bowel disease lead to symptoms that reduce quality of life, give rise to anxiety and depression, and lead to sleep disturbance.

4. Different species have different functions, so a broader gut flora confers a wider range of benefits. Their predominant function of the 500-plus, mainly bacterial, species is to protect their host from infection by other bacteria, by stimulating immunogenic cells in the intestinal mucosa, competing for nutrients and preventing attachment to the epithelium. They also synthesise short chain fatty acids from the breakdown of fibre and small amounts of vitamins including K and B_{12}.

5. Plaque acids, produced by bacteria in the mouth from food and drink, lead to tooth decay and gum disease. Saliva contains bicarbonate which neutralises the acids and also washes away some of the food that sticks to teeth after eating. It contains antibacterial agents such as IgA, defensins, lysozyme, thiocyanate and hydrogen peroxide. It also contains calcium and phosphate which help to strengthen the protective tooth enamel.

6. Food is broken down into smaller pieces by the teeth via their chewing, tearing and grinding actions. Saliva is also added which acts as a lubricant and contains amylase and lipase, which begin the process of digestion of sugars and fats. A bolus is formed which is pushed back by the tongue into the pharynx where it then passes in a coordinated manner through into the oesophagus.

7. The smell of food is one of several stimuli, including taste, sight and even the anticipation of eating, that causes the production of saliva by an involuntary reflex via the autonomic nervous system. The same sensory factors also stimulate the production

Answers *continued*

of gastric acid (via the cephalic phase of gastric secretion) as well as increasing peristaltic motility in the GI tract in the anticipation of the arrival of food.

8. Both food and fluid entering the oesophagus, and air entering the trachea, pass through the pharynx. An involuntary process during swallowing prevents food and fluid from entering the trachea; the hyoid bone and larynx elevate and the epiglottis (a flap of cartilage at the root of the tongue) moves downward to cover the entrance to the larynx. This allows food to pass down into the oesophagus, whilst the airway is temporarily closed off.

9. In peristalsis, food is propelled down the oesophagus and along the GI tract by a series of co-ordinated waves. The circular muscle behind the bolus contracts whilst the circular muscle directly in front of it relaxes. At the same time the longitudinal muscle in the region relaxes which pushes the food to the next segment where the sequence is rapidly repeated again. This process looks very much like an earthworm moving through soil, it too has an inner circular and outer longitudinal muscle layer.

10. Specialised cells in the stomach lining called columnar (goblet) epithelial cells produce mucous that forms a layer which protects the mucosa. These cells also produce a small amount of bicarbonate which helps to buffer the acid on the surface of the stomach. There is also precise regulation of acid secretion so it does not occur in excess. Acid production is increased by the hormone gastrin which is released when food is in the stomach (in the gastric phase of gastric secretion) as well as by stimulation by the vagus nerve endings on the sight, smell or taste of food (the cephalic phase).

11. The stomach is a muscular sac that varies in size to hold between approximately 45 mL and 2 L of food and fluid. There are three layers of muscle which allow this change in size and facilitates the breakdown of food. Distension of the stomach stimulates gastric acid secretion and helps enzyme function. This aids the partial breakdown of food into chyme, which is released slowly from the stomach, through the pylorus, into the duodenum. Depending on the size and nature of the meal this can take a few hours, following which the stomach will return to a small size again.

12. The noises of a 'rumbling stomach' – borborygmi – arise predominantly in the small intestine. They are heard in two situations: (1) in the hours after meals, due to movement of food and gas through the intestine by peristalsis. ; (2) with hunger or the thought or smell of food, by stimulation of motor activity by the vagus nerve.

13. The liver has a remarkable ability to regenerate after an acute injury or when a significant part is removed. It involves replication of liver cells including hepatocytes, biliary epithelial and sinusoidal endothelial cells, stimulated by cytokines, hormones and growth factors. The newly-divided cells then undergo restructuring and angiogenesis. A full-sized liver can regenerate from only 25% of a normal liver mass after a surgical hepatectomy or when part of a liver is transplanted. Recurrent damage to the liver by agents such as alcohol, fat or viruses leads to chronic inflammation, fibrosis and cirrhosis.

14. The liver's role in nutrition is crucial because it is the location of the metabolism, synthesis, storage and release of many nutrients. It stores glucose as glycogen, which is converted back to glucose and released into the circulation when blood glucose falls. It is the site of breakdown of amino acids into urea and of synthesis of proteins such as albumin, globulin and the clotting factors. In the liver, triacylglycerols are combined with proteins in to form lipoproteins which are transported in the blood.

Answers *continued*

The liver produces cholesterol and stores fats as well as vitamin B_{12}, iron, copper and the fat-soluble vitamins A,D, E and K. It also produces bile acids, which aid the digestion and absorption of fats from the small intestine.

15. The portal circulation is a venous system transporting nutrient-rich venous blood from the walls of the GI tract to the inferior vena cava via the liver. Travelling from the GI tract, the superior and inferior mesenteric veins join the splenic vein to form the portal vein, which enters the liver. Nutrients are then processed by the liver and enter the systemic circulation via the hepatic veins. In the same way, potential toxins are also delivered to the liver where they can be metabolised or eliminated. The portal circulation also facilitates the delivery of ingested drugs to the liver, where they are metabolised before reaching the systemic circulation.

16. The characteristic yellow–green colour of bile comes from bilirubin, a breakdown product of haemoglobin from red blood cells. Bilirubin is produced in the spleen and excreted in bile, and passes out of the body in stool and urine, giving them a yellow and brown colour, respectively.

17. The spleen has a role in immune function and removing ageing blood cells from the circulation; you can live without it but with reduced function. The spleen is sometimes removed (a 'splenectomy'), usually because of trauma but as a result of haematological disorders, e.g. some leukaemias and lymphomas, haemolytic conditions. A splenectomy increases the risk of infection with polysaccharide-encapsulated bacteria such as *Streptococcus pneumoniae* and *Haemophilus influenza*; patients are immunised against these and also given the influenza vaccine. Patients also become more prone to tropical diseases such as malaria and must take prophylaxis before travelling.

18. When the liver is inflamed or scarred there is increased 'back' pressure in the portal and then splenic veins (portal hypertension), causing the spleen to enlarge. The spleen normally functions as a 'sieve' removing old blood cells from the circulation, but when it enlarges it removes a greater number of cells. This reduces the platelet count (thrombocytopaenia), as well as the number of white blood and red blood cells (anaemia).

19. Gallstones are usually formed from cholesterol. Therefore a diet low in saturated fats – avoiding large amounts of processed foods such as meat pies and sausages as well food such as cream and hard cheeses – reduces the formation of gallstones. Weight loss also reduces the amount of cholesterol in the bile, which lowers the risk of stones; however sudden weight loss has a paradoxical association with a greater risk of gallstones, for reasons that are not known.

20. After its production in the liver, bile is stored in the gallbladder. When food enters the duodenum, particularly where fatty acids are present, the hormone cholecystokinin (CCK) is released by the endocrine cells in the mucosa. CCK stimulates the contraction of the gallbladder and relaxation of the sphincter of Oddi so a large amount of bile is delivered into the duodenum. The bile acids aid the digestion and absorption of fats by emulsifying them.

21. Proteolytic enzymes produced and secreted by the pancreatic acinar cells are released as inactive pro-enzymes, or zymogens. This prevents autodigestion of the pancreatic cells. The crypts of Lieberkuhn in the duodenum release the enzyme enterokinase which converts trypsinogen (a pro-enzyme) into trypsin once in the gut, which then activates the other enzymes.

Answers *continued*

22. Despite the pancreas' vital role in the GI system, its function can be replaced by taking certain medications. As insulin is produced in the pancreas, removal results in diabetes, which necessitates insulin therapy. Pancreatic enzyme supplements are also required before meals to replace the normal exocrine function and aid digestion of food.

23. The small intestine is the longest part of the GI tract and is approximately 7 metres in length. It has several features which contribute to increasing the surface area and this maximises its ability to absorb nutrients from the lumen by enterocyte cells. Circular folds in the intestinal wall help to slow the traction of food and, along with finger-like projections called villi, increase the surface area. Villi vary in size and shape across the small intestine, but are the longest in the jejunum. Microvilli are smaller projections on the luminal surface of enterocytes. These adaptions increase the surface area 600 fold, compared with a hollow, smooth-surfaced tube of the same length and diameter.

24. The enzymes produced by the small intestine and pancreas to facilitate the digestion of food function optimally at a neutral pH or in a more alkaline environment. When the pH in the duodenum falls to below 5.0, i.e. when gastric acid is present, the hormone secretin is released by the endocrine cells (S cells) of the mucosa. Secretin stimulates the release of bicarbonate from the pancreas. It is the bicarbonate that neutralises or buffers the gastric acid in the proximal small intestine.

25. The large intestine has a limited role in digestion; the vast majority of digestion occurs in the small intestine. The digestion that does take place in the large intestine is facilitated by its resident bacteria. Undigested fibre is converted by the bacteria to short chain fatty acids such as acetate, proprionate and butyrate. These fatty acids enter the mucosal cell of the large intestine where they are used as an energy source. Bacteria in the large intestine produce small amounts of vitamin K, vitamin B_{12} and thiamine. They also convert bile salts into secondary bile acids.

26. The large intestine has the ability to increase the amount of water absorbed from it in response to dehydration. It typically reabsorbs 1.0–1.5 L of water per day, as it converts fluid received from the small intestine into stool. In health, only 100 mL or so of water is lost in the stool each day. During dehydration, the amount of water entering from the small intestine is reduced; the volume reabsorbed in the large intestine is increased, leading to harder stools and constipation.

27. The external anal sphincter is a striated muscle and is under voluntary control. It is in a constant state of contraction to keep the anal canal closed. When straining to defaecate, an increase in intra-abdominal pressure relaxes the puborectalis muscle that forms a sling around the anorectal junction. This causes a reduction in the angle between the anus and rectum facilitating evacuation of faeces from the rectum.

28. The anus has two different blood supplied because, like the rest of the gut, it develops from two different embryological layers. The inferior section develops from proctoderm, the posterior part of the ectoderm and the superior part develops from endoderm and mesoderm. The anus has both separate blood and lymph supplies: the superior rectal artery above, and the middle and inferior rectal arteries below. The pectinate (or dentate) line is at the junction of these areas, with columnar epithelium above and stratified squamous epithelium below.

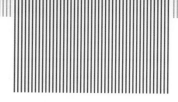

Chapter 2
Clinical essentials

Introduction

At the initial clinical encounter with a patient a history is taken and an examination performed with the aim of establishing the differential diagnoses, so that appropriate investigations can be undertaken in a structured way, usually starting with the least invasive, i.e. blood and stool tests. This approach minimises the need for unnecessary investigations, thereby reducing patient anxiety and discomfort and avoiding the cost of unnecessary tests and their potential for harm, for example perforation or bleeding during endoscopy.

This chapter discusses the full range of clinical and investigative tools and reviews the therapies used in gastrointestinal (GI) medicine. Treatments for GI disorders span a wide range of medications, psychological therapies and endoscopic interventions, for example cauterisation of a bleeding stomach ulcer.

Common symptoms and how to take a history

Starter questions

Answers to the following questions are on page 158.

1. When is abdominal pain likely to have a serious underlying cause?
2. Why do pale stools and dark urine occur in obstructive jaundice?

Symptoms of GI disease are a frequent cause of presentation both in general practice and the hospital. Knowing the function of the different regions of the GI system helps to understand which symptoms occur where; this knowledge informs choice of investigations and suggests possible diagnoses. As summarised in **Figure 2.1**, some symptoms suggest specific anatomical sites, for example with dysphagia the oesophagus is the likely

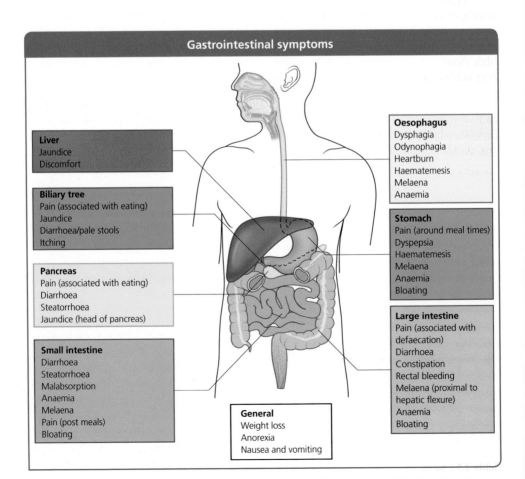

Gastrointestinal symptoms

Liver
Jaundice
Discomfort

Biliary tree
Pain (associated with eating)
Jaundice
Diarrhoea/pale stools
Itching

Pancreas
Pain (associated with eating)
Diarrhoea
Steatorrhoea
Jaundice (head of pancreas)

Small intestine
Diarrhoea
Steatorrhoea
Malabsorption
Anaemia
Melaena
Pain (post meals)
Bloating

Oesophagus
Dysphagia
Odynophagia
Heartburn
Haematemesis
Melaena
Anaemia

Stomach
Pain (around meal times)
Dyspepsia
Haematemesis
Melaena
Anaemia
Bloating

Large intestine
Pain (associated with defaecation)
Diarrhoea
Constipation
Rectal bleeding
Melaena (proximal to hepatic flexure)
Anaemia
Bloating

General
Weight loss
Anorexia
Nausea and vomiting

Figure 2.1 Gastrointestinal symptoms: the main symptoms from different regions of the GI system are shown.

site of disease; others do not, for example on their own neither weight loss nor anorexia help to specify a location.

Combinations of symptoms and signs gathered from the clinical history and examination are helpful in narrowing down the list of causes and therefore directing management. For example, loose stool with blood commonly signifies colonic pathology, whereas stool described as fatty and difficult to flush (steatorrhoea) by an individual with a history of alcohol excess suggests a pancreatic cause.

Common symptoms

Dysphagia

Dysphagia is difficulty swallowing. It is caused by disorders of the pharynx and oesophagus or by neuromuscular conditions (**Table 2.1**). In addition, central nervous system conditions sometimes affect the nerves controlling swallowing. Dysphagia at the level of the mouth or throat is termed high dysphagia, whereas dysphagia occurring behind the centre of the chest is called

Causes of dysphagia	
Site affected	Cause
Oesophageal	Oesophageal cancer
	Benign stricture
	Oesophagitis
	Achalasia
	Oesophageal dysmotility
Oropharyngeal	Pharyngeal pouch
	Pharyngitis or tonsillitis
	Painful mouth ulcers
	Mouth cancer
	Abscess (peritonsillar)
Neurological	Cerebrovascular accident
	Bulbar or pseudobulbar palsy
	Myasthenia gravis
Other	External compression, e.g. from lung cancer
	Systemic sclerosis
	Impacted foreign body

Table 2.1 Causes of dysphagia

retrosternal dysphagia and is usually due to oesophageal pathology.

Information about the onset and course of dysphagia and whether it occurs with liquids, solids or both, narrows down the list of potential causes. Problems with liquids only, which provoke coughing, suggest a neuromuscular cause. Conversely, narrowing of the oesophagus initially causes difficulty swallowing large pieces of solid food.

Progressive dysphagia is an 'alarm symptom' that merits urgent investigation due to the potential for a malignant cause. However, it is also caused by benign conditions such as strictures or motility disorders in which the peristaltic function is disturbed.

Dysphagia is often associated with symptoms of regurgitation or vomiting. Pain on swallowing is called odynophagia and is suggestive of an ulcerated or very inflamed oesophagus.

> **Alarm symptoms that suggest serious underlying pathology in the GI tract** include unintentional weight loss, progressive dysphagia and a new, persistent change in bowel habit.

Heartburn (gastro-oesophageal reflux or acid reflux)

Heartburn is a retrosternal burning discomfort in the oesophageal region. It is often described as a sensation rising from the lower chest to the mouth. Reflux is typically worse at night when patients lie flat, or when they bend over, and in 80% of cases is associated with regurgitation of contents from the stomach and the overproduction of saliva (water brash). Other symptoms associated with reflux are nausea and vomiting. Heartburn is often difficult to distinguish from cardiac chest pain.

Dyspepsia

This describes burning or pain occurring in the upper abdomen. Functional dyspepsia is often associated with bloating, belching and a feeling of fullness after meals. It is sometimes difficult to distinguish dyspepsia from cardiac, pancreatic and biliary disorders, due to the similar nature and site of the symptoms.

Early satiety is the feeling of fullness after eating small amounts of food. It is caused by disorders causing delayed stomach emptying (e.g. gastroparesis) or stomach cancer.

Haematemesis and melaena

Haematemesis is the vomiting of blood. This is fresh, i.e. bright red in colour, darker red and clotted, or has a 'coffee-ground' appearance in which small flecks of dark brown, altered blood are visible. It relates to bleeding from the proximal GI tract (oesophagus, stomach, duodenum).

A similar presentation occurs when swallowed blood originating from the nose, mouth or pharynx is vomited.

> Take care not to confuse the following terms:
> - **Haematemesis** – vomiting blood
> - **Haemoptysis** – coughing up blood from the airways
> - **Dysphagia** – difficulty swallowing
> - **Dysphasia** – difficulty speaking

Melaena describes a shiny black and tarry stool that is characteristically sticky and very smelly, due to the digestion of the blood by intestinal enzymes and bacteria. For it to be produced, blood has to remain in the GI tract for more than 12 hours so that the iron in the haemoglobin becomes oxidised, forming black-coloured haematin. Melaena is usually caused by bleeding in the upper GI tract. It less commonly originates from the small intestine or occasionally the right side of the large intestine.

Oral iron supplements almost always make the stool black but it does not smell as offensive. Blood loss below the level of the hepatic flexure in the colon presents as darker red blood loss per rectum, rather than melaena.

> It takes only 50 mL of blood loss into the GI tract to cause melaena.

Nausea and vomiting

Nausea is the sensation of wanting to vomit. Vomiting is the forceful ejection of stomach contents through the mouth. They often result from GI disorders, most commonly of the upper GI tract. However, pancreatic and biliary tree conditions, as well as acute intestinal obstruction also cause them.

Causes outside the GI tract should also be considered (see Chapter 4, page 185). Therefore a thorough clinical history, including a systems review, is required to establish the cause and need for further investigation.

Abdominal pain

Abdominal pain is a common symptom and has a wide range of causes (**Table 2.2**). The site and nature of the pain, as well as other features help to narrow down this list. The mnemonic SOCRATES is used to remember the relevant questions to ask:

- Site – described according to the quadrant or abdominal region affected (**Figure 2.2**)
- Onset – how long has it been present and did the pain come on suddenly or build up gradually? A gradual onset is often seen with inflammatory conditions affecting the GI tract, whereas pain from a perforated or ischaemic organ is usually more acute
- Character – used to describe the nature of the pain. Is it sharp, dull, burning or colicky? Colicky pain comes and goes in waves. It results from smooth muscle contraction and sometimes indicates obstruction of a hollow organ, e.g. the gallbladder, bile ducts or intestine. The character of pain can vary over time
- Radiation – does it travel from one area to another? For example, gallbladder pain is sometimes referred to the shoulder tip and pancreatic pain often travels through to the back
- Associated features – e.g. nausea or vomiting, a change in bowel habit, fever

Characteristic abdominal pains		
Cause	Location	Characteristics
Oesophageal	Retrosternal	Burning
Peptic ulcer disease	Epigastric	Burning/dull Exacerbated by eating
Pancreatic	Epigastric radiating to the back	Constant May be preceded by alcohol consumption
Biliary colic	Right upper quadrant or epigastric pain radiating to the back and shoulder tip	Severe and colicky Worse after eating, especially fatty foods
Small intestine	Central	Colicky Worse after meals (may occur several hours later if more distal small intestine)
Large intestine	Most commonly left lower quadrant, but can occur in other quadrants	Colicky Can improve with defaecation
Intestinal obstruction	Central	Colicky Abdominal distension and vomiting
Intestinal ischaemia	Central	Constant severe pain Exacerbated by eating
Appendicitis	Initially periumbilical, migrating to right iliac fossa	Constant
Peritonitic	Generalised throughout abdomen	Severe pain – patient lies still
Renal colic	Flanks and radiating to groins	Severe pain – patient unable to lie still
Bladder	Suprapubic	Diffuse and severe
Abdominal aortic aneurysm	Abdominal or back pain	Severe sudden-onset pain

Table 2.2 Characteristic abdominal pains

or urinary symptoms. Certain associations narrow down the list of possible causes

- Timing – does the pain follow any pattern, such as after eating or defaecation? Is it worse at certain times of day?
- Exacerbating or relieving factors – things that make the pain worse or better, such as coughing, moving or eating
- Severity – how bad is the pain? A pain score of 0–10 is often used, with 0 indicating no pain and 10 the worst pain imaginable

Patients often find it difficult to indicate the location of pain. Asking the patient to point to the area of worst pain with one finger helps to pinpoint it.

Abdominal pain also arises from organs outside the GI tract:

- Urological causes (kidney, ureter and bladder) – the causes are usually associated with urinary symptoms
- Gynaecological causes – pain is particularly common in young women and girls, almost always associated with menstruation or other gynaecological symptoms, such as vaginal discharge
- Musculoskeletal causes – pain from the abdominal wall or spine is usually worse with movement and is not associated with other GI symptoms
- Angina, pneumonia and pulmonary emboli sometimes present with acute upper abdominal pain

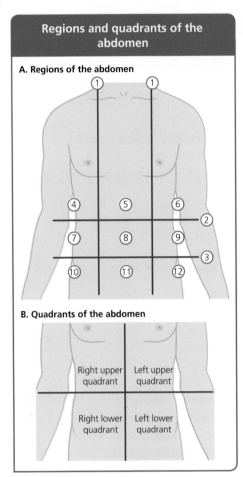

Regions and quadrants of the abdomen

A. Regions of the abdomen

B. Quadrants of the abdomen

Right upper quadrant | Left upper quadrant

Right lower quadrant | Left lower quadrant

Figure 2.2 Regions and quadrants of the abdomen. ① Midclavicular lines. ② Subcostal plane. ③ Transtubercular plane. ④ Right hypochondrium. ⑤ Epigastrium. ⑥ Left hypochondrium. ⑦ Right lumbar region. ⑧ Central/umbilical region. ⑨ Left lumbar region. ⑩ Right iliac fossa. ⑪ Suprapubic region/hypogastrium. ⑫ Left iliac fossa.

With lower abdominal pain in the left or right iliac fossa, it is often difficult to distinguish between intestinal and gynaecological causes in women. A change in bowel habit and relief after defaecation suggest an intestinal cause, whereas pain occurring cyclically with menstruation indicates a gynaecological origin.

Unintentional weight loss

On its own, this is a non-specific symptom caused by nearly any physical or psychiatric condition. It occurs with disorders of any part of the GI tract and is often associated with other symptoms that help direct the management plan. It is a worrying symptom when it occurs rapidly and particularly with increasing age, and merits further investigation.

Jaundice

Jaundice is a yellow discoloration that is usually seen initially in the whites of the eyes (sclerae) (see Figure 7.2). In more severe cases, the skin often becomes discoloured as well.

Jaundice is either categorised in terms of the anatomical site it arises from: pre-hepatic, hepatic or post-hepatic (**Figure 2.3**), or according to conditions affecting the liver cells (hepatitis/hepatocellular) or biliary tree (obstructive/cholestatic).

Pale stool, dark urine colour and itching (pruritus) occur in cholestatic jaundice.

Depending upon the underlying cause, patients sometimes also describe pain. Hepatocellular causes, such as viral infection and alcohol misuse are sometimes associated with right upper quadrant discomfort due to inflammation of the liver, as well as more general symptoms, for example lethargy, muscle aches and sweats. Gallstones blocking the common bile duct often cause colicky right upper quadrant pain radiating to the back. Pancreatic pathology commonly causes pain in the epigastric region and back.

Bloating

Bloating is the sensation of abdominal fullness and distension. It is sometimes associated with visible abdominal distension. It most commonly occurs in patients with functional GI disorders such as functional dyspepsia and irritable bowel syndrome. Other causes of bloating are bacterial overgrowth and carbohydrate intolerances, for instance lactose intolerance.

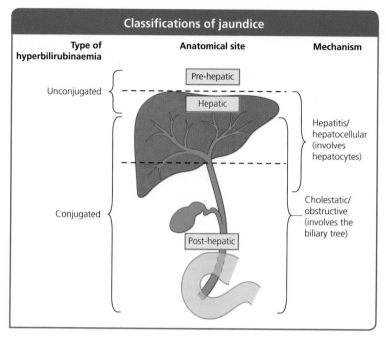

Figure 2.3
Classifications of jaundice according to the type of hyperbilirubinaemia, anatomical site and mechanism.

> Borborygmi are audible rumbling or gurgling noises caused by the movement of fluid and gas through the intestine.

Abdominal distension

The causes of visible distension of the abdomen are described by the '5 Fs'.

Ascites is the accumulation of fluid in the peritoneal cavity. It results in mild to gross abdominal distension, usually occurring over weeks to months. Patients often report swelling at the umbilicus due to a paraumbilical hernia, in addition to ankle swelling when suffering from ascites. Ascites usually results from failure of the liver, heart or kidneys, or from malignancy (**Table 2.3**). Chest pain, palpitations and shortness of breath suggest a cardiac source, whereas rapid unintentional weight loss with upper or lower GI symptoms usually indicates a malignancy.

Common causes of ascites	
Cause	Features
Liver cirrhosis	Clinical features of chronic liver disease, e.g. spider naevi (see Figure 7.1) SAAG >11 g/L
Abdominal or pelvic malignancy	Ascitic fluid may be bloodstained and cytology sometimes reveals malignant cells
Nephrotic syndrome	Proteinuria and low serum albumin SAAG <11 g/L
Heart failure	Clinical features, e.g. raised JVP, bibasal chest crepitations SAAG > 11 g/L
JVP, jugular venous pressure; SAAG, serum–ascites albumin gradient.	

Table 2.3 Common causes of ascites. Uncommon causes include Budd–Chiari syndrome, tuberculosis, restrictive pericarditis, pancreatic and biliary causes.

Causes of abdominal distension are the '5 Fs':

■ Fat – if the patient is overweight

■ Flatus – excess intestinal gas

■ Faeces

■ Fluid (ascites)

■ Fetus

Constipation

This is a reduced frequency of stool passage or firmer than normal stool that is difficult to pass. It is often associated with bloating, which gets better after defaecation. Symptoms of colicky abdominal pain suggest constipation-predominant irritable bowel syndrome. Obstructive defaecation occurs when there is a problem emptying the rectum, causing a feeling of incomplete evacuation or a need to remove stool using a finger (digitation). Ask about a potential history of injury to the anal muscles including obstetric trauma during childbirth or assisted delivery, for example the use of forceps.

A new change in bowel habit warrants urgent investigation to exclude malignancy, particularly when there are other alarm symptoms such as unintentional weight loss or rectal bleeding.

However, most patients describe chronic symptoms that are related to dietary factors, inadequate fluid intake or constipating analgesics (painkillers) such as codeine phosphate.

Diarrhoea

Diarrhoea is described as looser stool, increased stool frequency or a combination of the two. The Bristol stool chart (**Figure 2.4**) is widely used to accurately report stool consistency, which is alternatively broadly categorised as liquid, semi-formed or formed.

Patients also describe symptoms of faecal urgency (a need to rush to the toilet) and faecal incontinence (accidents). Incontinence occurs if individuals fail to make it to the toilet in time or due to disorders of the anus or rectum causing the leakage of stool.

Diarrhoeal symptoms that predominantly occur in the morning and occur with bloating and colicky abdominal pain that improves with defaecation are suggestive of irritable bowel syndrome (IBS). Nocturnal symptoms are particularly worrying and almost always indicate conditions other than IBS, for example inflammatory bowel disease.

Patients with infective diarrhoea describe offensive stool with a change in colour that usually resolves over a couple of days. Diarrhoea occurring after the ingestion of food

Bristol stool chart		
Type	Appearance	Description
1	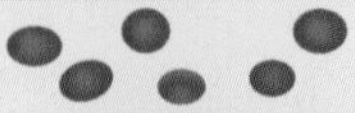	Separate lumps, like nuts (hard to pass)
2	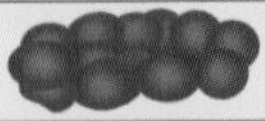	Sausage-shaped, but lumpy
3	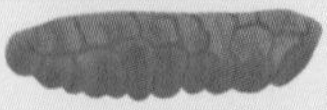	Like a sausage, but with cracks on the surface
4	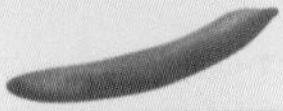	Like a sausage or snake, smooth and soft
5	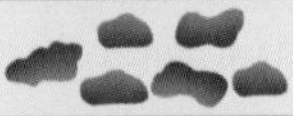	Soft blobs with clear-cut edges (passed easily)
6	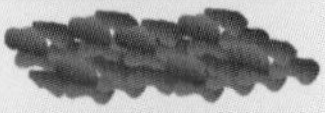	Fluffy pieces with ragged edges, a mushy stool
7	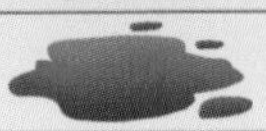	Watery or entirely liquid, no solid pieces

Figure 2.4 Bristol stool chart.

when digestive enzymes and bile are released suggests exocrine pancreatic insufficiency or bile salt malabsorption. Steatorrhoea describes pale, smelly stool with an oily appearance that is difficult to flush away – this is due to excess fat that is not absorbed because of disease of the small intestine or pancreas. The presence of blood and mucus suggests a source in the large intestine. A new onset of persistent diarrhoea and unintentional weight loss raises the possibility of an underlying malignancy and warrants urgent investigation.

> **Diarrhoea lasting for over 4 weeks is unlikely to be secondary to infection.**

Rectal bleeding

Fresh blood is suggestive of bleeding from the low rectum or anal region, for example from haemorrhoids. Bleeding from higher up the large intestine is darker red in colour. Patients may describe spotting of blood on the toilet paper, splattering in the pan or larger volumes. This is quantified by comparing the volume of blood with an eggcup or teacup full. When occurring with a change in bowel habit, causes such as malignancy or inflammatory bowel disease should be considered.

Most causes of rectal bleeding are painless. Pain and bleeding experienced during defaecation suggests an anal fissure (a tear in the skin of the anal canal) or haemorrhoids.

Taking a gastrointestinal history

A good clinical history provides a detailed assessment of the presenting symptoms (complaint), including their severity and how they have evolved over time. Any additional GI or other symptoms are also recorded. A combination of open followed by closed questions is usually required to elicit the history. Open questions allow the patient to answer in their own words using more than single word responses (e.g. 'What problems do you experience with your bowels?') compared with closed questions (e.g. 'Do you take NSAIDs?'), which are only answered by a 'yes' or 'no' response.

Relevant components of the past medical or surgical history, medications, family and social history help to suggest potential differential diagnoses (**Table 2.4**).

Presenting complaint

Following introductions, it is good practice to start the consultation with an open question such as: 'Your GP has asked me to see you due to problems with your swallowing. Please can you tell me about this?' A short sentence

Components of a GI history	
History	Key points
Presenting complaint and history of presenting complaint	Heartburn and reflux
	Dysphagia and odynophagia
	Haematemesis and melaena
	Dyspepsia
	Nausea and vomiting
	Loss of weight or appetite
	Abdominal pain, mass or swelling
	Jaundice
	Change in bowel habit (diarrhoea or constipation)
	Rectal bleeding
Past medical history	Previous operations
	Relevant medical conditions, e.g. diabetes
	Previous anaemia or jaundice
Medication history	All medications including analgesics and anti-inflammatory drugs
	Allergies
	Over-the-counter medicines
Family history	GI malignancy
	Autoimmune conditions
	Inflammatory bowel disease
Social history	Occupation
	Smoking (quantify in pack-years)
	Alcohol use
	Illicit drug use
Nutritional history	Number of meals per day
	Relationship of food types (e.g. fatty foods) to symptoms
Systems review	Overview of other systems, e.g. respiratory and cardiovascular

Table 2.4 Components of a GI history

is used to document the main presenting complaint in the medical records.

History of presenting complaint

This allows patients to describe their presenting symptom(s) in detail, such as:

- Location of the symptoms
- Onset of the symptoms – the timescale should be quantified in seconds, minutes or days, or as constant
- History of similar previous episodes – frequency, length of symptoms
- Exacerbating and relieving factors
- Associated symptoms experienced during the period of illness should be enquired about, for example symptoms of heartburn in patients with dysphagia
- Impact of the symptoms on the patient's daily activities

> **Abdominal pain** is occasionally caused by conditions affecting other parts of the body, for example pneumonia, pulmonary emboli, ischaemic heart disease and diabetic ketoacidosis.

In patients presenting with abdominal symptoms, positive and negative responses to questions relating to the GI system are recorded in the history of presenting complaint. For example, the absence of melaena is important to note in patients with GI haemorrhage, as it is used as part of a scoring system to determine the timing of an upper GI endoscopy.

Past medical history

This includes relevant surgical procedures, significant medical conditions and previous hospital admissions. For example, a history of diarrhoea in a patient with diabetes raises the possibility of pancreatic insufficiency.

> **A current list of medication, obtained from medical records or relatives, provides clues to the past medical history if the patient is unable to give details,** for instance due to confusion. Go through the list drug by drug, and think why each one has been prescribed.

Medication history and allergies

The medication history considers the following:

- Prescribed medications – patients may carry a list with them
- Over-the-counter medications
- Complementary or herbal medications and dietary supplements
- Illicit drug use – this is a potential risk factor for hepatitis B and C

Many drugs have GI side effects, including nausea, diarrhoea and cause abnormal liver function blood tests (**Table 2.5**). Medications should also be reviewed in patients with specific conditions. For example antibiotic and proton pump inhibitor treatment is associated with *Clostridium difficile* diarrhoea and should be reviewed and discontinued where possible.

Confirm any allergies when prescribing new medications or undertaking procedures that use local anaesthetic or sedation such as

Medication-related GI symptoms	
Symptoms	Medication
Diarrhoea	Antibiotics
	Colchicine
	Metformin
	Proton pump inhibitors
Constipation	Opioids
Nausea and vomiting	Antibiotics
	NSAIDs, e.g. ibuprofen
	Antiepileptics, e.g. gabapentin (page 186)
	Antidepressants
Jaundice	Antibiotics (flucloxacillin, co-amoxiclav)
	Paracetamol (in overdose)
	Rifampicin
	Isoniazid
GI bleeding and dyspepsia	NSAIDs and aspirin
	Calcium channel antagonists
	Selective serotonin reuptake inhibitors

NSAID, Non-steroidal anti-inflammatory drug.

Table 2.5 Examples of common medication-related GI symptoms

endoscopy, to ensure that the patient does not have an adverse reaction.

Family history

This documents any family history of GI malignancy, coeliac disease, inflammatory bowel disease, haemochromatosis and autoimmune conditions. The age and sex of affected relatives is often used to determine an individual's risk of GI malignancy and whether surveillance endoscopy or radiological imaging is required. For example, the risk of colorectal cancer increases with the number and younger age of relatives affected.

Social history

This has several components, which are used to determine the potential underlying aetiology and plan management:

- Occupation – this raises the possibility of certain potential causes, e.g. liver cancer in industrial workers due to chemical exposure
- Family support – review this when considering treatments such as liver transplantation, where patients require considerable help from friends and relatives during the recovery period
- Travel/vaccination history – this is particularly necessary for patients with diarrhoea or jaundice. It often points towards an infectious aetiology, e.g. hepatitis A
- Smoking history – smoking is a risk factor for certain malignancies, such as oesophageal cancer and increases the

need for escalation of medical treatment and surgery in patients with Crohn's disease
- Alcohol history – this is relevant for many GI presentations, e.g. cirrhosis
- Sexual history – this is relevant when considering hepatitis B and C

> **To assess a patient's smoking, calculate the pack–year history:**
>
> Pack–years = number of packs of 20 cigarettes smoked per day × number of years the person has smoked

A patient's functional status is particularly important when considering treatment options. For example, for a patient who has cardiovascular disease that is sufficiently severe to limit activities of daily living, the risks of anaesthesia are sometimes so high that surgery is contraindicated irrespective of the stage of a malignancy. In this situation, alternative treatments such as chemo-radio-therapy should be considered.

Alcohol history

A history of current and previous alcohol intake should be taken, recording the average number of units consumed per week (**Figure 2.5**). Alcohol excess is associated with an increased risk of a range of conditions (**Table 2.6**).

The screening questionnaires most commonly used to diagnose alcohol abuse and dependence are the 4-question CAGE (**Table 2.7**)

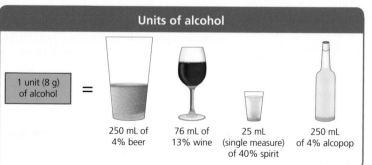

Figure 2.5 Units of alcohol.

Units of alcohol

1 unit (8 g) of alcohol =

250 mL of 4% beer

76 mL of 13% wine

25 mL (single measure) of 40% spirit

250 mL of 4% alcopop

Consequences of chronic alcohol consumption	
GI consequences	**Non-GI consequences**
Oesophagus	**Brain**
Oesophageal reflux	Wernicke's encephalopathy
Barrett's oesophagus	Korsakoff's psychosis
Cancer	Seizures
	Mood disturbance, e.g.
Stomach	depression
Gastritis	Ataxia
Liver	**Pharynx and larynx**
Alcoholic hepatitis	Cancer
Alcoholic steatohepatitis	
Cirrhosis	**Heart**
	Cardiomyopathy
Pancreas	Abnormal heart rhythms,
Pancreatitis (acute and chronic)	e.g. atrial fibrillation
	Blood
	Macrocytic anaemia
	Thrombocytopenia
	Genitalia
	Hypogonadism
	Erectile dysfunction
	Joints
	Gout

Table 2.6 Consequences of chronic alcohol consumption

The CAGE questionnaire to assess alcohol dependence
2 positive responses raise the possibility of alcohol dependence, which should be investigated further:
■ Have you ever felt you needed to **C**ut down on your drinking?
■ Have people **A**nnoyed you by criticising your drinking?
■ Have you ever felt **G**uilty about drinking?
■ Have you ever felt you needed a drink first thing in the morning (**E**ye-opener)?

Table 2.7 The CAGE questionnaire to assess alcohol dependence

Guideline daily amounts		
Component	**Men**	**Women***
Calories (kcal)	2,500	2,000
Protein (g)	55	45
Total fat (g)	95	70
Saturated fats (g)	30	20
Carbohydrates (g)	300	230
Fibre (g)	24	24
Salt (g)	6	6
Fluid (L)	2	1.6
Alcohol	< 14 units/week	< 14 units/week

*In Europe and the UK, on food labels the daily guidance on energy and nutrient intake is called the reference intake and the values given are for women.

Table 2.8 Guideline daily intake of energy, nutrients, fluids and alcohol for healthy living

and 10-question AUDIT (Alcohol Use Disorders Identification Test) tools.

Nutritional history

The history should incorporate the amounts and types of food consumed (**Table 2.8**). Poor nutrition plays a significant role in patient morbidity and mortality. The consequences of a poor diet range from undernutrition and vitamin deficiencies to obesity and resulting metabolic syndrome and fatty liver disease.

Around a third of hospital inpatients are undernourished due to reduced oral intake secondary to their symptoms and diseases. These include nausea or dysphagia, conditions causing malabsorption (diseases of the pancreas or small intestine) and diseases resulting in increased calorie consumption, for example chronic liver disease. Hospital patients also have periods of being nil by mouth during investigation.

Healthy eating recommendations:

- Plenty of fruit and vegetables – at least five portions a day

- Plenty of starchy foods – bread, rice, pasta (preferably wholegrain) and potatoes

- Some milk and dairy products – reduced-fat versions

- Some protein-rich foods, e.g. meat, fish, eggs, beans, nuts and pulses

- Small amounts of saturated fats, salt and sugar

Systems review

The systems review provides a brief overview of all body systems, for example cardiovascular and respiratory. In gastroenterology, the systems review is essential, as a patient's symptoms sometimes arise from one of several different organs. For example, a history of chest pain occurring during exertion is more suggestive of cardiac rather than GI cause.

Differential diagnoses

The information contained in the history should be used to develop a list of differential diagnoses. Potential causes are considered using the mnemonic VITAMIN CDEF:

- Vascular
- Infection/Inflammatory
- Trauma
- Autoimmune
- Metabolic
- Idiopathic (unknown cause)/Iatrogenic (illness caused by medical treatment)
- Neoplastic
- Congenital
- Drugs/Degenerative/Developmental
- Endocrine/Environment
- Functional (psychological)

Common signs and how to examine a patient

Starter questions

Answers to the following questions are on page 158.

3. How is ascites detected?
4. What is palpable in a normal abdomen?
5. What should be done before starting an abdominal examination?

The aim of the physical examination is to identify signs to support the differential diagnoses suggested by the history. Complications of disease are also assessed, for example the presence of ascites in chronic liver disease. A systematic approach is required so that components are not missed. This should follow the sequence (**Figure 2.6**):

- Inspection (look)
- Palpation (feel)
- Percussion (tap)
- Auscultation (listen using a stethoscope)

Before any examination, wash your hands using soap and water or clean them with alcohol gel. Basic observations such as blood pressure, height and weight should be recorded. These are used to calculate a patient's body mass index (BMI):

$$BMI = weight\ (kg)/height\ (m^2)$$

BMI is used to interpret whether the patient is of appropriate weight:

- Underweight <18.5 kg/m^2
- Normal range 18.5–24.9 kg/m^2
- Overweight >25 kg/m^2
- Obese >30 kg/m^2
- Morbidly obese >40 kg/m^2

The main problem with using BMI as an indicator of whether a patient's weight is appropriate is that it does not distinguish between fat and lean body (muscle) mass. For example, an athlete often has an increased BMI due to a high muscle mass rather than being overweight.

> **Inpatients should routinely be assessed for their risk of malnutrition**. Screening tools assess BMI, unintentional weight loss, co-morbidities and ability to maintain oral intake. The findings determine whether food monitoring and referral to a dietician are necessary.

General inspection

Begin the examination by taking a step back and making a general assessment from the end of the bed (**Figure 2.6**) to observe:

- Bedside clues, e.g. nil-by-mouth signs, medications, dark urine in a catheter bag
- Whether they look well or unwell
- Whether they appear comfortable or are in pain
- Body habitus (physical build), looking for signs of malnutrition, muscle wasting or obesity
- Their general appearance – e.g. pallor, jaundice or bruising secondary to underlying liver disease

The patient is conventionally examined from the right side of the bed, lying flat with their head supported by a single pillow. The abdomen should be fully exposed while maintaining the patient's dignity by keeping the groin covered until it is examined.

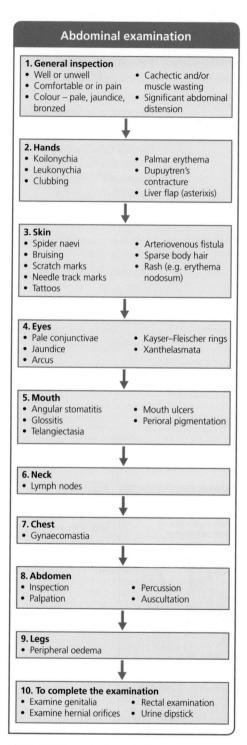

Abdominal examination

1. General inspection
- Well or unwell
- Comfortable or in pain
- Colour – pale, jaundice, bronzed
- Cachectic and/or muscle wasting
- Significant abdominal distension

2. Hands
- Koilonychia
- Leukonychia
- Clubbing
- Palmar erythema
- Dupuytren's contracture
- Liver flap (asterixis)

3. Skin
- Spider naevi
- Bruising
- Scratch marks
- Needle track marks
- Tattoos
- Arteriovenous fistula
- Sparse body hair
- Rash (e.g. erythema nodosum)

4. Eyes
- Pale conjunctivae
- Jaundice
- Arcus
- Kayser–Fleischer rings
- Xanthelasmata

5. Mouth
- Angular stomatitis
- Glossitis
- Telangiectasia
- Mouth ulcers
- Perioral pigmentation

6. Neck
- Lymph nodes

7. Chest
- Gynaecomastia

8. Abdomen
- Inspection
- Palpation
- Percussion
- Auscultation

9. Legs
- Peripheral oedema

10. To complete the examination
- Examine genitalia
- Examine hernial orifices
- Rectal examination
- Urine dipstick

Figure 2.6 Abdominal examination.

Patients should always be offered the option of a chaperone during intimate examinations, including rectal examination. It is good practice to document the identity of the chaperone in the medical records.

Hands

The examination starts by assessing for peripheral stigmata of abdominal disease. First, the patient should be asked to hold their hands out in front of them. A tremor is sometimes seen with alcohol withdrawal, anxiety or hyperthyroidism.

Nails

Signs observed in the nails:

- **Clubbing (Figure 2.7)** – this is a loss of the angle between the nail and nail bed, with increased curvature of the nails and increased fluctuance (sponginess) of the nail upon the nail bed. The underlying mechanism is unknown. Most cases are due to non-GI diseases (**Table 2.9**)
- **Leukonychia** – whitening of the nail bed due to hypoalbuminaemia (low albumin level). It occurs in liver disease, malabsorption and nephrotic syndrome
- **Koilonychia** – spoon-shaped nails seen in iron deficiency

Palms

Patients should be asked to turn their hands palm upwards (**Figure 2.8**) to assess for:

- **Palmar erythema** – reddening of the palms (of the thenar and hypothenar eminences). This is seen in chronic liver disease, as well as pregnancy, thyrotoxicosis and rheumatoid arthritis
- **Dupuytren's contracture** – thickening and contraction of the palmar fascia, which sometimes leads to a flexion deformity of the fingers. In the early stages, thickening of the fascia is felt by running a finger over the palm, especially overlying the

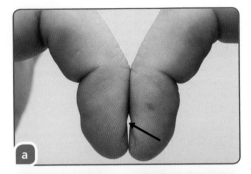

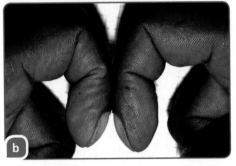

Figure 2.7 Clubbing. Schamroth's sign of clubbing. (a) In the normal nail, there is a diamond-shaped window between nail beds, Schamroth's window (arrowed). (b) In clubbing, there is obliteration of this window (a positive Schamroth's sign), increased curvature of the nails, increased fluctuance (sponginess) of the nail bed and bulbous enlargement of the fingers.

Causes of clubbing	
Site of pathology	Aetiology
Gastrointestinal	Inflammatory bowel disease
	Cirrhosis
	Malabsorption, e.g. coeliac disease
Respiratory	Lung cancer
	Interstitial lung disease, e.g. fibrosing alveolitis
	Suppurative lung disease, e.g. abscess, cystic fibrosis, bronchiectasis
	Complicated tuberculosis
Cardiovascular	Congenital cyanotic heart disease, e.g. tetralogy of Fallot
	Subacute bacterial endocarditis
	Atrial myxoma
Other	Graves' disease
	Familial
	Idiopathic

Table 2.9 Causes of clubbing

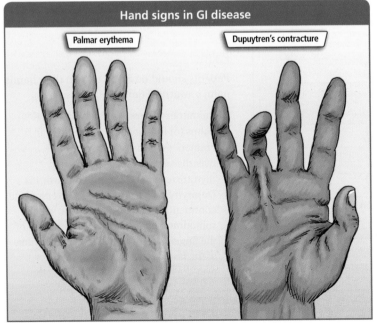

Hand signs in GI disease

Palmar erythema

Dupuytren's contracture

Figure 2.8 Hand signs in GI disease: palmar erythema and Dupuytren's contracture.

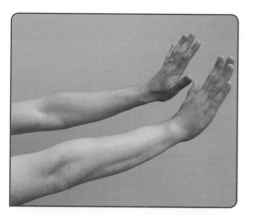

Figure 2.9 Testing for liver flap (asterixis). The patient is asked to hold arms outstretched with hands hyperextended at the wrist for at least 15 seconds. Liver flap is present if there are repetitive jerky and irregular flexion/extension movements at the wrist.

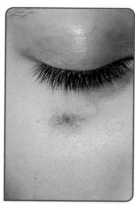

Figure 2.10 Spider naevus.

of circulating oestrogen in chronic liver disease, thought to occur due to reduced extraction of the steroid hormone androstenedione by the liver also arise in pregnancy.

fourth and fifth metacarpals. It occurs in chronic liver disease, manual workers or is sometimes idiopathic

Liver flap (asterixis)

This is assessed by asking patients to hold their arms straight out in front of them and then dorsiflexing their hands at the wrists (**Figure 2.9**). If a flap is present, there will be jerky, irregular flexion/extension movements at the wrist.

> Liver flap is seen in the early stages of hepatic encephalopathy (accumulation of liver toxins affecting brain function). It is caused by a loss of transmission of sense of joint position (proprioception) to the brain.

Skin

The arms should be examined for the signs outlined in **Figure 2.6**. Spider naevi are characterised by a central red spot from which small extensions radiate out like spider legs (**Figure 2.10**). They disappear when pressure is applied to the centre and refill from the centre when the pressure is removed.

Spider naevi occur in the drainage distribution of the superior vena cava (arms, face, chest, upper back). They are due to an increased level

> Presence of more than five spider naevi suggests underlying liver disease. Many people have fewer than this in the absence of an underlying disorder.

Eyes

The following signs may be visible in and around the eyes (**Figure 2.11**):

- **Jaundice** – a yellow discoloration of the sclerae
- **Arcus** – a white, grey or blue opaque ring at the corneal margin. It is caused by high cholesterol and old age (arcus senilis)
- **Kayser–Fleischer ring** – a yellowish-green ring around the outer edge of the cornea. It results from copper deposition in untreated Wilson's disease. A slit lamp is usually required to identify it
- **Pale conjunctivae** – this occurs with anaemia
- **Xanthelasmata** – raised yellow lesions seen around the nasal aspect of the eye that are caused by an accumulation of lipids under the skin. They are not specific to GI disease, however they are sometimes seen in patients with hypercholesterolaemia and associated fatty liver disease or primary biliary cholangitis who have chronic cholestasis

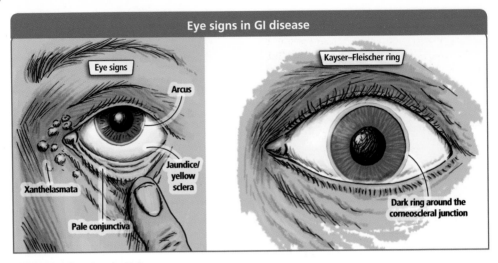

Figure 2.11 Eye signs in GI disease.

and reduced cholesterol excretion into the biliary tree

Mouth and tongue

Appearances to seek around the oral cavity (**Figure 2.12**) are:

- **Mouth ulcers** – these are due to inflammatory bowel disease, Behçet's disease, coeliac disease or poorly fitting dentures
- **Glossitis** – this is a smooth or reddened tongue seen in iron, vitamin B$_{12}$ or folate deficiency
- **Angular stomatitis (cheilitis)** – this is reddening and cracking at the corners of the mouth due to deficiency of iron and most B vitamins
- **Brown perioral pigmentation** – this is seen in Peutz–Jeghers syndrome, an autosomal dominant condition also characterised by benign polyps of the GI tract
- **Telangiectasia** – this is dilation of blood vessels, visible on the lips and in the mouth

> Hereditary haemorrhagic telangiectasia (Osler–Weber–Rendu syndrome) causes telangiectasia of the mucous membranes. The telangiectasia bleed resulting in chronic GI blood loss and iron deficiency anaemia.

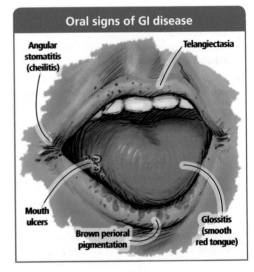

Figure 2.12 Oral signs of GI disease.

Neck and back

The patient is asked to sit forward to allow palpation of the neck for enlarged cervical and supraclavicular lymph nodes. A palpable left supraclavicular node is sometimes a sign of a metastatic gastric malignancy; this is called Virchow's node (Troisier's sign).

While the patient is leaning forwards, the back is inspected for scars (e.g. renal surgery), spider naevi and sacral oedema.

Chest

Gynaecomastia is benign enlargement of the breast tissue in males. It is a normal finding during puberty. It is also seen in chronic liver disease or secondary to medications, for example spironolactone and cimetidine.

Abdominal inspection

The abdomen is inspected for:

- **Abdominal distension** – causes include any one of the '5 Fs' (see page 90)
- **Surgical scars (Figure 2.13)**
- **Striae (stretch marks)** – these are whitish-pink streaky lines caused by rapid changes in abdominal wall tension; they are normal in pre-pubescent teens and are also seen as a result of pregnancy, obesity, steroid usage and ascites
- **Bruising** – this sometimes occurs in pancreatitis (e.g. Cullen's or Grey Turner's sign; see Figure 8.3) or after trauma
- **Obvious masses** – examples include enlarged organs and intra-abdominal tumours causing asymmetrical distension of the abdominal wall
- **Stoma** – these are surgically created openings that connect the intestine (e.g. ileostomy, colostomy) or urinary tract (e.g. urostomy) to the skin (**Table 2.10**)
- **Divarication of the recti** – this is lateral separation of the rectus abdominis muscles causing a bulge to appear between them; it is elicited by asking the patient to lift the head off the bed or sit up slightly and is not of any clinical significance
- **Abdominal wall hernia** – e.g. incisional at sites of previous surgery or paraumbilical. Herniation is more prominent when the patient sits forwards or coughs

Types of stoma		
	Ileostomy	Colostomy
Connection	Small intestine (ileum) to abdominal wall	Large intestine to abdominal wall
Indication	After resection of whole large intestine, e.g. inflammatory bowel disease, familial adenomatous polyposis	After resection of part of large intestine, e.g. Hartmann's procedure for colonic cancer or perforated diverticular disease, or after colovaginal fistula
Position	Usually in right iliac fossa	Usually in left iliac fossa
Characteristics	Has a spout	Flush with skin
Contents	Liquid	Semi solid

Table 2.10 Types of stoma

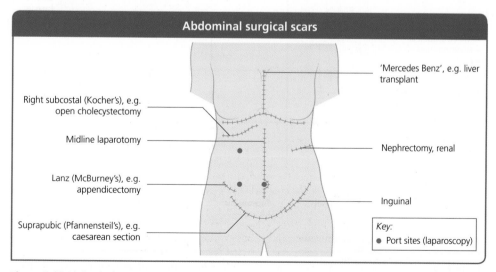

Abdominal surgical scars

- 'Mercedes Benz', e.g. liver transplant
- Right subcostal (Kocher's), e.g. open cholecystectomy
- Midline laparotomy
- Nephrectomy, renal
- Lanz (McBurney's), e.g. appendicectomy
- Inguinal
- Suprapubic (Pfannensteil's), e.g. caesarean section

Key:
● Port sites (laparoscopy)

Figure 2.13 Abdominal surgical scars.

- **Distended abdominal wall veins** – these occur over the upper abdominal wall and chest wall as a result of superior vena cava obstruction. Distended veins over the lower abdominal wall are secondary to inferior vena cava obstruction
- **Caput medusae** – these are prominent veins over the anterior abdominal wall that radiate out from the umbilicus. Portal hypertension causes the umbilical vein to become re-canalised resulting in engorgement of the superficial epigastric veins (see Figure 7.3).

Abdominal palpation

Palpation is use of the hands to feel for organs and abnormalities (**Figure 2.14**). If the patient has pain, palpation should commence in the opposite area of the abdomen. Initial superficial palpation of each of the four quadrants identifies areas of discomfort. Deeper palpation is then performed to identify any masses, and this is followed by examination for the individual organs (**Table 2.11**).

Masses are described by their site, size, shape, consistency and relationship to other structures.

Potential findings during abdominal palpation are:

- **Rebound tenderness** – acute pain experienced by the patient when the hand is removed from the abdominal wall during palpation. It occurs in peritonitis
- **Guarding** – involuntary tension in the abdominal muscles in patients with peritonitis
- **Murphy's sign** – pain on palpation of the gallbladder (right upper quadrant) during deep inspiration. It is a sign of cholecystitis
- **McBurney's point tenderness** – pain located one third of the distance from the right superior iliac spine to the umbilicus. It is suggestive of appendicitis

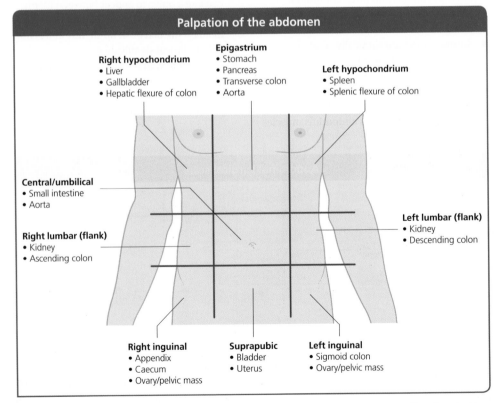

Palpation of the abdomen

Epigastrium
- Stomach
- Pancreas
- Transverse colon
- Aorta

Right hypochondrium
- Liver
- Gallbladder
- Hepatic flexure of colon

Left hypochondrium
- Spleen
- Splenic flexure of colon

Central/umbilical
- Small intestine
- Aorta

Right lumbar (flank)
- Kidney
- Ascending colon

Left lumbar (flank)
- Kidney
- Descending colon

Right inguinal
- Appendix
- Caecum
- Ovary/pelvic mass

Suprapubic
- Bladder
- Uterus

Left inguinal
- Sigmoid colon
- Ovary/pelvic mass

Figure 2.14 Palpable structures in different regions of the abdomen. Structures are normally only palpable if there is an underlying pathology.

Examination features of liver, kidney and spleen			
Feature	Liver	Spleen	Kidney
Direction of enlargement	Towards right iliac fossa	Towards right iliac fossa	Towards flank
Able to palpate above?	No	No	Yes
Resonant percussion note	No	No	Sometimes (overlying bowel gas)
Other features	Moves downwards on inspiration	Has palpable notch Moves downwards on inspiration	No notch Ballotable

Table 2.11 Examination features of the liver, kidney and spleen

> **Before palpating the abdomen, always check whether the patient has any painful areas. In addition, make sure your hands are warm.**

Liver

The healthy liver is located underneath the ribs on the right side, extending from the 5th intercostal space down to the costal margin (see **Figure 1.2**). Enlargement of the liver is called hepatomegaly; its causes are outlined in **Table 2.12**.

To identify hepatomegaly, the flat of the hand is first placed in the right lower quadrant (**Figure 2.15**). It is then pushed upwards and inwards as the patient takes a deep breath in. The hand should be moved progressively up towards the right upper quadrant, repeating this movement until either the costal margin or the liver edge is felt. The liver moves downwards with inspiration and is felt moving against the index finger if enlarged. It is also often possible to palpate the liver edge just below the costal margin in thin people or patients with conditions such as chronic obstructive pulmonary disease in which the chest is hyperexpanded, pushing the diaphragm and liver downwards.

If the liver edge is palpable, it is described according to its:

- Size – number of fingerbreadths or centimetres below the costal margin
- Surface – smooth or irregular

Causes of hepatomegaly	
Cause	Examples
Acute or chronic liver disease*	Alcoholic liver disease
	Fatty liver disease
	Autoimmune hepatitis
	Viral infection
Malignancy	Secondary metastatic cancer
	Hepatocellular carcinoma
Cardiac causes	Right heart failure
Haematological disorders	Lymphoma
	Leukaemia
	Myelofibrosis
	Polycythaemia
Infection	Glandular fever
	Hydatid cyst
Rarer causes	Amyloidosis
	Budd–Chiari syndrome
	Sarcoidosis
	Glycogen storage disorders

*In chronic liver disease the liver is sometimes shrunken and is not palpable.

Table 2.12 Causes of hepatomegaly

- Consistency – soft or firm
- Pulsatile nature
- Tenderness

Spleen

The healthy spleen lies beneath the 9th and 11th ribs in the left mid-axillary line.

Enlargement of the spleen is called spleno-megaly. Its causes are outlined in **Table 2.13**.

Palpation is started in the right lower quadrant, then moving upwards towards the left upper quadrant. The technique is identical to liver palpation (**Figure 2.15**). The left hand can be used to support the rib cage posterolateral-

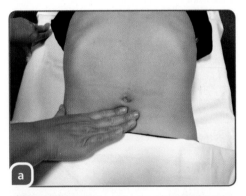

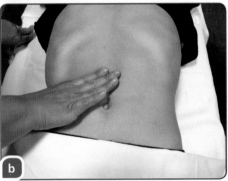

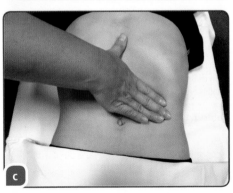

Figure 2.15 Palpation for the liver and spleen.
(a) Start palpation in the right lower quadrant to palpate for the liver and spleen. (b) Move the hand towards the right costal margin to palpate for the liver. (c) Move the hand towards the left upper quadrant to palpate for the spleen.

Causes of splenomegaly	
Cause	Examples
Haematological disease	Chronic leukaemia
	Myeloproliferative diseases
	Lymphoma
	Haemolytic anaemia
Portal hypertension	Cirrhosis with portal hypertension
	Portal or splenic vein thrombosis
Infection	Epstein–Barr virus
	Malaria
	Leishmaniasis
	Tuberculosis
Systemic disease	Sarcoidosis
	Amyloidosis
	Glycogen storage disorders
	Rheumatoid arthritis (as part of Felty's syndrome)

Table 2.13 Causes of splenomegaly

ly. If the spleen is palpable, its size is measured in the same way as the liver.

> **The spleen must treble in size before it becomes palpable. Therefore a palpable spleen always indicates splenomegaly.**

Kidneys

The kidneys are located retroperitoneally (potential space in the abdominal cavity behind the peritoneum) and are therefore difficult to palpate unless they are significantly enlarged (e.g. polycystic kidney disease).

The kidneys are examined by bimanual palpation (**Figure 2.16**). One of the examiner's hands is placed in the lumbar region behind the patient's back and pushes upwards. The other hand is placed on the anterior abdominal wall and pushes downwards. Flexion of the fingers of the hand in the lumbar region aims to float the kidney upwards towards the other hand, a manoeuvre called 'balloting'.

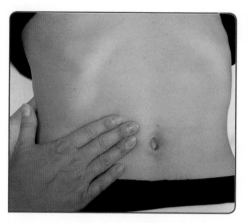

Figure 2.16 Bimanual examination of the right kidney.

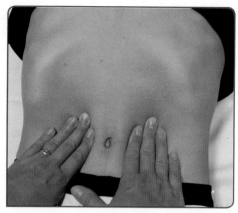

Figure 2.17 Palpation for the abdominal aorta.

> **A transplanted kidney forms an easily palpable mass in the iliac fossa.** An overlying scar is seen. The presence of an arteriovenous fistula in the arm indicates previous dialysis.

Aorta

This is the body's main artery and runs in the midline of the abdomen. It is often palpable in thin people or when there is localised swelling of its wall, termed an aneurysm. Placing a hand either side of the aorta determines its size (**Figure 2.17**).

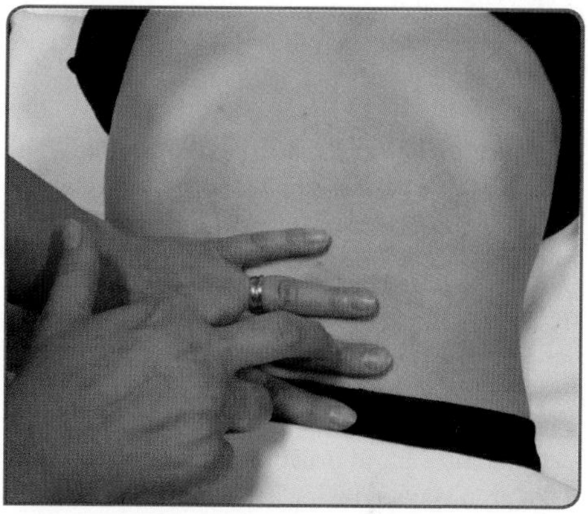

Figure 2.18 Percussion of the abdomen.

Abdominal percussion

Percussion (or tapping) is used to identify underlying abdominal structures and the presence of fluid (**Figure 2.18**). One hand is placed flat on the abdominal wall and its middle finger tapped by the tip of the middle finger of other hand. A sound will be elicited that will be either:

- Resonant (tympanic) – because of underlying intestinal gas
- Dull – due to underlying liquid, e.g. ascites, or solid structures such as the liver or an abdominal mass

The upper and lower borders of the liver and spleen are defined by percussion, starting in the right iliac fossa.

With the patient lying on their back, the presence of ascites is detected in two ways:

- **Shifting dullness (Figure 2.19)** – percuss from the midline out towards the flank, noting where the percussion sound changes from resonant to dull. Place a finger vertically on the abdominal wall at this point. Ask the patient to turn onto the side opposite to the finger. Wait for a few seconds to allow the ascites to gravitate downwards and then percuss again. If the area of dullness marked by the finger now sounds resonant, the sign of shifting dullness is present

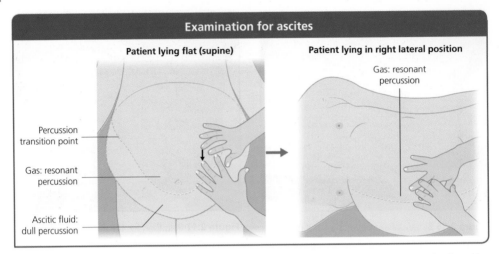

Examination for ascites

Patient lying flat (supine)

Percussion
transition point

Gas: resonant
percussion

Ascitic fluid:
dull percussion

Patient lying in right lateral position

Gas: resonant
percussion

Figure 2.19 Examination for ascites, eliciting shifting dullness. In a positive test percussion starting from the centre of the abdomen and moving out towards the flank identifies a transition point from resonant to dull which reverts to being resonant a few seconds after the patient turns onto their side.

- **Fluid thrill (Figure 2.20)** – this is only detectable if gross ascites is present. Ask the patient or another person to place the lateral edge of their hand down the midline of the abdomen. Placing the palm of your left hand against the left abdominal wall, flick a finger of your right hand against the right abdominal wall. The assistant's hand prevents the transmission of an impulse through the skin. If your left hand feels a ripple, ascites is present.

> For ascites to be detectable on clinical examination, at least 1500 mL of fluid must be present.

Abdominal auscultation

Auscultation is the process of listening to the body's internal sounds using a stethoscope. The diaphragm part of the stethoscope should be placed on the abdominal wall for at least 30 seconds to listen for characteristic 'gurgling' bowel sounds and if not heard, this time period is extended to 1 minute.

It is sometimes possible to hear a bruit (or 'whirring' noise) when listening over the aorta or other blood vessels. This is a sign of arterial narrowing, such as renal artery stenosis.

> **Bowel sounds vary in different conditions:**
> - Absent – paralytic ileus, perforation, peritonitis
> - High pitched or 'tinkling' – intestinal obstruction

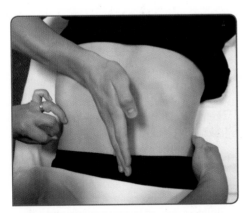

Figure 2.20 Examination for ascites: fluid thrill (see text for description of technique).

Several additional components of the examination should be considered after auscultation (**Figure 2.6**).

Rectal examination

Rectal examination is an embarrassing and intimate examination for patients, but is an important part of the GI examination to exclude abnormalities of the anus and lower rectum. The patient is often put at ease by a clear explanation of the reasons for performing the examination and what is involved in it. Unless declined by the patient, a chaperone must be present during the examination.

The technique is shown in **Figure 2.21** and is:

- The patient is positioned on their left side on the bed, with their knees bent up towards their chest. A sheet is used to cover the patient before the examination
- Using a gloved hand, inspect the anus and surrounding skin for scars, masses, skin tags, external haemorrhoids, redness and the external openings of a fistula (a hollow tract between the skin and lower bowel)

- Tell the patient what will happen next. Then insert a well-lubricated gloved finger into the anus to assess the anal tone. In patients with an anal fissure, this is usually very painful and sometimes proves impossible, in which case the examination might be delayed or performed under a short general anaesthetic
- All four walls of the rectum should be examined systematically for masses. The position of any abnormalities is described using a clock face, e.g. a mass is palpable in the 11 o'clock position. The prostate is felt anteriorly (3 o'clock position when lying on the left side) in men, and the cervix in women. The size and surface texture of abnormalities is also noted. Stool is also commonly present in the rectum
- After removal of the gloved finger, it should be inspected for the presence of blood or melaena. The patient is provided with some tissue to wipe away any remaining lubricant gel

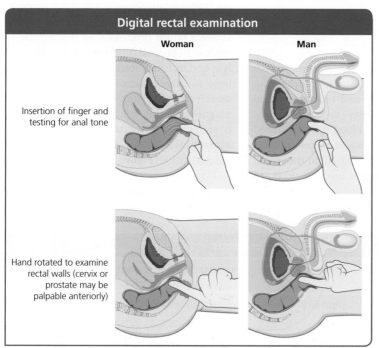

Digital rectal examination

Woman   **Man**

Insertion of finger and testing for anal tone

Hand rotated to examine rectal walls (cervix or prostate may be palpable anteriorly)

Figure 2.21 Digital rectal examination.

Investigations

Starter questions

Answers to the following questions are on page pages 158–159.

6. What can blood tests tell you about GI function?
7. How are investigations influenced by comorbidities?
8. Which presentations require further investigation?
9. How is the small bowel investigated, given that it is relatively difficult to reach?

Investigations are performed to confirm a diagnosis. The choice of tests is guided by factors including the clinical history and examination, patient's choice, patient's age and co-morbidities. Less invasive investigations, such as blood and stool tests, are usually undertaken first. The benefits of performing invasive tests, for example endoscopy or radiological investigations (because of exposure to ionising radiation), should outweigh the potential risks.

Blood tests

Samples of blood are taken from a vein to help diagnose conditions, monitor the response to treatment and to monitor and identify adverse effects to medications. Commonly performed blood tests are listed in **Table 2.14** and discussed below (normal values for these tests are listed on the inside back cover). More specific investigations are outlined in individual chapters.

Full blood count

The full blood count records cell counts and other parameters that help evaluate patients with GI disorders (**Table 2.15**).

Urea and electrolytes

These assess the function of the kidneys and record the sodium and potassium levels (**Table 2.16**). Surgical resection or damage to the small intestine sometimes results in short bowel syndrome, as it is unable to achieve its normal function of water, electrolyte and nutrient absorption (see Chapter 1, page 16). This results in excessive fluid loss and electrolyte disturbance, for example low magnesium and calcium levels. Cirrhosis is sometimes associated with a dilutional hyponatraemia (low sodium level) due to fluid retention (**Figure 2.22**).

Plasma urea is elevated in cases of upper GI bleeding, although the exact cause is

Blood tests			
Full blood count	Urea and electrolytes	Liver function test	Other investigations
Haemoglobin	Sodium	Bilirubin	Prothrombin time
Platelet count	Potassium	Aspartate transaminase	International normalised ratio
Mean corpuscular haemoglobin	Urea	Alanine transaminase	C-reactive protein
Mean corpuscular volume	Creatinine	Alkaline phosphatase	Erythrocyte sedimentation rate
White cell count		γ-Glutamyl transferase	
		Albumin	

Table 2.14 Blood tests commonly performed in gastroenterology

GI-related causes of an abnormal full blood count		
Test	Low	High
Haemoglobin	Anaemia, e.g. iron deficiency	Polycythaemia
Platelet count	Hypersplenism, e.g. portal hypertension Bone marrow suppression, e.g. alcohol misuse	Infective and inflammatory conditions, e.g. Crohn's disease
Mean corpuscular volume and mean corpuscular haemoglobin	Iron deficiency Blood disorders, e.g. thalassaemia	Alcohol misuse Vitamin B_{12} or folate deficiency Haemolysis secondary to liver disease Medications, e.g. azathioprine
White cell count	Medications, e.g. azathioprine	Infective or inflammatory conditions

Table 2.15 Components of the full blood count and common GI causes of abnormal results

GI-related causes of abnormal urea and electrolytes		
Test	Low	High
Sodium	Decompensated liver disease (dilutional) Fluid loss, e.g. diarrhoea, severe vomiting Diuretics used to treat decompensated liver disease Syndrome of inappropriate antidiuretic hormone secretion secondary to malignancy	Fluid loss, e.g. diarrhoea, severe vomiting
Potassium	Fluid loss, e.g. diarrhoea, severe vomiting Diuretics used to treat decompensated liver disease	Potassium-sparing diuretics, e.g. spironolactone
Urea	Alcohol misuse	Fluid loss, e.g. diarrhoea, severe vomiting Hepatorenal syndrome (see Table 7.4) Upper GI bleeding
Creatinine	Advanced liver disease	Dehydration secondary to fluid loss Hepatorenal syndrome (Table 7.4)

Table 2.16 Gastrointestinal causes of abnormal urea and electrolyte parameters

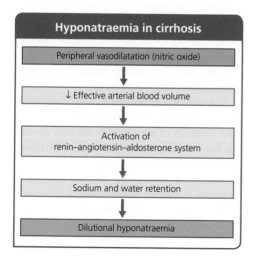

Figure 2.22 Development of hyponatraemia in cirrhosis.

unknown. It is thought that it might occur either due to the haemoglobin protein component of blood being digested in the GI tract to form amino acids, which are absorbed and broken down in the urea cycle to form the excretion product urea (see Chapter 1, page 49), or as a result of reduced kidney perfusion secondary to acute blood loss. A low level of urea often occurs with alcohol misuse due to inhibition of enzymes in the urea cycle.

Liver function tests

In liver function tests (LFTs), a single blood sample is used by the laboratory to determine levels of a series of enzymes and other proteins produced in the liver. The normal liver does not release its enzymes into the circulation: raised levels therefore indicate liver injury or malfunction. Changes in the level of albumin (a plasma protein) produced in the liver also suggest liver disease.

Similarly, a raised level of bilirubin, a product of hepatic breakdown of red blood cells, suggests hepatic malfunction.

> Among LFT results, elevated levels are considered abnormal for all components except for albumin, which is only of significance in GI diseases when the level falls.

The individual components are:

- Bilirubin – this is formed from the haem component of haemoglobin during hepatic breakdown of red blood cells (**Figure 1.38**). Elevated bilirubin level occurs in disorders that cause increased red cell breakdown and disorders of the liver and biliary tree.
- Aspartate transaminase (AST) and alanine transaminase (ALT) – these enzymes are present in hepatocytes and leak into the blood when hepatocytes are inflamed or damaged. This is called a 'hepatocellular picture' (or hepatitis) on blood testing. These enzymes catalyse the transfer of amino groups from asparate or alanine to ketoacids during glycogenesis (the metabolic pathway that forms glucose). ALT and AST are also found in other body tissues including (in descending frequency) skeletal muscle, heart muscle, kidney, brain, pancreas and red blood cells. ALT is found predominantly in the liver with lesser quantities than AST in the other body tissues. As a result, ALT is a more specific indicator than AST of hepatocellular disorders; AST is also elevated in conditions such as musculoskeletal damage, myocardial infarction, acute pancreatitis and haemolytic anaemia.
- Alkaline phosphatase (ALP) – this enzyme is mainly found on the membranes of hepatocytes adjacent to the biliary canaliculi and is released into the blood in conditions that affect the biliary tree, a so-called 'cholestatic (or obstructive) picture' on blood testing. It is a hydrolyse enzyme which removes phosphate from molecules in the body. It is also present in the bone, placenta, white blood cells, kidney and small intestine, and is elevated in conditions such as Paget's disease, osteomalacia, secondary malignancies in the bone and pregnancy.
- γ-glutamyl transferase (GGT) – this is present in the bile duct and hepatocytes with much smaller amounts elsewhere, e.g. in the pancreas and lymphocytes. It is a transferase enzyme which catalyses the transfer of γ-glutamyl groups of peptides to other amino acids. It is elevated in both hepatocellular damage and cholestasis, and it is therefore helpful to determine if a raised AST or ALP blood level is from the liver (where GGT will also be elevated) or elsewhere (where it will not).
- Albumin – this is the predominant plasma protein synthesised by hepatocytes and transports bilirubin, ions, metals, fatty acids, hormones and drugs around the body. Its blood level falls with damage to the liver, but because it has a long half life of around 20 days it takes a while to reduce in the blood after acute damage, e.g. a paracetamol overdose or hepatitis A. Low levels can also occur due to protein losses from the body, e.g. nephrotic syndrome, extensive small bowel Crohn's disease and where it is consumed in acute or chronic inflammatory disorders, e.g. sepsis.

Other plasma proteins synthesised by the liver but not included as components of LFTs include caeruloplasmin, alpha fetoprotein and alpha-1-antitrypsin levels.

The causes of abnormal levels of individual LFT components are summarised in **Table 2.17**. Patterns of abnormality are also revealing. For example, a rise of both alkaline phosphatase and γ-glutamyl transferase indicate cholestasis or obstruction of the biliary tree. Elevation of all liver enzymes is described as a 'mixed picture', due to several causes, e.g. systemic sepsis or the side effects of medications. It occurs when there is ballooning (swelling)

Abnormal liver function tests		
Abnormal result	Principal site(s) of production	Causes of abnormal results
Bilirubin: raised	Liver	Pre-hepatic, e.g. haemolysis
	Spleen	Hepatic, e.g. acute hepatitis, chronic liver disease
		Post-hepatic, e.g. common bile duct stones, pancreatic carcinoma
Aspartate transaminase (AST): raised	Liver	Alcohol misuse
	Cardiac and skeletal muscle	Drug induced, e.g. paracetamol, NSAIDs
		Ischaemic hepatitis
		Acute and chronic liver diseases
		Non-GI causes, e.g. myocardial infarction, myositis
Alanine transaminase (ALT): raised	Liver	Alcohol misuse
		Drug induced, e.g. paracetamol, NSAIDs
		Ischaemic hepatitis
		Acute and chronic liver diseases
		Non-GI causes, e.g. myositis
Alkaline phosphatase (ALP): raised	Liver	Cholestatic liver disease, e.g. PBC, PSC
	Bones	Biliary obstruction, e.g. gallstones
	Placenta	Drugs
		Non-GI causes, e.g. heart failure, bone disease or metastases
γ-Glutamyl transferase (GGT): raised	Liver	Drugs
		Fatty liver disease
		Alcohol misuse
Albumin: reduced	Liver	Chronic liver disease
		Non-GI causes, e.g. nephrotic syndrome, sepsis

NSAID, non-steroidal anti-inflammatory drug; PBC, primary biliary cholangitis; PSC, primary sclerosing cholangitis.

Table 2.17 Causes of abnormal liver function test results. The causes listed for each test result in elevated levels, except for albumin which falls in GI disease

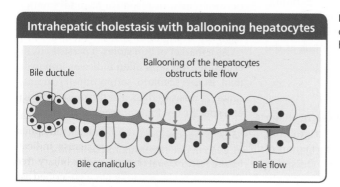

Intrahepatic cholestasis with ballooning hepatocytes

Bile ductule

Ballooning of the hepatocytes obstructs bile flow

Bile canaliculus

Bile flow

Figure 2.23 Intrahepatic cholestasis secondary to ballooning hepatocytes.

of the hepatocytes secondary to inflammation (causing a hepatocellular picture), which causes compression of the small bile canaliculi and obstruction of the flow of bile (**Figure 2.23**), producing an added cholestatic picture to the liver function tests. A mixed picture is also caused by the coexistence of several different conditions such as primary biliary cholangitis (PBC) and autoimmune hepatitis.

Coagulation tests are often done alongside LFTs, as described below, because they demonstrate aspects of liver function.

> **Alkaline phosphatase (ALP) is also produced by cells in the bone and placenta and less commonly by white blood cells and cells in the intestine and kidneys.** Elevated ALP with normal γ-glutamyl transferase suggests the ALP is of bony origin and investigation of the liver is not required.

Inflammatory markers

The inflammatory markers C-reactive protein (CRP) and erythrocyte sedimentation rate (ESR) are elevated by infection (e.g. gastroenteritis, biliary sepsis and abscesses), inflammation (e.g. inflammatory bowel disease and inflammation of blood vessels) and malignancy (e.g. lymphoma) in any part of the body including the GI tract. CRP is produced by the liver. Liver failure may interfere with the production of CRP. CRP and ESR are also markers of disease activity, useful in evaluating conditions such as inflammatory bowel disease. These are monitored to assess for an improvement in the underlying inflammation or infection, falling as the underlying cause is treated.

Coagulation screen

The liver is the site of the synthesis of all but one of the coagulation factors, a group of proteins that are essential for formation of blood clots and thus haemostasis (cessation of bleeding at a site of injury). Accordingly, measures of coagulation can be used to assess the liver's synthetic function. The main components of a coagulation screen relevant to GI diseases are:

- Prothrombin time (PT), a measure of how long it takes blood plasma to clot and
- International normalised ratio (INR), a ratio of the patient's PT to a control sample, used to standardise results across laboratories

These are both prolonged in liver disease. In acute liver failure predefined elevations of PT and INR also form part of the referral criteria for transplantation.

An INR is also required in patients who are taking warfarin, prior to invasive procedures such as therapeutic endoscopy, because warfarin increases the risk of bleeding. The warfarin is stopped prior to the procedure, which is only undertaken once the INR has fallen to <1.4 (normal <1.3).

Haematinics

Haematinics are the nutrients required for the formation of blood cells. Haematinic tests are done in the haematology laboratory and measure:

- ferritin or iron level
- vitamin B_{12}
- folate

Ferritin

Ferritin is a protein that stores and transports iron. Its level corresponds with the body's iron stores: a low level indicates iron deficiency. Ferritin is an acute-phase protein, a type of protein for which the plasma concentration increases in response to inflammation and underlying infection, for example acute hepatitis or inflammatory bowel disease.

As a marker of iron stores, a persistently elevated ferritin level often indicates iron overload. In this scenario, serum transferrin saturation is measured, as it is the most sensitive and specific test for iron accumulation.

> **Even in patients with iron deficiency, the ferritin level is often normal if there is coexisting inflammation (e.g. alcoholic hepatitis) or infection.** However, other clues of iron deficiency will also be present, such as microcytosis (unusually small red blood cell volume).

Vitamin B$_{12}$ (cobalamin) and folate

Vitamin B$_{12}$ (cobalamin) is bound by intrinsic factor produced by the gastric parietal cells, to form a vitamin B$_{12}$-intrinsic factor complex that is later absorbed in the terminal ileum. It is needed for enzyme reactions, in which it acts as a co-enzyme, including the formation of red blood cells. Folate (vitamin B$_9$) is absorbed from the proximal small intestine. It is needed for DNA and RNA synthesis, including the production of red blood cells. Deficiency of these vitamins is either dietary or due to GI disorders impairing absorption, such as coeliac disease.

Folate is sometimes elevated in people with bacterial overgrowth of the small intestine, because the bacteria produce it. Elevated folate is not harmful, however antibiotics are used to treat patients with symptomatic overgrowth.

Tumour markers

Tumour markers (**Table 2.18**) have a number of uses in GI medicine, for example:

- Surveillance of patients at increased risk of malignancy, for example 6-monthly monitoring of alpha-fetoprotein is done in patients with cirrhosis, because they are at increased risk for hepatocellular carcinoma
- Diagnosis of suspected cancer when a mass is identified in an organ on radiological imaging, for example CA19-9 is sought if a pancreatic mass is found
- Monitoring the response of malignancies to treatment, for example measuring carcinoembryonic antigen (CEA) in

patients receiving chemotherapy for cancer of the large intestine

Tumour markers are often non-specifically elevated with any malignancy. Carcinoembryonic antigen levels are sometimes slightly elevated in smokers, although the reason is uncertain. The tumour marker CA19-9 is often also elevated in benign causes of cholestasis.

CA125 is a tumour marker for ovarian malignancy. It is also commonly elevated in patients with ascites secondary to cirrhosis, although the cause of this is uncertain.

Immunoglobulins

Immunoglobulins (Ig) are proteins produced by white blood cells. Common reasons for raised Ig levels in GI conditions are:

- IgA – elevated in patients misusing alcohol. It also forms a component of coeliac disease serology testing (see below)
- IgM – elevated in primary biliary cholangitis and the early stages of infection
- IgG – elevated in autoimmune liver diseases (used as a marker of disease activity) and shows evidence of previous bacteria, viral or fungal infection
- IgE – elevated in patients who are having an allergic response, e.g. in parasitic infections, eosinophilic oesophagitis and drug reactions. The level falls to normal with treatment of the underlying condition

Coeliac serology

IgA anti-tissue transglutaminase antibodies are measured in individuals with suspected or risk factors for coeliac disease, for example osteoporosis (see Chapter 5, page 208). False-negative results sometimes occur in individuals with IgA deficiency and patients already on a gluten-free diet. In IgA deficiency, the IgG anti-tissue transglutaminase antibody is used instead.

Stool tests

When stool testing is required, a stool sample is collected in a specialised pot which

GI tumour markers		
Tumour marker	Abbreviation	Site of GI cancer
Alpha-fetoprotein	AFP	Liver primary
Cancer antigen 19-9	CA19-9	Pancreas
Carcinoembryonic antigen	CEA	Large intestine

Table 2.18 Markers of GI tumours

contains a scoop. Samples are sent to the microbiology laboratory if infection is suspected or to the biochemistry laboratory if faecal elastase or calprotectin levels are to be measured.

Infection

In patients with persistent diarrhoea microbiological analysis is required to exclude an infective cause. Stool microscopy is performed to examine for ova, cysts and parasites. Polymerase chain reaction (PCR) testing is used to screen for common bacterial infections including *Salmonella*, *Campylobacter, Shigella, Escherichia coli* and *Yersinia*. PCR testing for viral causes of infective diarrhoea, such as norovirus and rotavirus, is generally reserved for outbreaks in a hospital setting so that necessary infection control measures can be implemented.

Clostridium difficile

Two-stage testing is usually used. First a glutamate dehydrogenase (GDH) enzyme immunoassay is performed as a screening test to detect the presence of an antigen produced by *C. difficile*. If the result is positive, the more expensive and longer-to-perform toxin enzyme immunoassay is carried out to confirm infection (**Table 2.19**).

Helicobacter pylori

A faecal antigen enzyme immunoassay is used to diagnose *Helicobacter pylori* or

Clostridium difficile tests	
GDH enzyme immunoassay result	Toxin enzyme immunoassay
Negative	Testing not required: infection very unlikely
Positive	Positive: infection likely
Positive	Negative: *C. difficile* could be present. Repeat test advised if symptoms continue
GDH, glutamate dehydrogenase.	

Table 2.19 Interpretation of *Clostridium difficile* stool tests

provide evidence of its eradication after antibiotic therapy in patients with dyspepsia, peptic ulceration or gastric lymphoma. Proton pump inhibitor therapy is stopped 2 weeks before the test, as it suppresses *H. pylori*, leading to a false negative result.

Faecal elastase

Elastase is one of the enzymes secreted by the pancreatic exocrine cells into the duodenum to help in digestion. It is measured in the stool using an enzyme-linked immunosorbent assay kit.

Low faecal elastase suggests pancreatic exocrine insufficiency as a result of conditions such as diabetes mellitus, chronic pancreatitis or pancreatic cancer. A falsely low level can occur as a dilution effect secondary to watery diarrhoea due to other causes.

Faecal calprotectin

Calprotectin is a protein produced by neutrophil white blood cells and is elevated in intestinal inflammation. It is measured to distinguish irritable bowel syndrome from inflammatory bowel disease: the calprotectin level is normal in irritable bowel syndrome and high in active inflammatory bowel disease. The calprotectin level is also used to assess disease activity in patients with known inflammatory bowel disease.

An elevated level also occurs with infective diarrhoea, GI damage by non-steroidal anti-inflammatory drugs and colorectal malignancy. Falsely elevated results are also often observed with proton pump inhibitor use, although the cause is uncertain.

Faecal occult blood (FOB) testing

Faecal occult blood testing is used to detect non-visible blood in the stool, with the aim of identifying significant polyps and cancer of the large intestine. Positive results also occur in other conditions that result in GI blood loss such as inflammatory bowel disease or haemorrhoids. There are two FOB tests: guaiac and immunochemical. Guaiac stool testing is currently used most commonly. Three consecutive samples of stool are smeared onto guaiac paper and sent for analysis. In the laboratory, the application of hydrogen peroxide converts the sample blue if blood is present. False-positive results occur if the patient has ingested non-steroidal anti-inflammatory drugs, due to inflammation and blood loss from the stomach. Red meats and some vegetables, for example broccoli and parsnips, cause the same chemical reaction on the test kit as blood, also causing a false positive result.

In many countries, all individuals in a certain age range (60–74 years in the UK) are invited to complete faecal occult blood stool testing in a population-based bowel screening programme at set time intervals. Individuals with positive results are considered for further investigation such as CT imaging or colonoscopy (see pages 119 and 124). In some countries testing is also used in patients with unexplained abdominal symptoms and those with a change in bowel habit or iron deficiency anaemia.

If the guaiac test is equivocal, the more sensitive and specific faecal immunochemical test (FIT) is performed. Over the next few years FIT testing is planned as the initial bowel screening test in parts of the UK. It is expected that FIT testing, which was not widely available when evidence for population-based bowel screening was being collected, will eventually supersede guaiac as the initial bowel screening test.

Urine tests

A urine dipstick test is undertaken in patients with iron deficiency anaemia to exclude the presence of blood in the urine and a potential underlying urinary tract cause for the bleeding. It is performed as a bedside test in the GP surgery or hospital.

The following rare GI disorders are also diagnosed by urine testing. 5-hydroxyindole-actic acid (5-HIAA) is a metabolite of the neurotransmitter serotonin. A raised 24-hour urine level occurs with neuroendocrine tumours of the small intestine, which release serotonin. Porphyria is a rare set of hereditary conditions resulting from deficiencies in enzymes involved in haem synthesis, causing symptoms such as severe abdominal pain, nausea and constipation. Urine and stool samples are taken at the time of symptoms for porphyrin studies.

Breath tests

These are most commonly performed to diagnose lactose malabsorption and bacterial overgrowth (**Table 2.20**). Lactose malabsorption results from a deficiency of the enzyme lactase. This lines the microvilli of the small intestine and breaks lactose down into the sugars glucose and galactose. If lactose is not broken down, it passes into the large intestine where it is metabolised by

Common breath tests		
Breath test	Symptoms	Causes
Lactose	Abdominal bloating and distension Borborygmi Increased flatus Diarrhoea	Congenital lactase deficiency Primary lactase deficiency Secondary lactase deficiency
Bacterial overgrowth	Abdominal bloating and distension Borborygmi Increased flatus Diarrhoea or steatorrhoea Symptoms secondary to haematinic deficiency	Surgery Fistulas Proton pump inhibitor therapy Diverticular disease Diabetes Scleroderma Immunodeficiency conditions

Table 2.20 Commonly performed breath tests

bacteria to form hydrogen, methane and carbon dioxide.

A breath test is performed after an overnight fast and drink of lactose. Patients are asked to breathe into a mouthpiece at regular time intervals, which is connected to a machine that measures the level of hydrogen. Some devices also measure the level of methane. The test is positive if these readings rise by > 20 parts per million at any time point during the investigation above the lowest preceding reading. Fructose malabsorption causes similar symptoms to lactose intolerance and is tested for in the same way, but using a fructose drink.

Breath tests are also used to diagnose bacterial overgrowth (**Table 2.20**) in patients with symptoms such as bloating, diarrhoea and weight loss. In the small intestine, bacteria metabolise ingested carbohydrates to hydrogen and methane. A breath test is performed using the technique outlined above, but with a glucose or lactulose drink.

Helicobacter pylori

The urea breath test is a non-invasive way to test for active *H. pylori* infection. Proton pump inhibitor medications are stopped 2 weeks prior to the test, as these suppress the bacteria leading to a false negative result. It is used as an alternative to the *H. pylori* faecal antigen depending upon the local availability of each investigation.

H. pylori uses the enzyme urease to metabolise urea to form carbon dioxide and ammonia. Exhaled breath samples are collected after patients drink a radiolabelled urea compound to detect carbon dioxide, confirming the presence of *H. pylori* (Figure 4.1).

Imaging

Radiological tests are available to image different regions of the GI tract to investigate symptoms, abnormal blood test results and abnormal findings from the physical examination (**Table 2.21**). To identify the most appropriate investigation, several factors are considered:

- The question to be answered in the context of the differential diagnoses
- The risk from radiation exposure in comparison to the benefit of running the test (**Table 2.22**)
- Patient co-morbidity (including pregnancy and risk to the fetus)
- Patient choice

Plain films (radiographs)

X-ray beams are passed from a generator, through the part of the body being examined,

Visualising the GI tract		
	Endoscopy	Radiology
Oesophagus	Oesophagogastroduodenoscopy (OGD)	Barium swallow
Stomach	OGD	Barium meal
Small intestine	OGD (duodenum)	Barium follow-through
	Enteroscopy	CT enterogram
	Wireless capsule endoscopy	MR enterogram
Large intestine	Sigmoidoscopy (left colon)	Minimal-preparation CT of abdomen and pelvis
	Colonoscopy	CT pneumocolon
	Wireless capsule endoscopy	Barium enema*
Biliary tree	Endoscopic retrograde cholangiopancreatography (ERCP) – rarely performed as diagnostic procedure	Ultrasound
		MR cholangiopancreatography
		CT of abdomen

*Barium enema is being phased out due to its suboptimal detection rates for abnormalities of the large intestine compared to colonoscopy and CT pneumocolon (see page 122).

Table 2.21 Tests to visualise different parts of the GI tract

Radiation exposure from GI investigations		
Investigation	Radiation dose (mSv)*	Equivalent number of chest radiographs
Ultrasound	0	–
MRI	0	–
Chest radiograph	0.02	–
Abdominal radiograph	0.7	35
Barium swallow	1.5	75
Barium meal	3	150
Barium enema	7	350
CT abdomen and pelvis	10	500
CT pneumocolon	10	500

*The dose of ionising radiation is measured in millisieverts (mSv).

Table 2.22 Radiation exposure from radiological GI investigations. Naturally occurring radiation exposure, e.g. from cosmic radiation, is approximately 3 mSv/year

onto an X-ray-sensitive plate to produce a two-dimensional image. The appearance of tissues depends upon their density:

- Air – black
- Bones – white
- Soft tissue organs and structures – grey

Abdominal radiograph

An abdominal radiograph (**Figure 2.24**) is taken with the patient in a supine position. It is used to evaluate causes of abdominal pain and symptoms of constipation and diarrhoea (**Table 2.23**). Abdominal radiography also visualises:

- **Metal clips and wires** after previous surgery, for example laparoscopic cholecystectomy; these show up as bright white objects on radiographs.
- **Calcification**, for example due to gallbladder or renal stones (calculi), or appearing as a white outline to vessels such as the aorta and iliac arteries.

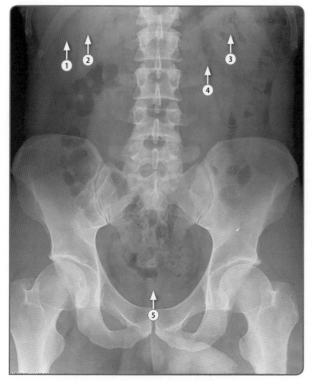

Figure 2.24 An abdominal radiograph is most commonly done to assess intestinal symptoms and acute abdominal pain. In addition to the small and large intestine, other structures that are sometimes visualised include: ① Liver. ② Gallbladder. ③ Kidney. ④ Psoas muscle shadow. ⑤ Bladder.

Features on abdominal radiographs

Condition	Radiological features	Causes
Perforation (pneumoperitoneum)	Rim of gas seen around organs, e.g. liver Rigler's sign – gas on both sides of the bowel wall Football sign – gas trapped within the peritoneal cavity	Malignancy Peptic ulcers Inflammatory bowel disease Diverticular disease Trauma
Small bowel obstruction	Small intestine dilated to >3 cm Small intestine lies in the centre of the abdomen and is identified by the valvulae conniventes (see page 61)	Adhesions Strictures secondary to Crohn's disease, radiation, ischaemia or NSAIDs
Large bowel obstruction	Transverse colon dilated to >6 cm Gas and stool is not seen below the level of the obstruction	Malignancy Hernias Foreign bodies
Volvulus	Sigmoid volvulus – coffee bean shape Caecal volvulus – the caecum is moved towards the midline	Excess mesentery
Mucosal inflammation	Thumb-printing – thumb-shaped indentations in the wall of the large intestine Lead pipe colon – straight colon due to mucosal oedema	Inflammatory bowel disease Infection
Toxic megacolon	Transverse colon dilated >6 cm	Inflammatory bowel disease Infection

Table 2.23 Radiological features seen on abdominal radiographs and potential causes

Other findings include:

■ Ileus – distension of the small intestine resulting from impaired peristalsis rather than obstruction
■ Pseudo-obstruction – distension of the large intestine; the radiological features are identical to those of large intestinal obstruction
■ Volvulus – part of the GI tract twists on its axis. This most commonly occurs in parts of the large intestine (sigmoid colon or caecum). The features are outlined in **Table 2.23**. It occurs less commonly with the stomach, which appears distended on an abdominal radiograph with collapsed small bowel

Chest radiograph

Appearances related to GI disorders include:

■ **Subphrenic gas**, i.e. air visible below the diaphragm: this is sometimes identified on an erect chest radiograph (i.e. one taken with the patient sitting upright) and is the result of perforation of a hollow abdominal organ, for example the intestine.
■ **Pneumomediastinum**, i.e. air surrounding structures in the chest cavity; this sometimes occur from oesophageal fistulas. It also caused by perforation resulting from endoscopic procedures, malignancy or Boerhaave's syndrome (oesophageal perforation due to vomiting)
■ **Pleural effusions** (fluid collections in the pleural cavity), which has the same causes as pneumomediastinum. It also occasionally occurs in patients with cirrhosis (Table 7.4)

Ultrasonography

This is a non-invasive investigation that does not involve exposure to ionising radiation. A probe is placed against the abdominal wall, using gel to transmit the sound waves to the tissue. Sound waves produced by the probe reflect off the abdominal organs before returning to the probe and being converted to an electrical signal, which is processed and converted into an image. The colour of the abdominal structures varies from dark to bright depending upon their echogenicity (ability to bounce an echo), for example the hepatic veins appear as hypoechoic (darker) structures.

Ultrasound is useful in assessing hepatobiliary pathology, such as stones in the gallbladder (**Figure 2.25**) and bile duct. However, visualisation of retroperitoneal structures, such as the pancreas, is sometimes limited by overlying intestinal gas.

Doppler ultrasonography visualises the flow of fluids by measuring the frequency of echo waves moving towards and away from the ultrasound probe. It is used to assess blood flow through organs such as the portal and hepatic veins in the liver.

Transient elastography is a type of ultrasonography that is used to assess liver fibrosis (thickening of the tissue). The probe is placed on the skin between the ribs on the right hand side, and the software calculates a fibrosis score indicating the liver 'stiffness'. Higher scores indicate more severe fibrosis.

Computed tomography

In computed tomography (CT) scanning, multiple two-dimensional cross-sectional X-ray images ('slices') are taken; these are sometimes reconstructed as three-dimensional images by the scanner software to examine organs such as the large intestine. The patient lies flat on a table which is advanced into a large static circular structure. Interpretation of pathology requires specialist knowledge and all images are reported by a radiologist.

CT is used to investigate abdominal symptoms (**Table 2.24**) and to stage malignancy (i.e. determine the extent to which a cancer has spread). Intravenous contrast is injected into a peripheral vein to highlight blood vessels and

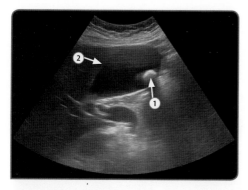

Figure 2.25 Ultrasound scan showing a gallstone ① in the gallbladder ②.

Abdominal CT imaging			
Type	Structure examined	Preparation	Indications
CT enterography	Principally the small intestine	Laxative bowel preparation IV contrast	Crohn's disease Tumours
CT liver/pancreas	Liver and pancreas	IV contrast	Benign and malignant liver and pancreatic lesions
Minimal preparation CT abdomen and pelvis	All abdominal organs	Low-residue diet Stool-tagging agent IV contrast	Colorectal malignancies large in size Weight loss Frailty Poor mobility
CT pneumocolon	Principally the large intestine	Low-residue diet Laxative bowel preparation IV contrast	Colorectal polyps and malignancy Reduced mobility
CT angiogram	Blood supply to the organs	IV contrast (fast infusion rate)	Significant GI bleeding
IV, intravenous			

Table 2.24 Types of abdominal CT imaging

help outline and diagnose any abnormalities identified. Because CT exposes the patient to radiation, the risk and benefits compared with alternative investigations are always considered, for example MRI enterography when investigating the small intestine.

CT pneumocolon

CT pneumocolon is performed by distending the large intestine with carbon dioxide passed through a plastic catheter that has been inserted into the rectum. A series of CT images is taken with the patient in the supine and prone positions. This moves the position of any remaining intestinal contents, allowing the radiologist to distinguish stool from polyps. The two-dimensional images are often reconstructed into a three-dimensional format, allowing a 'fly through' of the large intestine (**Figure 2.26**). The detection rates

for colorectal polyps and cancer are equivalent to those of colonoscopy but CT pneumocolon lacks the ability to biopsy or remove lesions. It is used:

- in patients who do not have the mobility required for colonoscopy (see page 123)
- following an incomplete colonoscopy procedure when it has not been possible for the endoscopist to reach the caecum, for example due to narrowing of the large intestine, or for patients who are unable to tolerate the procedure due to abdominal pain
- if the patient prefers this non-invasive test

Minimal-preparation CT scan

A minimal-preparation CT scan is used to exclude significant colorectal pathology (i.e. cancer) in patients who are frail, with

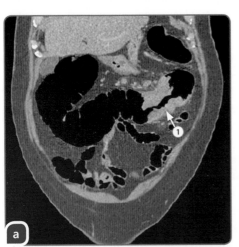

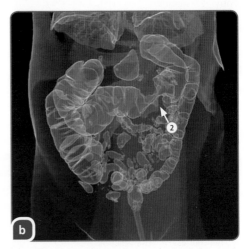

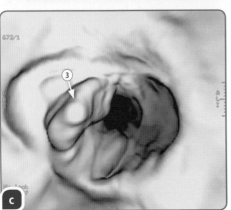

Figure 2.26 CT pneumocolon. (a) Coronal CT section on which the tumour can be identified ①. (b) Three-dimensional reconstruction with an 'apple core' lesion marked in the transverse colon ②. (c) CT 'fly through' showing an irregular colonic wall with narrowing ③.

significant comorbidity or limited life expectancy. A series of CT images is taken with the patient lying supine after drinking a faecal tagging agent (i.e. no laxative bowel preparation required) that highlights the stool. The detection rate for polyps is lower than with CT pneumocolon.

CT angiography

CT angiography is used to investigate patients with significant GI bleeding of unknown origin. Intravenous contrast is injected through a cannula in a peripheral vein. The contrast passes through the heart into the arterial system. Scans are taken to show the site where the contrast is leaking from the blood vessels into the lumen of the GI tract. This localises the point of blood loss and identifies the potential underlying cause. Further investigations (e.g. endoscopy) and treatments (e.g. therapeutic endoscopy or surgery) are then undertaken.

Magnetic resonance imaging

Magnetic resonance imaging (MRI) uses strong magnetic fields and radiowaves. Nuclei within the body absorb and emit radiofrequency energy when placed in this field, which creates a series of two-dimensional cross-sectional images. The patient lies flat on a table, which is advanced into a tightly enclosed tube. MRI is contraindicated in some patients with certain types of metal implants, for example pacemakers, and often limited in patients with claustrophobia. Its main advantage is that it does not involve exposure to radiation.

Several types of MRI imaging are used in GI disorders (Table 2.25).

In magnetic resonance cholangiopancreatography (MRCP), the biliary and pancreatic fluid appears bright in comparison to the solid surrounding tissues such as the bile ducts, highlighting biliary tract pathology such as stones or strictures. Intravenous contrast is not required. Magnetic resonance enterography (MRE) is used to examine the small intestine, to assess for the presence of strictures or inflammation. The preparation for the scan is identical to CT enterography (Table 2.24).

Positron emission tomography (PET)

A PET scan is a nuclear medicine scan used to detect metastases in patients with GI malignancy. A radioactive analogue of glucose (the 'tracer') is injected into the venous circulation; it is absorbed by cells with a high glucose uptake, for example some normal tissues (e.g. the brain and liver) and cancers. The scanner assesses metabolic activity by detecting gamma rays emitted by the tracer. Three-dimensional images are constructed using computer software.

Abdominal MRI		
Type	Structure examined	Indications
Magnetic resonance cholangiopancreatography (MRCP)	Biliary tree	Biliary and pancreatic duct pathology, e.g. gallstones
MR of liver or pancreas	Liver	Benign and malignant liver and pancreatic lesions, e.g. hepatocellular carcinoma
	Pancreas	
MR of pelvis	Rectum	Staging rectal polyps or cancers
	Anus	Perianal disease, e.g. fistula
MR enterography	Small intestine	Crohn's disease
		Tumours

Table 2.25 Types of abdominal MRI

White cell scan

This is a type of nuclear medicine scan used to identify areas of inflammation or infection. In gastroenterology, it is occasionally used to search for evidence of inflammatory bowel disease. White blood cells (mainly neutrophils) are removed from the patient and a radioactive label is attached. After they have been re-injected into the venous system, a scan is performed to highlight any abnormal tissue where they localise.

Barium studies

In a barium study radiodense barium sulphate liquid or paste is swallowed or is inserted into the colon through a rectal tube to coat the lining of the GI tract. The patient is moved into different positions to provide an adequate coating of the area of the GI tract being examined. Real-time radiography, a technique called fluoroscopy, is then used to assess for any structural abnormalities. As the images are taken in real time, they also provide information about motility disorders.

There are several types of barium study:

- Barium swallow – for the oesophagus
- Barium meal – for the stomach and duodenum
- Barium follow-through – for the small intestine
- Barium enema – for the large intestine and terminal ileum

Barium studies are being phased out in many centres because they are suboptimal for detecting pathology when compared with endoscopy and other radiological investigations such as CT pneumocolon. They should therefore be largely reserved for patients who decline alternative tests.

Contrast studies

Barium occasionally leads to an obstruction of the intestine by making the bowel contents more viscous; if it leaks into the abdominal cavity, mediastinum or the airways it commonly causes severe irritation. As a result, water-soluble contrast agents are preferred if obstruction, perforation or oropharyngeal aspiration is suspected because they are safer. The water-soluble contrast agent can be seen on CT scans and during fluoroscopy. It is swallowed to assess for suspected oesophageal perforation and, during video fluoroscopy, to assess the swallowing mechanism in patients thought to be at risk of aspiration. Water-soluble contrast is also inserted as an enema to assess for a leak between surgical connections (anastomoses) of the large intestine after colorectal surgery, and to outline the anatomy when a large bowel obstruction occurs from a cancer on the left side of the colon and a metal stent is being considered to relieve symptoms.

Endoscopic studies

An endoscope is a flexible tube inserted through the mouth or anus into the GI tract (**Figure 2.27**). Light passed down the endoscope is reflected off the lining of the GI tract and passes down fibre-optic cables in the endoscope, to a processor which generates an image on a television monitor. To allow better visualisation, the lumen is distended using air or carbon dioxide. An accessory channel runs down the length of the endoscope through which biopsy forceps and therapeutic devices are inserted.

Endoscopy is used both in diagnosis, through direct visualisation and via tissue biopsy, and in therapeutic intervention (**Table 2.26**). The main endoscopic procedures are described below:

- Oesophagogastroduodenoscopy
- Sigmoidoscopy
- Colonoscopy
- Wireless capsule endoscopy
- Endoscopic retrograde cholangiopancreatography
- Endoscopic ultrasonography

The general risks of endoscopy are perforation, bleeding and the cardiopulmonary consequences of sedation, for example respiratory depression. These risks are increased with therapeutic endoscopy procedures such as the removal of polyps and cauterisation of stomach ulcers. Oesophagogastroduodenoscopy, sigmoidoscopy and colonoscopy are some of the most commonly performed endoscopic procedures.

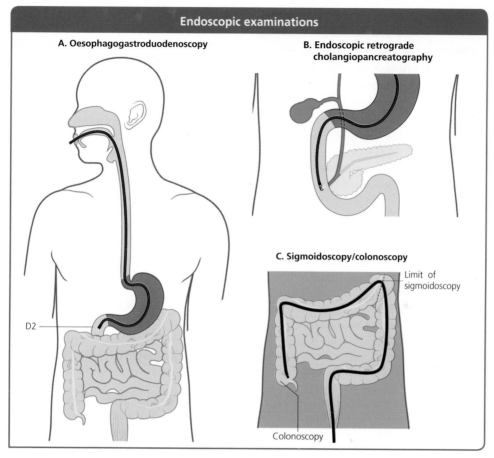

Figure 2.27 Endoscopic examinations. D2 is the second part of the duodenum.

The principal contraindications to endoscopy are:

- For all types: significant comorbidity (e.g. severe cardiorespiratory disease)
- For lower GI endoscopy: an inability to tolerate laxative bowel preparation or to change position on the trolley

Oesophagogastro-duodenoscopy (OGD)

This procedure is also referred to as an upper GI endoscopy or gastroscopy. The patient fasts for 6 hours before the procedure so that the oesophagus, stomach and duodenum are empty to ensure clear views. A topical xylocaine local anaesthetic throat spray is used to numb the back of the throat or an intravenous benzodiazepine such as midazolam is used to achieve conscious sedation, i.e. the patient is in a relaxed state but able to maintain communication. The patient lies in the left lateral position so that they are facing the endoscopist (person performing the endoscopy procedure), before an endoscope is passed through the mouth to examine the oesophagus, stomach and proximal duodenum.

The principal complications are perforation (0.03% of patients), bleeding, the risk from sedation (if used) and aspiration pneumonitis.

> **In conscious sedation, sedative medication is given to induce a relaxed state.** Some patients ask to be 'knocked out' but heavy sedation sometimes results in complications such as respiratory depression or aspiration.

Indications for diagnostic endoscopy	
Procedure	Principal indications
Oesophagogastro-duodenoscopy (upper GI endoscopy)	Dysphagia
	Dyspepsia
	GI bleeding
	Iron deficiency anaemia
	Confirmation of coeliac disease
	Abnormal radiological imaging, e.g. barium swallow
	Surveillance or follow-up in Barrett's oesophagus or gastric ulcers
Sigmoidoscopy	Rectal bleeding
	Abnormal radiology identifying pathology in the left colon
Colonoscopy	Change in bowel habit
	GI bleeding, e.g. rectal bleeding, melaena
	Iron deficiency anaemia
	Abnormal radiological imaging, e.g. CT pneumocolon
	Bowel cancer screening
	Surveillance or follow-up of colorectal polyps, IBD or moderate-to- strong family history of colorectal cancer

IBD, inflammatory bowel disease.

Table 2.26 Diagnostic indications for endoscopic procedures

Sigmoidoscopy

A laxative enema is first administered to evacuate the descending colon, sigmoid colon and rectum of stool. With the patient lying on the left side, the endoscope is passed through the anus up to the region of the splenic flexure, visualising the left side of the large intestine.

The principal complications of sigmoidoscopy are perforation (0.11% of patients), bleeding (0.24%), electrolyte disturbance with some types of bowel preparation, and the risk from sedation (if used).

Colonoscopy

The patient is put on a low-fibre diet several days before the procedure, followed by an oral bowel preparation (a strong laxative) in the 24 hours prior to the colonoscopy to evacuate stool from the large intestine. The procedure is performed without sedation or with conscious sedation (a combination of opiates, e.g. fentanyl, and benzodiazepines, e.g. midazolam).

With the patient lying on their left side, the endoscope is passed through the anus up to the caecum and sometimes through the ileocaecal valve into the terminal ileum. During the test the patient is repositioned several times so that the endoscope is more easily moved around the bowel and to provide optimal visualisation of its lining. If this is not possible, for example because of immobility due to arthritis, an alternative investigation is performed, such as CT pneumocolon.

The principal complications of colonoscopy are the same as for sigmoidoscopy (see above).

Wireless capsule endoscopy

Technique

A capsule the size of a large vitamin tablet is swallowed. This contains a camera that takes multiple pictures as it travels along the GI tract. The pictures are transmitted to sensors located in a belt worn around the patient's abdomen, which in turn transfer the information to a data recorder that stores the images. The images are converted into a video for viewing.

Wireless capsule endoscopy is most commonly used to examine the small intestine. It is also sometimes used to visualise the large intestine. Oral bowel preparation is given to clear the contents of the small and large intestine to improve the views.

Indications

- Gastrointestinal bleeding that is either overt (e.g. melaena) or occult (i.e. iron deficiency anaemia)
- Suspected Crohn's disease
- Abnormal radiological findings
- Suspected complications of coeliac disease (e.g. lymphoma)
- Polyposis syndromes (e.g. familial adenomatous polyposis)

Contraindications

- Pregnancy
- Oesophageal strictures – as the capsule is unable to pass the narrowing into the small intestine
- Known strictures of the small intestine

Complications

The main risk is retention of the capsule if it is unable to pass small intestinal lesions, such as strictures. If the capsule becomes trapped it is retrieved by an enteroscope (see below) or at surgery.

> **In wireless capsule endoscopy the risk of capsule retention rises from 1.4% to about 15% in patients who have Crohn's disease which has caused small intestinal narrowing (strictures).**

Enteroscopy

An enteroscope is an endoscope with a longer shaft than standard endoscopes, allowing it to move further into the GI tract.

Technique

Double-balloon enteroscopes have a balloon attached both to the end of the scope and a plastic overtube. The balloons are repeatedly inflated and deflated to concertina the small intestine, allowing deeper insertion of the scope. Enteroscopy is usually performed after abnormalities are identified by wireless capsule endoscopy.

Depending on the location within the small intestine, the enteroscope is inserted through the mouth (oral approach) or terminal ileum (retrograde approach) under conscious sedation with intravenous opiate and benzodiapezine medication or deep sedation with propofol. Oral bowel preparation is required to clear the contents of the small intestine.

Indications

- Treatment of vascular abnormalities e.g. angioectasia (dilated blood vessels)
- Biopsy and tattoo ink marking of tumours of the small intestine and of abnormalities prior to surgery

- Resection of polyps
- Dilatation and/or stenting of benign and malignant strictures

Contraindications

Enteroscopy is contraindicated if there is significant cardiopulmonary disease that precludes sedation.

Complications

In addition to the standard risks of upper GI endoscopy such as perforation and bleeding, there is a small risk of pancreatitis with oral approach enteroscopy, although the exact cause of this is uncertain.

Endoscopic retrograde cholangiopancreatography

Technique

Endoscopic retrograde cholangiopancreatography (ERCP) is performed under conscious sedation. The endoscope is inserted through the mouth and down to the second part of the duodenum.

ERCP uses a side-viewing endoscope to look at right angles into the ampulla of Vater and the biliary tree. Contrast is injected through a plastic catheter into the bile and pancreatic ducts under fluoroscopy imaging to detect pathology, including gallstones and strictures.

Instruments are inserted through a channel in the endoscope to carry out treatment in the bile and pancreatic ducts.

Since the introduction of MRCP as a non-invasive diagnostic test to visualise the biliary tree, ERCP is now principally considered a therapeutic procedure.

Indications

- Diagnosis and treatment of biliary strictures
- Biliary sepsis or jaundice occurring secondary to gallstones in the bile ducts
- Gallstone pancreatitis
- Assessment and treatment of sphincter of Oddi dysfunction
- Assessment of ampullary lesions

Contraindications

- Significant cardiopulmonary disease precluding sedation
- Coagulopathy unless it has been corrected

Complications

In addition to the standard risks of upper GI endoscopy, there is a small risk of pancreatitis (< 5%) and infection.

Endoscopic ultrasonography

Technique

Endoscopic ultrasonography (EUS) uses an endoscope that has been modified to incorporate an ultrasound device into its tip. It is most commonly used in the staging of cancer, to assess the layers of the GI tract and establish the depth of invasion of a lesion.

Conscious sedation is commonly used for upper GI examinations. A laxative enema is required to prepare for anorectal endoscopic ultrasonography.

Indications

- Staging of oesophageal and rectal malignancy
- Assessment of gastric, duodenal, pancreatic and hepatobiliary pathology (benign and malignant) with the option of fine-needle aspiration
- Assessment of the anal sphincter muscles in patients with faecal incontinence (e.g. secondary to obstetric trauma)

Contraindications

- Significant cardiopulmonary disease in upper GI tract EUS, due to the risks of sedation
- Significant oesophageal stricture due to the risk of perforation and inability to pass the endoscope through this area

Complications

These are the same as for oesophagogastroduodenoscopy and sigmoidoscopy, such as perforation and bleeding.

Pathology

A biopsy is a sample of tissue taken from an organ to help diagnose underlying disorders. The GI sites most commonly biopsied are the mucosa of the GI tract (oesophagus, stomach, duodenum and large intestine, using biopsy forceps during endoscopy procedures) and the liver (using a specialised needle) (see page 127). These specimens are placed in a formalin pot to fix and preserve the tissue for transfer to the histopathology laboratory. After preparation and staining of sections of the tissue samples, they are placed on a glass slide for review by a histopathologist.

Samples taken from gastrointestinal organs (e.g. pancreas) by fine-needle aspiration and samples of ascitic fluid are studied by cytopathology. This refers to the study of individual cells under a microscope to assess for malignant or benign cells.

> **Tissue samples are described by their appearance:**
>
> **Macroscopic** – the appearance observed by the naked eye
>
> **Microscopic** – the appearance under a microscope

Larger samples of tissue are studied after they have been removed at endoscopy (e.g. polyps) or during surgical procedures (e.g. sections of intestine or liver). After the macroscopic appearance has been examined, the tissue is cut into thin sections for viewing under a microscope.

In the context of malignancy, this information is used to stage the disease. This is described using the TNM staging system (**Figure 2.28**).

> **The TNM classification of malignant tumours is used for cancer staging in all parts of the GI tract:**
>
> - T = the size of the primary tumour
> - N = lymph node involvement
> - M = the presence of metastases

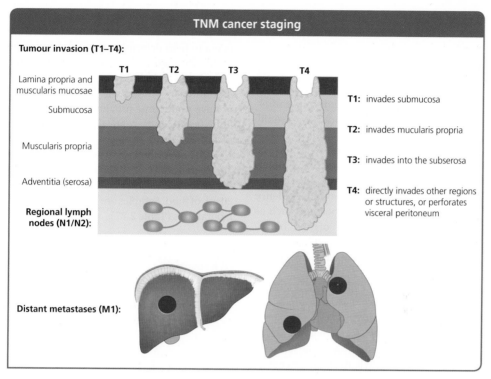

Figure 2.28 TNM cancer staging. T describes tumour depth, for example as shown here for tumours of the gut wall, and M denotes the existence of metastases. The N classifications describe lymph node involvement. N1: regional node; N3, multiple or distant nodes; N2, spread between N1 and N3.

Other investigations

Oesophageal pH and manometry studies

A plastic catheter containing pressure sensors and pH electrodes is inserted through the nose into the oesophagus. This is attached to an ambulatory device that records information as patients go about their normal daily activities. The manometry component measures the pressures of the lower oesophageal sphincter and in the oesophagus.

This test is performed to assess for oesophageal dysmotility disorders (e.g. achalasia) and reflux symptoms not responding to medical therapy or prior to consideration of anti-reflux surgery.

Gastric emptying studies

These are used to investigate patients with symptoms of delayed gastric emptying.

Medications that affect gastric motility, for example opioids, should be discontinued at least two days prior to the test. Patients are kept nil by mouth for 4 hours, after which they ingest technetium-radiolabelled scrambled egg (used to standardise the test, as different food types affect gastric emptying differently). Gamma camera images are taken for up to 4 hours after the egg is ingested. Delayed emptying of the stomach indicates gastroparesis.

SeHCAT scan

SeHCAT   (23-seleno-25-homotaurocholic acid, a synthetic bile acid) testing is used to diagnose bile salt malabsorption. A radiolabelled SeHCAT preparation is swallowed with water and a baseline scan performed in the medical physics department. This labelled bile acid is incorporated into the bile and enters the enterohepatic circulation. A further scan is performed 7 days later to calculate the percentage SeHCAT retention. Values of less than 15% indicate bile salt malabsorption.

Liver biopsy

Liver biopsy is used to identify the cause of impaired liver function or abnormal radiology, including tumours. Samples are usually taken through the abdominal wall.

After injecting local anaesthetic into the skin and soft tissue between the ribs, a biopsy needle is passed into the liver. This is usually performed under ultrasound guidance to reduce the risks of the procedure such as bleeding, puncture of other organs, biliary peritonitis and infection, by highlighting local structures (e.g. bile ducts and liver blood vessels).

Samples are also obtainable via the transjugular route if patients have abnormal clotting (e.g. high INR), large-volume ascites or morbid obesity, where it is not possible for the needle to reach the liver through the abdominal wall. In this approach, the biopsy needle is inserted through the jugular (neck) vein under fluoroscopy to the hepatic vein. Samples of the liver are taken through the vein wall.

Samples are placed in formalin to fix and preserve the tissue for transport to the histopathology laboratory, prior to analysis. Depending upon the clinical picture, special stains are used to confirm a diagnosis, for example Perls' stain to assess for iron overload.

Ascitic tap

The presence of ascites is initially established by clinical examination (see page 106). If there is any doubt, an abdominal ultrasound is performed. Fluid samples are taken to help determine the aetiology of the ascites through calculation of the SAAG (see below), and to exclude spontaneous bacterial peritonitis in patients who have liver disease or have undergone previous drainage of the fluid (ascitic paracentesis). Ascitic fluid is usually sterile.

Local anaesthetic is used to infiltrate the abdominal wall. A needle is then passed into the peritoneal cavity to take approximately 10–20 mL of fluid. Samples are sent to the relevant laboratories (**Table 2.27**).

> **If spontaneous bacterial peritonitis is suspected**, samples are also sent in blood culture bottles. The presence of media promotes reproduction of organisms, which increases the rate of detection.

The serum–ascites albumin gradient (SAAG) is used to determine whether the ascites is due to portal hypertension. It is calculated by:

$$SAAG = \left[\frac{serum}{albumin} \right] - \left[\frac{ascitic\ fluid}{albumin} \right]$$

A value over 11 g/L indicates that the ascites is the result of portal hypertension secondary to a hepatic cause (e.g. cirrhosis, fulminant liver failure, or hepatic or portal vein thrombosis) or a non-hepatic cause (e.g. heart failure). A value of < 11 g/L indicates that portal hypertension is unlikely.

Ascitic fluid analysis		
Test	Laboratory department	Positive result
Albumin	Biochemistry – universal container	Used to calculate SAAG
White cell count (WCC)	Microbiology – universal container	>250/mm³ (polymorphs) indicates SBP
Microscopy, culture and sensitivity (M,C&S)	Microbiology – blood culture bottles	Any growth is abnormal and indicates SBP
Cytology	Cytology or pathology – universal container	Presence of malignant cells
SBP, spontaneous bacterial peritonitis.		

Table 2.27 Ascitic fluid analysis

Anorectal manometry

This is used to assess causes of faecal incontinence and constipation.

First, a laxative enema is administered to clear the lower part of the large intestine of stool. With the patient awake and lying in the left lateral position, a lubricated flexible tube containing a series of sensors and a balloon attached to the end is inserted into the anus and rectum. Local anaesthetic is not usually required as the test is not painful. This tube is connected to a machine that records the pressure of the anal sphincters. Measurements are taken of the resting anal pressure and as the patient is asked to squeeze the anus. The balloon is inflated in the rectum to assess sensation and the recto-anal inhibitory reflux (involuntary relaxation of the internal anal sphincter due to rectal distension). Failure of the sphincter muscles to relax is a cause of constipation. Weak anal sphincter muscles or poor rectal sensation sometimes results in faecal incontinence.

Biofeedback therapy is also provided using this equipment, by teaching the patient to relax the anal sphincters in cases of constipation and pelvic floor exercises to strengthen the muscles for faecal incontinence.

Management options

Starter questions

Answers to the following questions are on page pages 159–160.

10. What determines the most appropriate treatment for a patient with a GI disorder?
11. How are medications chosen when treating a GI condition?
12. How can the nutritional status of patients with GI disease and weight loss be improved?

Medications

Although some GI disorders are self-limiting (e.g. gastroenteritis) or improve with lifestyle or dietary modifications (e.g. gastro-oesophageal reflux), many require drug treatment. Whereas some drugs provide symptomatic relief (e.g. for nausea or constipation), others treat specific conditions (e.g. viral hepatitis).

Most drugs used in gastroenterology are administered orally. Other routes of delivery include per rectum (rectally or 'PR'), intravenously or subcutaneously. When a patient has to remain nil by mouth, for example before surgery, oral drugs can nevertheless usually be given with a sip of water. If there are significant problems with swallowing, a nasogastric tube is often used for medications as well as nutritional support.

The sections below concentrate on the clinically most significant drugs that are commonly used in GI conditions. However other medications are sometimes required to manage complications and symptoms, such as diuretics in decompensated liver disease or analgesics and antidepressants for functional abdominal pain.

> **Most medications are absorbed systemically but some are also formulated for topical release at the disease site**. For example oral and rectal formulations of mesalazine are both available for colitis.

Antacids

Antacids treat the symptoms of indigestion and are available without prescription.

Drugs in this group

- Magnesium carbonate
- Aluminium hydroxide
- Calcium carbonate
- Sodium bicarbonate

In some preparations more than one of these is combined.

Mode of action

Antacids are weak bases that partly buffer gastric acid and therefore raise the gastric pH, reducing the symptoms of stomach acid (e.g. dyspepsia or heartburn). The increase in pH also reduces the activity of pepsin (see page 41), which is inactivated by a pH of more than 4.

Some formulations include sodium alginate, which produces a protective 'raft' over the oesophageal and gastric lining.

Indications

- Dyspepsia
- Gastro-oesophageal reflux

Adverse effects

- Constipation (aluminium formulations)
- Diarrhoea (magnesium formulations)
- Excess use of calcium-containing preparations sometimes results in its systemic absorption

- Excess consumption of magnesium- and aluminium-containing antacids sometimes cause hypophosphataemia

Aluminium (can cause constipation) and magnesium (can cause diarrhoea) containing antacids are often used together to counteract their opposite effects on the large intestine.

Sucralfate is a mixture of aluminium hydroxide and sulphated sucrose that has minimal antacid affect and is therefore only occasionally used in the treatment of dyspepsia. It is also used with caution due to its potential adverse effect of bezoar (mass trapped within the GI system) formation. It protects the mucosa from gastric acid but does not affect gastric pH.

H₂ receptor antagonists

H₂ receptor antagonists are used to treat dyspepsia or heartburn and are more effective than antacids.

Drugs in this group

- Cimetidine
- Ranitidine

Mode of action

These block the action of histamine on the H_2 receptors of the gastric parietal cells and thereby reduce gastric acid production (**Figure 2.29**).

Indications

- Dyspepsia
- Gastro-oesophageal reflux
- Gastric and duodenal ulcers

Adverse effects

- Diarrhoea
- Headache
- Dizziness

Because it has fewer side effects and drug interactions, ranitidine is generally favoured over cimetidine. Cimetidine has anti-androgenic effects that sometimes cause impotence and gynaecomastia in men. It is also a cytochrome p450 inhibitor and impairs the metabolism of some drugs, for example warfarin and phenytoin.

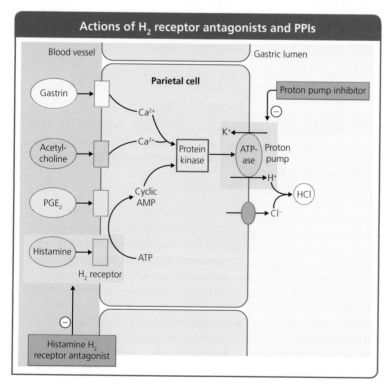

Actions of H₂ receptor antagonists and PPIs

Blood vessel — Gastric lumen

Parietal cell

Gastrin

Ca²⁺

Proton pump inhibitor

Acetyl-choline

Ca²⁺

K⁺

Protein kinase

ATP-ase

Proton pump

H⁺

PGE₂

Cyclic AMP

HCl

Cl⁻

Histamine

ATP

H₂ receptor

Histamine H₂ receptor antagonist

Figure 2.29 Actions of proton pump inhibitors and H₂ receptor antagonists on the gastric parietal cell. PGE2, prostaglandin E2.

Proton pump inhibitors

Proton pump inhibitors are more potent acid suppressants than H_2 receptor antagonists.

Drugs in this group

- Omeprazole
- Lansoprazole
- Pantoprazole
- Rabeprazole
- Esomeprazole

Mode of action

These block the hydrogen/potassium ATP pump (proton pump) on the gastric parietal cells and so reduce acid secretion (**Figure 2.29**).

Indications

- Dyspepsia
- Gastro-oesophageal reflux
- Gastric and duodenal ulcers
- *Helicobacter pylori* eradication (in combination with antibiotics)
- Prevention of peptic ulcers caused by non-steroidal anti-inflammatory drugs

Adverse effects

- Diarrhoea
- Nausea
- Flatulence
- Headache
- Increased risk of *C. difficile* infection (see page 223–226)
- Increased incidence of osteoporosis and associated fractures with long-term usage, particularly in the elderly. The cause for this is uncertain.

Antiemetics

Identifying the underlying cause of nausea and vomiting means that the best drug treatment is determined. A number of drug options are used (**Table 2.28**). These work on different receptors and at different sites in the GI tract or the brain (**Figure 2.30**).

If drugs cannot be taken orally, for example due to severe vomiting or intestinal obstruction, they are administered intravenously intramuscularly, rectally, sublingually (e.g. prochlorperazine) or via a transdermal patch (e.g. hyoscine).

Terlipressin

Mode of action

Terlipressin is a synthetic derivative of antidiuretic hormone (vasopressin). It causes vasoconstriction, thereby reducing blood flow and pressure in the portal system. It is administered intravenously

Indications

- Bleeding from varices (see page 261)
- Hepatorenal syndrome

Adverse effects

- Abdominal pain
- Diarrhoea
- Peripheral vasoconstriction
- Angina and arrhythmias (abnormal heart rhythms)

Terlipressin is contraindicated in patients with severe ischaemic heart disease, because it commonly causes coronary artery vasoconstriction.

Ursodeoxycholic acid

Mode of action

Ursodeoxycholic acid reduces the biliary secretion and absorption of cholesterol, as well as increasing the solubility of cholesterol.

Indications

- Primary biliary cholangitis (PBC) – ursodeoxycholic acid helps to improve the bilirubin, alkaline phosphatase and γ-glutamyl transferase liver function tests and sometimes delays the progression of early PBC, but there is no evidence that it improves survival
- Treatment of cholesterol gallstones – ursodeoxycholic acid has a very limited benefit and has been superseded by laparoscopic cholecystectomy and ERCP

Commonly used antiemetics			
Mode of action	Example	Indications	Adverse effects and cautions
Antihistamine (H_1 receptor)	Cyclizine (PO, PR, IV, IM, SC)	Most causes of nausea and vomiting First-line in pregnancy and postoperatively Motion sickness	Drowsiness, headache, blurred vision, dry mouth, urinary retention Avoid in severe ischaemic heart disease
Serotonin (5-HT_3) receptor antagonist	Ondansetron (PO, PR, IV, IM)	Chemotherapy and radiotherapy induced vomiting Second line postoperatively	Constipation, headaches, flushing Avoid in long QT syndrome; correct low K^+ and Mg^{2+} levels beforehand (to reduce arrhythmia risk)
Dopamine (D_2) antagonists	Metoclopramide (PO, IV, IM, SC)*	GI causes Drug side effects, migraines	Galactorrhoea (spontaneous production of milk from the breast) High prolactin Extrapyramidal side-effects: ■ parkinsonism ■ tardive dyskinesia (with long-term use)
	Domperidone (PO)*	Parkinson's disease	
	Prochlorperazine (PO, IV, IM)	Vestibular causes 2nd line in pregnancy, drug side effects, post operatively and chemo- or radiotherapy	
	Haloperidol (PO, IV, IM, SC)	Palliative care	
	Levomepromazine (PO, IV, IM, SC)	Most causes – useful in refractory symptoms	
Antimuscarinic	Hyoscine (PO, TOP)	Motion sickness	Antimuscarinic side effects especially in elderly – dry mouth, urinary retention and pupillary dilation Avoid in severe ischaemic heart disease and glaucoma
Steroids	Dexamethasone (PO, IV, IM, SC)	Raised intracranial pressure Chemo- or radiotherapy	See Table 2.32 (most significantly osteoporosis, adrenal cortex suppression and hyperglycaemia)

*Short-term use only: metoclopramide has CNS effects and in the elderly domperidone raises arrhythmia risk.

Abbreviations: PO, oral; PR, rectal; IV, intravenous; IM, intramuscular; SC, subcutaneous; TOP, topical.

Table 2.28 Commonly used antiemetics

Adverse effects

- Diarrhoea
- Abdominal pain
- Nausea

Bile acid sequestrants

These drugs are used in the treatment of bile salt malabsorption.

Drugs in this group

- Colestyramine – in many countries this is the only bile acid sequestrant with a license for GI symptoms
- Colestipol
- Colesevelam

Mode of action

These drugs bind to bile acids in the large

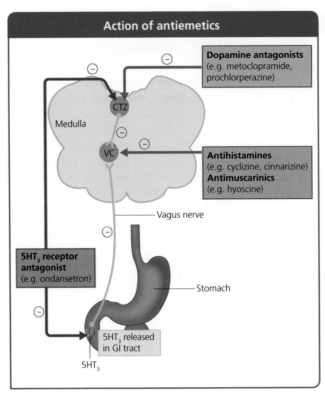

Action of antiemetics

- Dopamine antagonists (e.g. metoclopramide, prochlorperazine)
- CTZ
- Medulla
- VC
- Antihistamines (e.g. cyclizine, cinnarizine)
  Antimuscarinics (e.g. hyoscine)
- Vagus nerve
- 5HT₃ receptor antagonist (e.g. ondansetron)
- Stomach
- 5HT₃ released in GI tract
- 5HT₃

Figure 2.30 Action of antiemetics. 5HT3, 5-hydroxytryptamine type 3; CTZ, chemoreceptor trigger zone (drugs, toxins, movement via the vestibular centre); GI, gastrointestinal; VC, vomiting centre (odour, smell, taste).

intestine to form insoluble complexes which are excreted in the stool, rather than being reabsorbed into the enterohepatic circulation.

Indications

- Pruritus (itching) in cholestatic liver disease
- Bile salt malabsorption, e.g. after surgery in which the terminal ileum has been removed

Adverse effects

- Nausea and vomiting
- Abdominal pain
- Reduced absorption of medications and fat-soluble vitamins; the mechanism for this is uncertain

Because of the latter effect, patients are advised to avoid taking other medications for 1 hour before and 4 hours after taking sequestrants. Individuals on long-term treatment require monitoring of fat-soluble vitamin

(A, D, E) levels and international normalised ratio (a marker of vitamin K deficiency) at least annually. Vitamin supplements should be given if these levels are low.

> **Colestyramine is a resin and is not very palatable.** It is better tolerated by adding a small amount of fruit juice.

Pancreatin (pancreatic enzyme formulations)

These replace the enzymes that are usually produced by the pancreas to aid digestion. They are taken at the same time as each meal and snack. The preparations have an enteric coating to prevent the enzymes being denatured by the gastric acid. The enzymes are then released in the duodenum.

Patients with pancreatic exocrine insufficiency often have low pancreatic bicarbonate secretion, which is insufficient to increase the pH of the chyme entering the duodenum from the stomach, affecting the action of the enzyme supplements. H_2 receptor antagonists or proton pump inhibitors are sometimes co-prescribed to increase the gastric pH.

Drugs in this group

There are multiple preparations available that contain different ratios of protease, lipase and amylase enzymes.

Mode of action

They contain replacement enzymes (outlined above) that are normally produced by the pancreas.

Indications

Pancreatic exocrine insufficiency in:

- Cystic fibrosis
- Chronic pancreatitis
- After pancreatectomy
- Pancreatic cancer

Adverse effects

- Nausea and vomiting
- Abdominal pain
- Oral irritation if left in the mouth

The dosage should be varied in line with the fat content and size of the patient's meals to improve the number and consistency of stools.

Antispasmodics

These cause smooth muscle relaxation and are used to reduce abdominal pain. They are well tolerated with few side effects. Therefore many preparations are available to buy without prescription.

Drugs in this group

Of the many different drugs available, commonly used examples are mebeverine, peppermint oil and hyoscine butylbromide.

Mode of action

Some medications have a direct action on the smooth muscle of the GI tract, e.g. alverine, mebeverine and peppermint oil. Others reduce intestinal motility through their antimuscarinic effect, inhibiting the action of acetylcholine, a neurotransmitter in the parasympathetic nervous system, e.g. hyoscine and dicycloverine.

Indications

- Irritable bowel syndrome
- Diverticular disease

Adverse effects

- Nausea
- Headache
- Dizziness
- For antimuscarinic drugs – constipation, bradycardia, urinary urgency or retention, dilation of the pupils and dry mouth sometimes occur due to inhibition of the acetylcholine neurotransmitter in other organs

Antidiarrhoeal agents

These are obtained 'over the counter' as well as being prescribed. Packs contain advice to consult a doctor if the symptoms continue for more than a few days so that an underlying cause can be determined.

Drugs in this group

- Loperamide
- Co-phenotrope
- Codeine phosphate

Mode of action

These opioid drugs act on opioid receptors in the intestine to reduce its motility.

Indications

They provide symptomatic relief in acute diarrhoea. They also have a role in some causes of chronic diarrhoea as an adjunct to targeted treatment such as diarrhoea predominant IBS, bile salt diarrhoea and short bowel syndrome.

Adverse effects

- Constipation
- Nausea
- Dizziness

These drugs should be avoided in patients with suspected or active inflammatory bowel disease due to the risk of colonic dilatation. Codeine phosphate is used with caution and only for short periods of time because of tolerance and the risk of dependency. This does not occur with loperamide and co-phenotrope as they are not absorbed from the gut.

Laxatives

There are broadly two types of laxatives:

- laxatives that affect the gut motility, i.e. act as stimulants
- laxatives that change the physical characteristics of the intestinal contents, for example by drawing water into the intestine

Laxatives are used to treat constipation either as a single symptom or as a component of irritable bowel syndrome or diverticular disease (**Table 2.29**). They also prevent constipation in patients with anal fissures, fistulae and haemorrhoids, to help healing and reduce symptoms such as pain and bleeding due to straining. Laxatives are used in combination with other treatments for constipation including adequate water and fibre intake.

Oral formulations of the laxatives magnesium citrate, polyethylene glycol, sodium phosphate and sodium picosulfate are principally used to clean out the large bowel before colonoscopy, CT colonography or surgery, but are also occasionally used for severe constipation. However, they sometimes cause hypovolaemia and electrolyte disturbances by drawing large volumes of water into the bowel and so must be used with caution in patients who have significant cardiac or renal co-morbidity.

Laxatives				
Group	Examples	Mode of action	Indications	Adverse effects
Bulk-forming	Dietary fibre, wheat or oat bran, ispaghula husk, methylcellulose, sterculia	Retain water in stool Increase bulk and make peristalsis easier (e.g. diverticular disease)	Chronic constipation (1st-line treatment)	Bloating, excess flatus, abdominal discomfort
Osmotic	Oral – lactulose, polyethylene glycols, magnesium hydroxide or citrate Enema – sodium acid phosphate or sodium citrate	Osmotic effect drawing water into the large intestine Stool becomes softer and easier to pass	Chronic constipation (2nd-line instead of or as well as bulk-forming agent) Hepatic encephalopathy: lactulose decreases release of ammonia by bacteria resident in the large intestine	Nausea, bloating, abdominal discomfort, flatus
Stimulant	Senna, bisacodyl, sodium picosulfate Glycerol (suppository)	Stimulate peristalsis at myenteric plexus Decrease water absorption in colon	Acute constipation Chronic constipation with intermittent use	Abdominal cramps, diarrhoea, nausea and vomiting, low K$^+$ (if used in excess)
Stool-softening	Docusate sodium, liquid paraffin, arachis oil (enema)	Detergent action traps water in stool and makes it 'slippery'	Used occasionally in chronic constipation Helpful with Haemorrhoids and anal fissures	Diarrhoea, anal irritation

Table 2.29 Laxatives (all examples are oral, unless stated otherwise)

Laxative enemas are usually used as a preparation prior to sigmoidoscopy or surgical procedures, but are sometimes used to treat severe constipation or patients with hepatic encephalopathy who are unable to take oral medications (see page 260). Through a soft rectal catheter attached to a small plastic bottle, fluid is introduced into the left colon to stimulate the expulsion of stool from the large intestine.

New agents that target receptors in the GI tract have recently been developed to treat patients who have ongoing constipation (either alone or in conjunction with irritable bowel syndrome) despite lifestyle modifications and laxative use (**Table 2.30**).

> **Long-term use of the laxative senna sometimes results in melanosis coli,** caused by deposition of a brown pigment in the lamina propria of the colon. It is visible at colonoscopy (**Figure 2.31**); however, it does not cause any problems.

Aminosalicylates

Sulphasalazine was the first aminosalicylate developed, however its use is often limited by intolerance to the sulphapyridine component, especially in higher dosages. 5-aminosalicylic acid (5-ASA) drugs do not contain this element and are therefore generally used in clinical practice.

Oral 5-ASA formulations have been designed to provide topical (i.e. local) release in the distal GI tract utilising different mechanisms (**Figure 2.32**). 5-aminosalicylates are also given rectally as suppositories or as foam or liquid enemas applied topically to the rectum and left colon.

Drugs in this group

- Mesalazine
- Sulphasalazine

Mode of action

These drugs inhibit the synthesis of proinflammatory cytokines, prostaglandins and

Newer agents to treat constipation				
Group	Examples	Mode of action	Indication	Adverse effects
Guanylate cyclase-C receptor agonist	Linaclotide	↑ Peristalsis, ↑ fluid secretion into the intestine, ↓ visceral pain	Irritable bowel syndrome with constipation	Diarrhoea, flatus, abdominal pain, nausea, headache, dizziness
Chloride channel activator	Lubiprostone	↑ Intestinal fluid secretion, ↑ motility	Chronic constipation not responsive to lifestyle changes	
Serotonin (5-HT$_4$) agonist	Prucalopride	↑ Peristalsis	Chronic constipation not responsive to laxatives	

Table 2.30 Newer agents used to treat constipation. All of these agents are given orally.

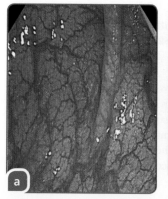
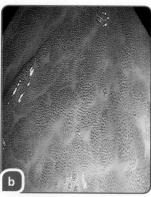

Figure 2.31 Endoscopic image of (a) normal mucosa in the large intestine and (b) melanosis coli.

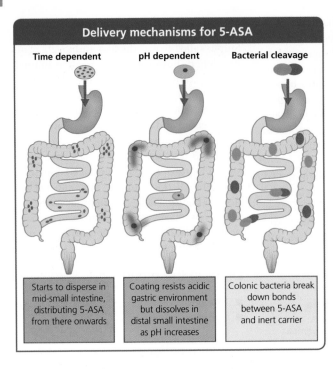

Delivery mechanisms for 5-ASA

Time dependent	pH dependent	Bacterial cleavage
Starts to disperse in mid-small intestine, distributing 5-ASA from there onwards	Coating resists acidic gastric environment but dissolves in distal small intestine as pH increases	Colonic bacteria break down bonds between 5-ASA and inert carrier

Figure 2.32 Mechanisms for oral delivery of 5-ASA (mesalazine) drugs.

leukotrienes and act as free radical scavengers (unstable molecules that cause cell damage).

Indications

They are used in ulcerative colitis to treat active disease and maintain remission. They also reduce the risk of cancer in long-standing extensive colitis. These drugs have very little benefit in Crohn's disease, especially small bowel disease.

Adverse effects

- Diarrhoea
- Nausea
- Hypersensitivity, e.g. rash (especially sulphasalazine)
- Rarely renal impairment, bone marrow suppression and pancreatitis

Patients taking 5-aminosalicylates should undergo full blood count and urea and electrolyte monitoring at least annually to monitor for these side effects.

Immunosuppressive drugs

Immunosuppressive drugs work by suppressing the immune system or supress its responses. They are frequently used in gastrointestinal medicine to treat chronic inflammatory disorders.

Drugs in this group

Four types of immunosuppressive drug are used in gastrointestinal medicine:

- Corticosteroids: prednisolone, hydrocortisone and budesonide
- Thiopurines: azathioprine and 6-mercaptopurine (6MP)
- A dihydrofolate reductase inhibitor: methotrexate
- Ciclosporin

Mode of action

This varies with the type of drug and is outlined in **Table 2.31**.

Indications

Immunosuppressants have a valuable role in both induction and maintenance of remission in conditions such as inflammatory bowel disease, autoimmune hepatitis and pancreatitis (**Table 2.31**). They are also used after transplantation, to reduce the chance of organ rejection.

Immunosuppressant drugs			
Drug	Mode of action	Indication	Adverse effects and cautions
Corticosteroids: Prednisolone (oral, rectal) Hydrocortisone (IV, rectal), Budesonide (oral, rectal)	Anti-inflammatory by suppressing multiple genes: ↓ Leucocyte infiltration ↓ Inflammatory mediators ↓ Humoral immune responses	Active inflammatory disorders: ulcerative colitis, Crohn's disease*, microscopic colitis, autoimmune hepatitis and pancreatitis After liver transplant Eosinophilic oesophagitis (swallow inhaled steroid)	See **Table 2.32**; the most significant effects are: ■ osteoporosis ■ adrenal cortex suppression ■ hyperglycaemia
Thiopurines†: Azathioprine (oral) 6-mercaptopurine (oral)	Blocks purine metabolism and therefore DNA synthesis Particularly affects cell-mediated and antibody-mediated immune reactions	Induction and maintenance of remission in ulcerative colitis, Crohn's disease and autoimmune hepatitis or pancreatitis After liver transplant Steroid reduction or cessation in these patient groups	Hypersensitivity, e.g. nausea, fevers, myalgia, arthralgia Dose-related bone marrow suppression, particularly neutropenia (leading to infections); also anaemia and ↓ platelets Hepatotoxicity and pancreatitis Non-Hodgkin's lymphoma (relative risk = 4)
Dihydrofolate reductase inhibitor: methotrexate (oral or IM)	↓ Conversion of folic acid into active form required for purine and pyrimidines synthesis, causing ↓ DNA replication Especially targets rapidly dividing cells, e.g. bone marrow	Crohn's disease: induction of remission and maintenance	Neutropenia and thrombocytopenia, GI symptoms, hepatotoxicity, renal toxicity, rash, alopecia, pulmonary fibrosis Congenital deformities and miscarriage: used with extreme caution in women of child-bearing age; folic acid is co-prescribed to reduce toxicities
Ciclosporin (IV initially, then oral)	Fungal derivative that reduces immune system activity, predominantly by affecting T cells	Severe acute active ulcerative colitis After liver transplant	Anorexia, nausea, renal impairment, hypertension, hepatotoxicity, tremor

IM, intramuscularly; IV, intravenously.

*Oral budesonide specifically for distal small intestine and proximal colonic Crohn's disease. Extensive metabolism by the liver after absorption helps to minimise adverse effects. † Dosage reduced if taking allopurinol because this interferes with thiopurine metabolism.

Table 2.31 Immunosuppressant drugs used in gastroenterology

Adverse effects

These are outlined in **Tables 2.31** and **2.32**. Patients are counselled on the nature and adverse effects of these drugs prior to starting, so that they understand the potential side effects and need for regular blood monitoring. The major concern is infection. Prior to therapy, patients should be up to date with nationally recommended vaccinations and should be alerted to the need to report to a doctor if they develop symptoms of sepsis, such as a high temperature and sore throat.

Regular blood monitoring (full blood count and biochemistry) is required for all immunosuppressants, except steroids, to monitor for potential toxicity. If evidence of toxicity is found, the dose is reduced or the drug is stopped.

Side-effects of corticosteroids	
System/type	Side effect
Cardiovascular	Hypertension
Musculoskeletal	Osteoporosis
	Aseptic necrosis
	Myopathy (especially proximal)
Neurological	Neuropathy
Ophthalmic	Cataracts
	Glaucoma
Immunological	Immunosuppression
	Lymphocytopenia
Endocrine	Diabetes
	Adrenal cortex suppression
Developmental	Growth retardation (children)
Psychiatric	Mood disturbance (depression or euphoria)
	Psychosis
	Sleep disturbance
Skin	Acne
	Hirsutism
	Oedema
	Striae (abdomen)
'Cushingoid' features	Moon face
	Buffalo hump
	Weight gain

Table 2.32 Side-effects of corticosteroids.

> **Giving steroids topically reduces their side effects, because systemic absorption is lower.** For example, steroids can be given as enemas.

> **A patient's thiopurine methyl transferase (TPMT) activity should be checked before starting azathioprine or 6-mercaptopurine.** TPMT catalyses the methylation of these drugs to form less toxic metabolites; low activity due to enzyme defects results in accumulation of more toxic metabolites, which causes bone marrow suppression. There is ethnic variation in TPMT activity; in 10% of people it is low and in <1% it is zero.

Biologic agents

These drugs are cytokine modulators. In gastrointestinal medicine they are used in the treatment of inflammatory bowel disease. They are also widely used in other specialities such as rheumatology and dermatology.

Drugs in this group

- Infliximab
- Adalimumab
- Golimumab
- Vedolizumab
- Ustekinumab

Mode of action

These drugs either have an anti-TNFα action or affect white blood cell function (**Table 2.33**). Newer 'biologics' targeting different mediators in the inflammatory cascade will become available in the near future.

Indications

Anti-TNFα agents are used in the induction and remission of both ulcerative colitis and Crohn's disease (**Table 2.33**). Vedolizumab and Ustekinumab are used as second-line treatments in patients who don't tolerate or fail to respond to immunosuppressant or anti-TNFα agents.

Adverse effects

Adverse effects are outlined in **Table 2.33**. An indirect adverse effect arises from the biological nature of the drugs, which means there is a risk they are recognised as foreign antigens and antibodies are raised against them, reducing their effectiveness. For this reason, patients treated with biologics are usually also commenced on azathioprine, 6MP or methotrexate to minimise the risk of antibody formation to these drugs and reduced effectiveness. Counselling and monitoring for adverse effects are required as outlined for immunosuppressants above.

Anorectal preparations

Anorectal discomfort, itching and soreness are treated by ensuring regular bowel habits

Cytokine modulators in gastroenterology			
Drug	Mode of action	Indication	Adverse effects
Anti-TNF drugs: Infliximab (IV) Adalimumab (SC) Golimumab (SC)	Bind to TNF-α and stop it binding to receptors ↓ Production of proinflammatory cytokines, e.g. interleukins 1 and 6	Ulcerative colitis and Crohn's disease: induction and maintenance of remission	Infections including opportunistic infection, tuberculosis and hepatitis B reactivation (screening required before starting drug) Nausea, hypersensitivity reactions, fevers, lupus-like syndrome, bone marrow suppression
Vedolizumab (IV)	Inhibits adhesion and migration of neutrophils by binding to α4β7 integrin, blocking interaction with adhesion molecules in blood vessels in the gut	Ulcerative colitis and Crohn's disease: induction and maintenance of remission (2nd line)	Headache, joint pain, nausea, fever, lethargy, sepsis, hepatotoxicity, allergic responses
Ustekinumab (IV)	Monoclonocal antibody against interleukin 12 and 23, which activate T-cells	Crohn's disease: induction and maintenance of remission (2nd line)	Headache, joint pain, nausea, sepsis, allergic responses

TNF, tumour necrosis factor; Abbreviations: IV, intravenous; SC, subcutaneous

Table 2.33 Cytokine modulators ('biologics') used in gastroenterology

to help healing and reduce symptoms such as pain and bleeding due to straining. This is done using dietary modifications and/or bulk-forming laxatives. Careful cleaning is also needed to remove sweat and any residual stool, which causes local irritation. Creams, ointments or suppositories are used to provide symptomatic benefit.

Drugs in this group

This group comprises local anaesthetics, for example lidocaine, corticosteroids and combinations of these.

Indications

- Anal irritation
- Haemorrhoids
- Anal fissures
- Fistulae

Adverse effects

Local anaesthetics are absorbed and cause sensitisation of the anal skin. It is therefore recommended that they are used sparingly.

Treatment for anal fissures

If regulation of bowel habit and topical anorectal formulations outlined above are

not effective, the majority of fissures will heal with a glyceryl trinitrate (GTN) or diltiazem ointment. These are applied in small amounts directly onto the fissure, twice a day for up to 8 weeks.

Drugs in this group

- Glyceryl trinitrate 0.4%
- Diltiazem 2% ointments

Mode of action

They cause vasodilation and reduce muscle spasm and ischaemia to promote healing.

Adverse effects

- Headache – usually resolves within 2–3 days of treatment
- Dizziness
- Perianal discomfort or itching

Antibiotics

Antibiotics have a range of indications in gastroenterology (**Table 2.34**). The choice of drug is governed by guidelines produced by the local microbiology department and based on patterns of antibiotic resistance. Guidelines specify the most appropriate empirical

Antibiotics in gastroenterology

Indication	Antibiotics
Helicobacter pylori eradication	Two antibiotics (amoxicillin, clarithromycin or metronidazole most commonly used) together with a proton pump inhibitor
Severe *Campylobacter* or *Salmonella* enteritis	Ciprofloxacin Clarithromycin
Clostridium difficile infection	Metronidazole Vancomycin (oral)
Biliary tract sepsis	Gentamicin + metronidazole Cephalosporin, (e.g. cefuroxime) + metronidazole Co-amoxiclav
Diverticulitis, peritonitis	Gentamicin, metronidazole + doxycycline Piperacillin–tazobactam + gentamicin (if systemic sepsis) Cephalosporin + metronidazole Co-amoxiclav
Perianal abscesses	Cephalosporin + metronidazole Co-amoxiclav
Perianal Crohn's disease	Metronidazole Ciprofloxacin
Spontaneous bacterial peritonitis	Cefotaxime Ciproflxacin
Small intestinal bacterial overgrowth	Doxycycline Ciprofloxacin Rifaxamin
Hepatic encephalopathy	Rifaxamin

*Choice of antibiotics and combinations depend on local microbiology guidelines (see text).

Table 2.34 Antibiotics and antibiotic combinations used in gastroenterology; '+' indicates combination

treatments and the most suitable antibiotic for confirmed organisms. They also rationalise the use of those broad-spectrum antibiotics that are particularly likely to cause *C. difficile* infection, for example co-amoxiclav, ciprofloxacin and the cephalosporins. These have been replaced by antibiotics such as co-trimoxazole throughout the UK.

The local microbiology department provides advice on whether treatment should be altered based on the patient's clinical response and antibiotic sensitivity results when bacteria have been isolated and identified.

Probiotics

These are living microorganisms used as therapy. The most commonly used are bacteria such as *Lactobacillus* and *Bifidobacterium*, and yeasts such as *Saccharomyces*.

Mode of action

The aim is to improve GI function by restoring the composition of the gut microflora. Probiotics are considered by many to be a 'natural' treatment and therefore often more acceptable to patients.

Indications

There is evidence that specific formulations have a minor benefit for some patients who have diarrhoea caused by antibiotic treatment, pouchitis (inflammation of a surgically formed artificial rectum made from the small intestine), irritable bowel syndrome or inflammatory bowel disease.

Adverse effects

Probiotics appear to be safe in healthy individuals. Only minor symptoms, such as abdominal bloating and flatus occur.

There are many different formulations of probiotics, for example capsules and yoghurts. Few have been evaluated: the optimal formulations, duration of treatment and mode of action are still unknown.

Diet and nutritional interventions

The number of calories required to maintain a patient's weight varies with factors such as their age, level of physical activity and medical conditions. The average diet in developed countries contains many processed foods with excessive amounts of calories, saturated fats and salt, but less fibre than recommended.

Food commonly provokes abdominal symptoms such as bloating and diarrhoea. The diet is modified to treat GI disorders as outlined below.

Weight loss or weight gain

Gastrointestinal conditions sometimes lead to unintentional weight loss because of reduced appetite, malabsorption or avoidance of food due to symptoms when eating. Rates of obesity have increased greatly over recent years and nearly two-thirds of UK adults are now overweight. Obesity increases the potential to develop certain conditions (**Table 2.35**).

The patient's current food and fluid intake is assessed and a diet suggested that details certain foods and portion sizes to lose or gain weight. Some patients who need to put on weight require high-calorie supplements in the form of fruit juices, milkshakes and powders. Where possible, oral feeding is always preferred to enteral tube feeding. Feeding routes are outlined in **Table 2.36**.

Ethical issues of nutritional support

Food and fluid should not be withheld from a patient who expresses a desire to eat and drink, unless there are contraindications, for example a risk of aspiration. In this situation the patient is initially reviewed by the speech and language team, to guide the safest consistency of fluids (powder is added to thicken if needed) and foods the patient can consume. The need for tube feeding is also considered. However, there are some scenarios in which the provision of artificial or

Complications of obesity	
System	Complication
Cardiovascular	Coronary heart disease
	Stroke
	Diabetes
Gastrointestinal	Non-alcoholic steato-hepatitis (NASH) (see page 270)
	NASH cirrhosis
Respiratory	Sleep apnoea
	Respiratory failure
Psychological	Depression
	Low self-esteem
Other	Gallstones
	Colorectal cancer
	Breast and uterine cancers
	Skin infections
	Osteoarthritis

Table 2.35 Complications of obesity

Types of nutritional support		
Route	Description	Indications
Oral:		
supplements	Supplementation of oral diet	Diet inadequate to meet nutritional needs, e.g. in elderly patients, malignancy
Enteral:		
Nasogastric	Feeding tube via nose into stomach	If oral supplementation unsafe, e.g. neurological illness with unsafe swallow
Nasojejunal	Feeding tube via nose into jejunum	Delayed gastric emptying
Gastrostomy*	Feeding tube through skin, directly into stomach	When >4 weeks of feeding required
Parenteral	Nutrition provided directly into vein (bypassing the gut) usually via tunnelled central feeding line	Intestinal failure

*Inserted endoscopically under radiographic guidance or surgically.

Table 2.36 Types of nutritional support

tube feeding is not appropriate, for example individuals with significant dementia, where prognosis and quality of life is not improved.

Refeeding syndrome

This is characterised by a metabolic disturbance caused by reinstating nutrition after a period of starvation or severe malnutrition. The reintroduction of nutrition causes a rapid conversion from a catabolic state (in which molecules in the body are broken down) to the opposite, an anabolic state. This is because the increased carbohydrate intake causes insulin release, which drives electrolytes such as potassium, glucose, magnesium and phosphate into cells, and reduces their levels in the blood. The resulting electrolyte imbalance occasionally has serious consequences including abnormal heart rhythms. Careful monitoring and replacement of electrolytes is important to prevent this. Nutrition is reintroduced slowly in those individuals deemed by a dietician to be at risk.

The level of thiamine (vitamin B_1) also falls with refeeding, leading to neurological complications such as Wernicke-Korsakoff syndrome (impaired vision, memory and unsteady gait). Therefore it should be administered intravenously to patients being refed.

Intestinal failure

This arises from a lack of working gut due to extensive intestinal resection or because of malabsorption associated with diseases such as small bowel Crohn's disease. It is characterised by the inability to maintain protein–energy, fluid or micronutrient balance resulting in weight loss, undernutrition and dehydration. Patients usually require parenteral nutritional support.

Specific diets

A number of specific diets are used in gastroenterology (**Table 2.37**). Many patients believe their abdominal symptoms are

Diets for GI disorders		
Diet	**Details**	**Indications**
Low fat	Decreased saturated fat Unsaturated fats not restricted, e.g. oily fish, sunflower seeds and olive oil (all good for health)	Obesity (weight loss beneficial in gastro-oesophageal reflux disease, etc.) High serum cholesterol Exocrine pancreatic insufficiency and bile salt malabsorption (lessens diarrhoeal symptoms)
High fibre	Insoluble fibre, e.g. brown bread or bran Soluble fibre, e.g. oats, root vegetables such as carrots (NB Too much fibre causes bloating and excess flatus)	Constipation Diverticular disease
Low residue*	Reduced fibre and foods which increase bowel activity, e.g. milk and prunes	Obstructive symptoms from strictures in the small intestine, e.g. in Crohn's disease
No added salt	Whole fresh foods with salt added sparingly in cooking but not at table: salt is reduced but food is still palatable Herbs and spices can be substituted to make food 'tasty'	Fluid overload in liver failure Hypertension
Gluten free	Omission of foods containing gluten, a protein in wheat, barley and rye	Coeliac disease IBS: some patients benefit, possibly because this diet avoids fructan (which is present in wheat and is a part of the FODMAP exclusion diet – see Table 2.38)

*A diet that reduces the frequency and volume of stool

Table 2.37 Diets for specific GI disorders

related to certain foods, which may or may not be true. However, when it is the case, almost anything in the diet is a potential cause.

There is no effective test to determine what food is causing problems. The only way of identifying it is by judging the symptomatic response from eliminating food groups. The most commonly implicated are dairy products (which contain lactose), spicy meals, alcohol, fats, caffeine, bread and other foods containing gluten.

The FODMAP (fermentable oligosaccharides, disaccharides, monosaccharides and polyols) diet is a recent advance in the treatment of functional abdominal conditions. FODMAPS are short-chain carbohydrates that are poorly absorbed in the small intestine and pass to the large intestine where they are fermented by bacteria to produce gas, sometimes resulting in symptoms of bloating and excess flatus.

The first stage in the FODMAP approach is to restrict all foods containing significant amounts of the FODMAP short-chain carbohydrates for up to 2 months (**Table 2.38**). After this period, the short-chain sugar groups are reintroduced one by one to see if the patient tolerates them. Up to 75% of patients with symptoms of irritable bowel syndrome, such as bloating, report a significant improvement in their symptoms with restriction of the trigger FODMAPs they identify. Dietetic input is advised to supervise the diet and ensure that adequate nutrition is maintained throughout.

FODMAP categorisation of common foods					
High or low FODMAP Category	Fructans (polysaccharide)	Galactans (oligosaccharide)	Lactose (disaccharide)	Fructose (monosaccharide)	Polyols (sugar alcohols)
High FODMAP	**Cereals:** wheat, rye **Vegetables:** garlic, onions, leek, asparagus, beetroot, Brussel sprouts, broccoli, cabbage	**Legumes:** lentils, baked beans, kidney beans, chickpeas	**Milk products:** Milk from cows, sheep and goats Yoghurt, custard, ice-cream Soft unripened cheeses	**Fruits:** apple, mango, watermelon **Sweeteners:** Containing fructose Honey	**Sweeteners:** ending in -ol: mannitol, sorbitol, xylitol, Isomalt **Stone fruits:** avocados, apricots, cherries, peaches, plums **Vegetables:** green peppers, cauliflower, mushrooms, sweetcorn
Low FODMAP	Carrots red peppers, potatoes, parsnips, swedes, green beans, celery, olives, lettuce, spinach, tomatoes, turnips **Herbs:** basil, chili, parsley, mint, thyme **Spices:** ginger	**Fruit:** bananas, strawberries, blueberries, grapes, grapefruit, lemons, oranges, raspberries, rhubarb, cranberries, honeydew or cantaloupe melon, kiwi fruit	**Milk and related products:** Lactose-free milk or yoghurt Soya or rice milk Olive oil spreads Sorbets Hard cheeses Butter	**Grain:** gluten-free products, rice, oats, polenta	**Various:** Glucose Sucrose Sweeteners not ending in -ol Golden syrup Maple syrup Treacle

FODMAP, fermentable oligosaccharides, disaccharides, monosaccharides and polyols.

Table 2.38 Examples of foods that have to be avoided in FODMAP diets and alternatives: on a FODMAP diet, high-FODMAP foods are avoided, but low-FODMAP foods are unrestricted

> **A food diary is helpful to determine which food groups are causing symptoms.** A record of every meal and snack together with abdominal symptoms at any time point is kept for several weeks.

Nasogastric tube

A nasogastric tube is a tube placed through the nose and down into the stomach. It provides a means of giving nutrition and medication to a patient who is unable to swallow safely or cannot meet their calorie requirements by mouth.

Technique

The tube is inserted through the nostril (**Figure 2.33**). Flexion of the head helps to open up the pharyngeal space and improves the chance of the tube passing into the oesophagus rather than the lungs. At least 50 cm of tube should be inserted. If the patient starts to cough or has evidence of respiratory compromise it suggests that the tube has been inserted into the lungs and should be withdrawn.

The tube is secured to the nose with tape. A device called a bridle is sometimes inserted if the tube is at risk of becoming inadvertently dislodged or removed, for example in patients with confusion. A ribbon is passed around the nasal septum, with each end fastened to the tube using a plastic clip.

> **To check a nasogastric tube is in the correct position in the stomach, aspirate some fluid and use pH strips to confirm it is acidic.** If this cannot be done, a radiograph of the chest and upper abdomen will identify whether the tube has entered the stomach.

Indications

Nasogastric tubes are used for patients who are unable to swallow and therefore at risk of aspiration, for example after a stroke, and in neurodegenerative conditions such as Parkinson's disease. They are also helpful for very drowsy patients, for example those with hepatic encephalopathy. Food supplements are sometimes administered to individuals who cannot eat enough to maintain or increase their weight when they are feeling unwell such as patients with Crohn's disease. Liquid and soluble or crushed medications are also given through the tube. Wider bore

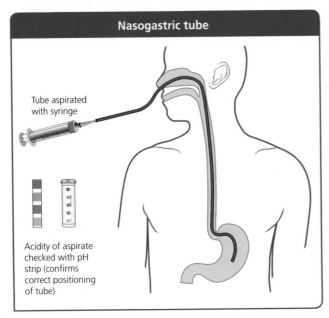

Nasogastric tube

Tube aspirated with syringe

Acidity of aspirate checked with pH strip (confirms correct positioning of tube)

Figure 2.33 A nasogastric tube positioned within the stomach. A syringe is attached to the end of the tube to aspirate secretions from the stomach. The pH of this fluid is tested to confirm correct placement of the tube (acidic on testing).

(Ryles) tubes are used to aspirate stomach contents to prevent vomiting and rest the gut, for example in intestinal obstruction.

Contraindications

The tube is sometimes difficult to insert. In addition, it may have to be removed quickly from patients with severe agitation or confusion.

Complications

Complications relate to the tube or the feed:

- Accidental insertion of the tube into the lungs is the most significant problem: subsequent introduction of feeding solution causes a chemical pneumonitis or pneumonia
- Increased gastro-oesophageal reflux, particularly if the patient is being fed while lying flat
- Tube blockage, which can be caused by medications that do not dissolve or crush easily for insertion through the tube. A carbonated drink is used to help unblock the tube

Percutaneous endoscopic gastrostomy

Percutaneous endoscopic gastrostomy (PEG) and nasogastric tubes are both used for patients who have a functioning GI tract. However, PEG is preferred for those needing long-term nutritional support, as it less visible and not as likely to become dislodged. With good care, percutaneous endoscopic gastrostomy tubes last for several years before they need to be replaced.

Technique

Upper GI endoscopy is used to provide direct vision during the procedure.

After infiltration of the skin of the abdominal wall in the epigastrium with local anaesthetic, a small incision is made using a scalpel. A trocar is passed through this incision and the anterior gastric wall into the stomach lumen. A nylon guidewire inserted through the trocar is grasped within the stomach by biopsy forceps that have been inserted through the

endoscope. The wire is then pulled up through the oesophagus and out through the mouth.

Next the gastrostomy feeding tube is attached to the upper end of the guidewire. As the lower end of the guidewire is pulled out through the skin insertion, the feeding tube is pulled through the mouth, down into the stomach and out through the abdominal wall. The tube is secured by a plastic 'button' or a balloon in the stomach (**Figure 2.34**). Antibiotic prophylaxis is routine because there is risk of infection at the skin entry site.

Indications

Indications for PEG tube insertion are:

- Long-term problems with swallowing, e.g. after a stroke or in neurological conditions such as Parkinson's disease and motor neurone disease
- Patients who are unable to meet their nutritional requirements through oral feeding, e.g. in head and neck cancer or cystic fibrosis

Contraindications

The principal contraindications to PEG insertion are:

- Large volume ascites
- Pregnancy
- Patients who have had extensive gastric surgery as insertion is often difficult
- Severe respiratory disease

Complications

The potential complications of PEG insertion are:

- Perforation of the small or large intestine
- Bleeding (into the skin or intra-abdominally)
- Infection at the skin site
- Blockage or splitting of the tube

> **In patients with cognitive impairment such as dementia, poor oral intake reflects an advanced condition with a very poor prognosis.** Feeding via a percutaneous endoscopic gastrostomy tube does not improve survival.

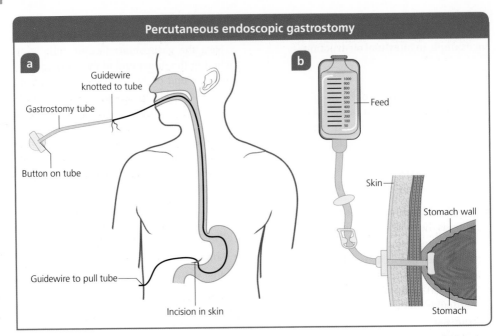

Figure 2.34 Insertion of a percutaneous endoscopic gastrostomy (PEG) tube. See text for methodological details. Part b shows the final position of the tube.

Parenteral nutrition

Parenteral nutrition bypasses the GI tract to provide nutrition intravenously. It is sometimes necessary for patients who cannot use the GI tract to ingest an adequate number of calories due to intestinal obstruction or following surgery. It is usually a temporary measure, but is occasionally required longer term for patients with short bowel syndrome occurring after extensive small bowel resection or enteritis due to Crohn's disease or radiotherapy.

Technique

Short-term nutritional support is sometimes provided via a long line inserted peripherally into an arm vein. Even with stringent aseptic nursing, however, these lines invariably cause phlebitis (inflammation of the vein) and infection at the insertion site.

For patients who require a longer period of intravenous nutrition, a central line is preferred. This is inserted into the jugular or subclavian vein using a strict aseptic technique, to minimise the risk of infection. The aseptic technique needs to be maintained whenever the line is used to attach the feed or take blood samples.

Indications

Short-term intravenous nutritional support is often required for prolonged ileus after surgery. Longer term or permanent treatment is necessary where large areas of the small intestine are not functioning or have been surgically removed. Examples of this are Crohn's disease, ischaemia or after abdominal radiotherapy.

Contraindications

Contraindications to the use of parenteral nutrition are:

- Functioning GI tract
- Treatment that is required for only a few days
- Limited prognosis of underlying disease (a relative contraindication) – the disease outcome or quality of life is not necessarily improved by parenteral nutrition

Complications

Complications relating to the feeding line and the consequences of parenteral nutrition are:

- Pneumothorax (a collection of air in the pleural cavity) as a complication of insertion
- Line sepsis
- Venous thrombosis
- Electrolyte disturbances
- Hepatic cholestasis
- Cholecystitis (inflammation of the gallbladder)
- Metabolic bone disease, e.g. osteopenia

> **Intravenous fluid, e.g. 0.9% ('normal') saline or dextrose, provides hydration but no significant nutrition.** If the patient cannot receive oral or nasogastric tube feeding for more than a few days due to intestinal obstruction or following surgery, parenteral (intravenous) nutrition is considered.

Alcohol reduction

Reduction of alcohol intake or abstinence is recommended in individuals with GI symptoms such as reflux or a history of excess intake, especially in those with concurrent liver disease to prevent disease progression. The minimum aim is to reduce alcohol intake to within the recommended level, with several alcohol-free days per week.

The key to success is the patient wanting to stop, and realising that the benefits that are gained. Alcohol support services are accessible through self-referral or referral from the GP or hospital. These provide individual or group counselling. If the patient is motivated, however, help from others is often not needed.

When patients stop drinking after a long and significant alcohol history, they often experience withdrawal symptoms such as tremor, sweats and vomiting. Benzodiazepines such as diazepam or chlordiazepoxide are given to reduce these symptoms. However, benzodiazepines are themselves addictive, so they are only given under close medical super-

vision and on a short-term basis, usually for no more than a couple of days.

Intravenous and oral vitamin B_1 (thiamine) is prescribed to reduce neurological complications of alcohol abuse, such as Wernicke's encephalopathy (see Chapter 7).

Acamprosate helps to reduce cravings when the patient is abstinent. It should be used alongside counselling as outlined above. The exact mode of action of acamprosate is uncertain. However, it is known to alter the disordered chemical balance in the brain that occurs in alcoholism; for example, it activates γ-aminobutyric acid receptors. Acamprosate sometimes cause headaches, insomnia and rarely allergic responses and arrhythmias.

Naltrexone, an opioid antagonist, reduces cravings and is given orally. Disulfiram (Antabuse) is given to encourage a patient to avoid alcohol, which causes symptoms of severe nausea when it is taken with this medication.

Psychological interventions

Cognitive–behavioural therapy

This is a type of psychotherapy that is frequently used to treat anxiety and depression and is performed with a trained individual. Over several sessions, the 'cognitive' part of the therapy is used to address unhelpful thinking and the behavioural therapy to change coping strategies.

Gut-centred hypnotherapy

Deep relaxation is induced by hypnosis before soothing images and sensations are suggested that focus on the specific abdominal symptoms experienced by the patient. They learn how to influence and control their gut function, which ultimately changes the way the brain modulates gut activity.

Relaxation techniques

These make patients feel more in control of their symptoms. Exercises involve deep and slow breathing using the diaphragm or tensing and then relaxing muscle groups progressively from the forehead to the feet.

Another technique is positive imagery, in which a relaxing place is visualised with the eyes closed.

> **Psychological interventions are effective for all functional GI disorders but** should be undertaken by experienced individuals.

Endoscopic treatments

As well as containing a viewing mechanism, an endoscope has a therapeutic channel that allows a range of accessories to be passed into the lumen of the GI tract such as biopsy forceps and injection needles (**Table 2.39**).

Dilation and stenting

These treatments open up lumens of the GI tract that are blocked due to disease. An example is a stricture, a narrowing of the lumen of the intestine. There are both malignant and benign causes of strictures in the intestinal tract or biliary tree. The symptoms vary depending on the location of the stricture, for example dysphagia if it is in the oesophagus and jaundice if it is in the biliary tree.

Dilation

Indications
Dilation is used for symptomatic strictures, most commonly performed in the oesophagus.

Technique
The stricture is widened by initially passing a wire and then a fine-bore catheter through it. This is usually performed under a combination of direct vision at endoscopy and X-ray guidance. The balloon on the catheter is inflated to stretch the narrowed area (**Figure 2.35**). This procedure is usually performed with analgesia and sedation, as it is often painful.

Complications
Complications occurring with dilation:

- Pain and bleeding often occur at the site of dilation, but these are usually transient

Therapeutic role of endoscopy	
Procedure	Application
OGD: oesophagus	Treatment of bleeding oesophageal lesions
	Banding of oesophageal varices
	Resection of dysplastic lesions and early oesophageal cancer
	Dilation of benign and malignant strictures
	Insertion of oesophageal stent
	Removal of food boluses
OGD: stomach	Resection of gastric polyps and early gastric cancers
	Injection of gastric varices
	Treatment of bleeding gastric ulcers
	Insertion of percutaneous endoscopic gastrostomy feeding tube
OGD: duodenum	Treatment of bleeding duodenal ulcer
	Resection of duodenal polyps and early duodenal cancers
Sigmoidoscopy and colonoscopy	Resection of colorectal polyps and early colorectal cancers
	Thermal ablation of vascular lesions, e.g. angioectasia
	Insertion of a colonic stent
	Banding of haemorrhoids
	Tattoo marking (to mark polyps and cancer)
ERCP	Sphincterotomy
	Dilation of strictures
	Removal of stones
	Insertion of stent into biliary or pancreatic duct to treat benign and malignant disease

ERCP, endoscopic retrograde cholangiopancreatography; OGD, oesophagogastroduodenoscopy.

Table 2.39 Examples of the therapeutic roles of endoscopic procedures

- The most significant complication is perforation. The risk of dilating benign oesophageal strictures is approximately 1 in 200, rising to as high as 1 in 20 for the dilatation of malignant strictures, due to more fragile tissue. If this occurs, the patient will require admission to hospital and sometimes requires surgery

Stents

Dilation provides only a temporary relief of malignant strictures. To prevent these closing up again and to give longer term palliation, a stent is inserted into the affected part of the oesophagus, pylorus, duodenum or large intestine. This is then left in situ. Stents are usually a metal mesh that expands when released (**Figure 2.35**).

Bile duct stents are used:

- For benign as well as malignant strictures of the duct
- To bypass stones that are not removable from the common bile duct

In both situations, stenting aids drainage and reduces the risk of biliary sepsis.

Complications

Complications of stent insertion are:

- Blockage by food in the oesophagus or solid stool in the large intestine
- Tumour overgrowth through or at either end of the stent
- Migration away from site of insertion
- Infection, particularly when they are in situ for a long period in the biliary tree

Removal of benign and early malignant lesions

In both the upper and lower GI tract, it is possible to completely remove lesions that are premalignant, for example colorectal adenomas, or show very early malignant change. All lesions must be carefully assessed. If there is any uncertainty whether they can be effectively and safely removed, biopsy and radiological imaging are required to exclude more advanced lesions and metastases.

Technique

With pedunculated polyps (lesions with a stalk), a snare loop is placed around the stalk and then a low-dose current is applied through the loop (**Figure 2.36**). This cuts the tissue and cauterises the blood vessels. Sessile (flat) polyps are usually removed by endoscopic mucosal resection (EMR). Fluid is injected into the submucosa using a needle to raise the polyp up on a fluid cushion before the snare is applied, to avoid trapping deeper layers of the intestinal wall, which leads to perforation.

This technique has recently been further developed with endoscopic submucosal

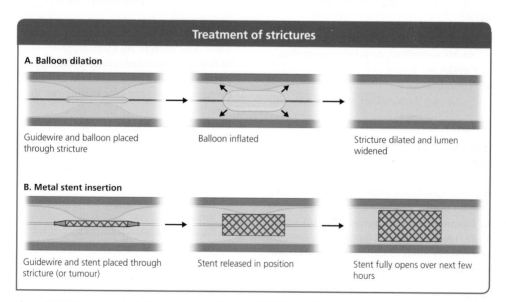

Figure 2.35 Endoscopic techniques to treat strictures – (a) balloon dilation and (b) stent insertion.

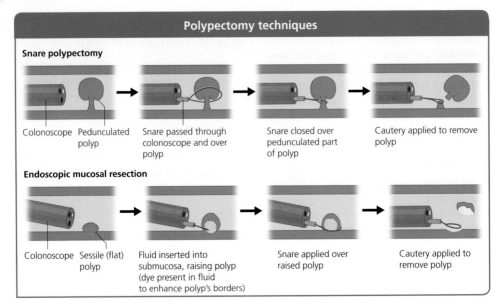

Figure 2.36 Polypectomy techniques.

dissection, allowing early malignancies to be carefully dissected out and removed in their entirety.

Complications

The complication rates vary depending on the size, morphology and location of the lesion:

■ Bleeding – usually at the time of removal but it is sometimes delayed by more than a week
■ Perforation

Haemostasis

Endoscopy allows the site and cause of GI bleeding to be determined. The outcome is stratified according to the presence of adverse features, for example active bleeding from an artery, and provides an opportunity for haemostasis. Haemostasis is also sometimes required when GI haemorrhage occurs as a complication of therapeutic endoscopy, for example polypectomy.

Technique

Haemostasis is achievable through a variety of endoscopic techniques (**Figure 2.37**):

■ **Dilute adrenaline (epinephrine) injection** close to the site of bleeding. This causes a degree of tamponade (pressure on surrounding blood vessels) and vasoconstriction to stop the bleeding. The effect lasts for only a few hours and so is always used with another form of haemostasis
■ **Cauterisation**, i.e. the application of either a low-dose current via a heater probe or argon plasma coagulation. Current is passed through a jet of argon gas delivered through a plastic catheter, to cauterise the bleeding area
■ **Mechanical techniques**, i.e. clips and bands.
  ■ Clips are applied to compress the tissue, including the bleeding vessels. Clips are also applied to close small perforations of the wall of the GI tract if they are recognised at the time of endoscopic therapy.
  ■ Bands are released onto oesophageal varices (dilated veins occurring due to portal hypertension) and haemorrhoids. They cause fibrosis and scarring around the vein to reduce the risk of further bleeding
■ **Sclerosants** such as ethanolamine are sometimes injected into varices. However,

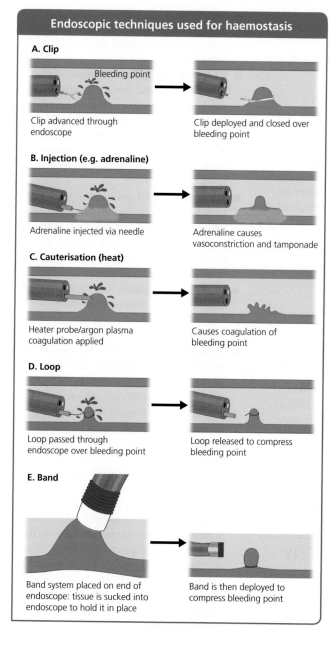

Endoscopic techniques used for haemostasis

A. Clip

Bleeding point

Clip advanced through endoscope

Clip deployed and closed over bleeding point

B. Injection (e.g. adrenaline)

Adrenaline injected via needle

Adrenaline causes vasoconstriction and tamponade

C. Cauterisation (heat)

Heater probe/argon plasma coagulation applied

Causes coagulation of bleeding point

D. Loop

Loop passed through endoscope over bleeding point

Loop released to compress bleeding point

E. Band

Band system placed on end of endoscope: tissue is sucked into endoscope to hold it in place

Band is then deployed to compress bleeding point

Figure 2.37 Haemostatic techniques at endoscopy.

this is less effective than banding and is not commonly used

- **Haemostatic powder** is sprayed onto an area of bleeding to form a barrier and enhance clot formation
- A **Sengstaken–Blakemore tube** (see Figure 10.2); this is inserted if a patient is exsanguinating from actively bleeding oesophageal or gastric varices. The plastic tube is passed through the mouth or nose into the stomach. A balloon attached to the end of the tube is inflated with air within the stomach and then pulled upwards to apply pressure to the gastro-oesophageal junction. This compresses (tamponades) the varices to stop the bleeding, as a short-term measure to stabilise the patient's condition until definitive endoscopy or a TIPS procedure is performed

Other endoscopic procedures

Other commonly performed endoscopic procedures are:

- **Oesophagogastroduodenoscopy** to remove ingested foreign bodies and food bolus
- **Radiofrequency ablation** to treat early oesophageal cancers and dysplasia in Barrett's oesophagus (see Chapter 3, page 170): high-frequency electrical currents are passed through an electrode to destroy the involved tissue
- **ERCP to extract stones** from the common bile duct: a catheter with a balloon attached to its tip is inserted into the bile duct. The balloon is inflated above the stone and the catheter is pulled down within the bile duct to bring the stone down the duct into the duodenum. Usually the ampulla of Vater is cut (a process called sphincterotomy) to increase the size of opening into the common bile duct, allowing subsequent stones to pass from the duct into the duodenum more easily
- **Drainage of pancreatic pseudocysts** through the gastric wall, under radiographic guidance or by using endoscopic ultrasonography
- **Sigmoidoscopy to correct a volvulus or decompress a pseudo-obstruction** (see page 118)

Interventional radiology

There is a wide range of interventional radiological techniques for treating various GI conditions, both electively and in an emergency setting:

- **Angiography** with embolisation (blocking) of an arterial bleeding point is used in patients with upper and lower GI bleeding (e.g. stomach ulcers or as a complication of diverticular disease) that cannot be stopped by endoscopy or where there is significant re-bleeding. It is also invaluable in stopping GI bleeds that cannot be controlled following endoscopic or surgical interventions

- **Fluoroscopy**, i.e. radiographic guidance, to place stents over guidewires into the upper or lower GI tract; this avoids the need for endoscopy
- **Radiologically guided insertion of a gastrostomy tube**: this is considered if a percutaneous endoscopic gastrostomy is not possible. It is also used in patients with medical conditions that preclude endoscopy due to the risks of sedation, such as a severe myopathy (muscle weakness)
- **Ultrasound- or CT-guided drainage** of cysts or abscesses in the liver or abdominal cavity
- **Chemo-embolisation**: small particles are inserted through a plastic catheter into the blood vessels supplying primary liver tumours to slow their growth
- **Radiofrequency ablation**: heat generated from a probe is used as a palliative treatment for primary liver tumours; the heat kills the cancerous cells
- **Transjugular intrahepatic portosystemic shunt (TIPS)**, i.e. placing a stent between the hepatic and portal veins in the liver, via the jugular vein, which causes a fall in portal pressure. It is used as an emergency treatment for variceal bleeding if not controlled endoscopically and electively to treat recurrent ascites that is refractory to diuretic treatment. TIPS allows stabilisation of a patient's condition prior to liver transplantation. The most significant adverse effect that sometimes occurs is encephalopathy, due to the passage of gut-derived toxins from the intestine directly into the systemic circulation. The stent can also thrombose.

Surgery

Abdominal surgery is undertaken for a wide variety of benign and malignant conditions both electively and in an emergency setting. Commonly used terms are outline in **Table 2.40**.

Minimally invasive surgery

Minimally invasive, i.e. laparoscopic, operations are preferred because of quicker recovery times and lower morbidity. If possible, all the disease should be removed but this may

Prefixes and suffixes in abdominal surgery	
Prefix	**Relating to**
Append-	Appendix
Caec-	Caecum
Cholecyst-	Gallbladder
Colono- (or col-)	Large intestine (often includes segment, e.g. 'sigmoid col-')
Duoden-	Duodenum
Gastr-	Stomach
Hepat-	Liver
Ile-	Ileum
Jejun-	Jejunum
Lapar-	Abdominal cavity
Pancreat-	Pancreas
Proct-	Rectum
Suffix	**Meaning**
-ectomy	Surgical removal
-oscopy	Looking at with a scope
-ostomy (or -stomy)	Creating a new hole (or stoma)
-otomy (or -tomy)	Surgical incision
-pexy	Securing or fixing
-plasty	Reshaping
-plication	Tightening by folding in and suturing
-rrhaphy	Strengthening (often with a suture)

Table 2.40 Common prefixes and suffixes in abdominal surgery

not be possible if there is a risk of significant consequences. For example, the removal of extensive areas of small bowel Crohn's disease usually leads to malabsorption (short bowel syndrome). A good knowledge of anatomy is essential, particularly in terms of the blood supply, to ensure that the remaining tissues are viable.

Liver surgery

Liver transplantation is undertaken at specialist centres. It is very successful in patients with end-stage liver disease and no other significant co-morbidity. Either a matched living or cadaveric donor is identified. After surgical removal of the diseased liver, either

a segment or all of the donor liver is transplanted into the recipient. Life-long immunosuppressant medications (e.g. steroids, azathioprine, ciclosporin) are required to minimise the risk of liver rejection. Five-year survival rates are over 90%.

Gastric surgery

Types of gastric surgery are shown in **Figure 2.38**. Bariatric surgery, to aid weight loss, is becoming increasingly common in developed countries. Techniques involve reducing the size of the stomach to limit the available space for food intake so that the patient feels full more quickly, and/or bypassing parts of the small intestine to reduce absorption.

Complications

Each operation has specific complications. However, abdominal surgery can in general be complicated by:

- Bleeding
- Perforation
- Infection
- Postoperative ileus
- Adhesions (scar tissue, within the abdominal cavity, which sometimes compresses the intestine and other organs, causing pain and obstruction)

Other interventions

Paracentesis

This is the therapeutic procedure used to drain ascites from the abdomen.

Technique

Local anaesthetic is injected into the abdominal wall. The drain is then inserted into the peritoneal cavity using an aseptic technique. It is placed in the low lateral part of the left or right side of the abdomen where the percussion note is dull (**Figure 2.39**).

Indications

Paracentesis is used when symptoms such as abdominal discomfort or shortness of breath are occurring as a result of large-volume ascites. It is used in patients with cirrhosis and intra-abdominal or pelvic malignancy.

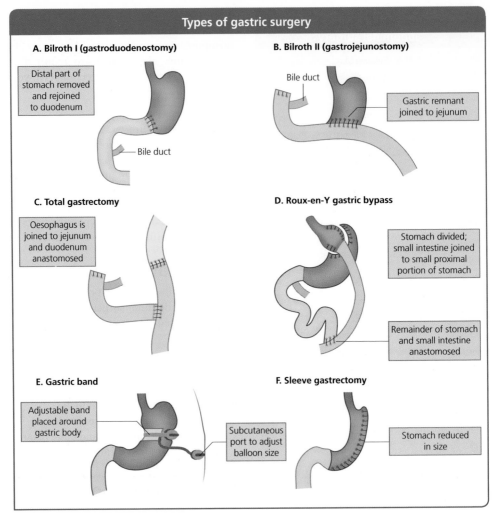

Figure 2.38 Types of gastric surgery. Bilroth I, Bilroth II and total gastrectomy are all used to treat ulcers and cancers. Roux-en-Y gastric bypass, gastric band and sleeve gastrectomy are types of bariatric surgery.

Contraindications

The contraindications of paracentesis are:

- Significant problems with coagulation
- Pregnancy

Complications

Complications result from the procedure of drain insertion or drainage of the ascitic fluid:

- Perforation of the intestine
- Bleeding either as a skin wall haematoma or intra-abdominal bleeding (haematoperitoneum)
- Sepsis at the puncture site or of the ascitic fluid (secondary bacterial peritonitis)

- Renal dysfunction due to rapid fluid loss; this is reduced by administering human albumin solution intravenously at the same time as the fluid is drained
- Leakage of fluid from the puncture site

The drain is removed after 6 hours to reduce the risk of infection, or earlier if all of the ascitic fluid has drained.

> When paracentesis rather than a diuretic is used to treat tense ascites, hospital stays are shorter and a lower incidence of renal dysfunction and encephalopathy are seen.

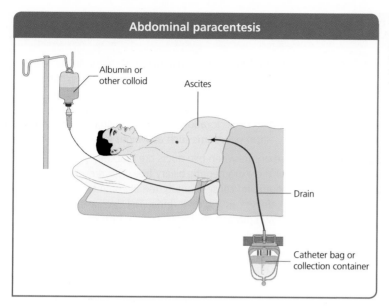

Abdominal paracentesis

Albumin or other colloid

Ascites

Drain

Catheter bag or collection container

Figure 2.39 Abdominal paracentesis. Albumin is delivered through a cannula inserted into the patient's vein.

Trans-anal rectal irrigation

This is instillation of fluid into the rectum. It helps patients with slow-transit constipation or faecal incontinence. It is also used with disorders of defaecation caused by significant neurological disease, for example spinal cord injury or multiple sclerosis.

Technique

A catheter is inserted into the rectum and held in place with a balloon. Warm water is slowly introduced through the catheter into the distal large intestine using a pump, to dislodge the stool. When the balloon is deflated, faecal matter from the intestine is evacuated with the water.

Biofeedback

This is used to retrain the pelvic floor muscles and anal sphincters in order to strengthen or relax them. It is used in both constipation and incontinence that does not respond to standard treatment.

A greater awareness of the process of defaecation is gained by using electrical sensors on the abdominal wall and in the anal canal to provide information on muscle activity during contraction and relaxation. This is displayed on a computer monitor for the patient to see. Several sessions in hospital, supported by practice at home, allows the patient to gain greater control of the bowel function.

Answers to starter questions

1. Abdominal pain is a very common symptom. In most instances it is minor, self limiting and not due to a serious cause. A detailed history using the 'SOCRATES' mnemonic (see page 86) helps to determine the likely cause, which will guide the subsequent investigations and treatment. Severe pain indicates emergency presentations such as acute pancreatitis, intestinal obstruction or perforation. When the pain is due to a GI cancer it is usually accompanied by alarm symptoms such as weight loss.

2. Obstructive (or cholestatic) jaundice occurs when bile ducts are blocked; either the smaller calibre intrahepatic ducts or the extra hepatic biliary tree. This reduces the flow of bile from the liver to the duodenum and causes conjugated bilirubin to enter the blood. Bilirubin is excreted by the kidneys causing dark urine. The decrease/absence of conjugated bilirubin and its breakdown products in the GI tract, which give the stool its characteristic brown colour, causes paler stools.

3. Ascites is free fluid in the abdominal cavity and presents as abdominal distension. Causes include chronic liver disease, malignancy and heart failure. In a supine patient, the fluid gravitates to both flanks and the pelvis. On percussion, this causes a resonant sound in the centre of the abdomen, due to a gas-filled bowel, and dullness in both flanks, due to the fluid. With the patient on their side, the dullness 'shifts' towards the central abdomen as the fluid moves. A large amount of ascites may also present with a fluid thrill, where flicking or tapping one side of the abdomen results in a wave of fluid felt at the opposite flank.

4. The aorta is often felt and may be seen as a pulsatile structure in the midline. The lower border of the liver may just be palpable in deep inspiration (when the diaphragm descends fully). If the bowel has not been opened recently, it is often possible to feel stool in the colon, particularly the sigmoid. A palpable spleen or gallbladder always represents an abnormality. The normal pancreas and kidneys are deep, retroperitoneal structures and are not palpable.

5. Before starting an examination, firstly, introduce yourself by name and role and confirm the patient's name. Next, gain verbal consent to proceed. The patient should be lying flat to relax their abdominal musculature and clothing exposed to the groin, which should be covered with a towel or blanket. The room should be warm, well-lit and private. Patients should always be offered the option of a chaperone being present during the examination. Before starting, wash your hands with alcohol gel or soap and water. Approach the patient from their right hand side.

6. Blood tests indicate how well the GI system is functioning to process food and then absorb nutrients into the circulation and remove waste from it. Thus they help determine the cause of abdominal symptoms and aid decisions on further investigation and treatment.

   In symptomatic GI disease, some tests pinpoint exact causes while others suggest a likely cause that requires investigation. For example, in epigastric pain a high level of amylase diagnoses acute pancreatitis whereas raised anti-tTG antibodies strongly suggests coeliac disease, which can then be confirmed by duodenal biopsy. In contrast, in the absence of symptoms, abnormal test results may reveal significant GI disease. For example, abnormal liver function tests suggest liver disease, and low iron in a man or a post-menopausal women suggests chronic GI blood loss.

   In some tests the blood level of the substance demonstrates the degree of malfunction. For example, synthetic problems in the liver prolong the prothrombin

Answers *continued*

time and reduce the albumin level; the more abnormal the results, the more severe the disease. In other tests, it is the pattern that matters. For example, in testing liver enzymes, alkaline phosphatase and gamma glutamyl transferase are raised in 'cholestatic' disorders affecting the biliary tree but raised alanine or aspartate transaminase function indicates a disorder affecting the hepatocytes.

7. Comorbidities often determine whether further investigation is appropriate and which test is most suitable. For example, the bowel preparation that is necessary before colonoscopy and CT pneumocolon has a strong laxative effect which means patients have to be mobile enough to get to the toilet. It also causes dehydration and electrolye disorders, which is sometimes a problem with severe cardiac or renal failure. Patients also need to be able to roll into different positions during colonoscopy and CT pneumocolon. Some conditions, e.g. severe cardiorespiratory disease, are associated with increased procedural risk and may contraindicate general anaesthetic or even intravenous sedation before colonoscopy, ERCP or oesophagogastroduodenoscopy. A newly presenting comorbidity may warrant further investigation itself.

8. The clinical history helps to establish a list of differential diagnoses, from which a decision is made as to whether further investigation is required. Less invasive investigations (e.g. blood and stool tests) are usually undertaken initially unless there are alarm features requiring more invasive tests, such as endoscopy. Some conditions may be diagnosed by the history and examination alone, e.g. gastro-oesophageal reflux, and require no further investigation before starting treatment.

9. The small intestine is the longest and least accessible section of the GI tract. Radiological investigations (e.g. magnetic resonance enterogram) can provide information about structural abnormalities, such as strictures and inflammatory change. Wireless capsule endoscopy (WCE) is a diagnostic test providing information about the mucosal surface, e.g. angioectasia and ulcers. Enteroscopy is a specialised endoscopic test used to take a biopsy and treat abnormalities detected on radiological or WCE investigation.

10. There are many factors to consider when deciding the best treatment for a patient, not least their own preference. Treatment options include simple reassurance, drugs, surgery, endoscopic therapy, dietary interventions, lifestyle changes and psychological treatments. For medical and surgical options, it helps to fully define the underlying cause and anatomical site of the condition. Comorbidity and concurrent treatments must be considered. In many cases, multidisciplinary discussions are critical to determine a management plan. The risks and benefits of any treatment must be clearly explained to the patient so they may make an informed decision on how to proceed.

11. Local and national prescribing guidelines will state which medications are favoured; this is particularly important with antibiotics, due to changes in their efficacy and, differing local patterns of resistance and the need to reduce the incidence of *Clostridium difficile* diarrhoea. The severity of the condition, e.g. inflammatory bowel disease, influences the most appropriate option and dosage. Patient choice also influences the form of medication, i.e. tablets, capsules, syrups, suspensions or enemas, when alternatives are available.

12. It is important to monitor a patient's nutritional status to maintain their health and prevent future complications. Assess the body mass index, food and fluid intake and

Answers *continued*

look for recent weight loss. A dietician can provide specific, tailored advice. Most patients only need a change in their meals, but some will require supplemental drinks or mousses. If a healthy state can't be reached through eating, a nasogastric (NG) tube can provide a temporary route for additional calories. Rarely (e.g. after a stroke), long term feeding is necessary via a percutaneous endoscopic gastrostomy. Enteral feeding, i.e. via the GI tract, is always preferred, but those who have little or no GI tract function may need parental, i.e. IV nutrition.

Chapter 3
Oesophageal disorders

Starter questions

Reading this chapter will enable you to answer the following questions. Answers are on page 180.

1. How does a hiatus hernia develop?
2. Is heartburn dangerous?
3. Why is the incidence of oesophageal cancer increasing?

Introduction

The characteristic symptoms of oesophageal conditions are difficulty in swallowing (dysphagia) and pain in the centre of the chest. Dysphagia is caused by a variety of benign and malignant diseases that affect the pharynx and oesophagus. Oesophageal pain is sometimes hard to distinguish from angina, so a clear history and appropriate investigations are important to ensure correct treatment. Gastro-oesophageal reflux disease (GORD) has a high worldwide prevalence and often causes significant symptoms that affect quality of life. It occasionally also leads to Barrett's oesophagus, a premalignant change. The incidence of oesophageal adenocarcinoma is increasing rapidly. Unfortunately, oesophageal cancer often presents with advanced disease where it is incurable.

Case 1 Heartburn

Presentation

Simon Rogers is a 46-year-old IT manager who visits his general practitioner (GP) with a history of retrosternal chest discomfort that has been present for several years. It has recently been getting worse, making him concerned.

Initial interpretation

Gastrointestinal (GI), cardiac and musculoskeletal causes (**Table 3.1**) must all be considered. Further questioning about the nature of the pain and any exacerbating and relieving factors will help narrow down the differential diagnoses, although these are sometimes challenging to distinguish from each other as they are frequently very similar.

History

Simon is experiencing almost daily burning chest discomfort. On one occasion the pain was so severe he thought he was having a heart attack. He called the paramedics, who gave him oral aspirin and a nitrate spray under his tongue. The spray helped the pain. An electrocardiogram showed no acute abnormalities and a troponin blood test was normal; this is elevated in acute coronary syndromes. He was later discharged home and subsequently had an exercise treadmill test which was also normal.

Simon describes the pain as feeling like a fire in his chest and usually he has a bitter taste in his mouth. It is worse whenever he eats spicy food, bends over to pick things up and is lying flat in bed at night. He finds that antacids help and he always keeps them nearby.

Interpretation of history

Oesophageal pain (from gastro-oesophageal reflux and spasm) is occasionally very similar to pain caused by ischaemic heart disease (**Table 3.1**).

Simon's history suggests GORD. However, associated symptoms must be identified, particularly 'alarm' symptoms that indicate a greater risk of serious underlying pathology such as malignancy (**Table 3.2**). These prompt a referral for urgent endos-

Differentiating between causes of central chest pain	
Cause	Clues from history
Oesophageal	'Burning' or occasionally 'heavy' (i.e. 'cardiac' like)
	Often radiates through to the back
	Occurs after meals (especially rich, spicy foods or alcohol) or on lying flat in bed
	Improved by antacids (NB: sublingual nitrates sometimes help)
Cardiac	'Heavy' or 'crushing'
	Often radiates to the neck or down the arm
	Occurs on exertion
	Improved by rest and sublingual nitrates
Musculoskeletal	'Sharp'
	Worse with breathing and movement
	Tender to touch
	Often a history of trauma, coughing or concurrent chest infection

Table 3.1 Differentiating between causes of central chest pain

Upper GI 'alarm' features	
Symptoms	Dysphagia
	Weight loss and new-onset dyspepsia if >55 years old
	Persistent vomiting
	GI bleeding
Signs	Epigastric mass
Investigations	Iron deficiency anaemia

Table 3.2 Upper GI tract 'alarm' features

Case 1 *continued*

copy. It is also important to ask about life-style habits such as diet, alcohol intake and smoking, because these increase the risk of gastro-oesophageal reflux (**Figure 3.1**).

Further history

On further questioning, Simon says that he has a persistent dry cough and his voice becomes hoarse at times. He reports no dysphagia, odynophagia (painful swallowing) or symptoms of GI bleeding.

Over the last 2 years he has put on around 12 kg in weight. Despite this, he tries to remain active and plays squash once a week without experiencing chest pain. He finds his job busy and stressful, often working long hours. He knows this has resulted in bad eating habits – he often relies on numerous cups of coffee a day be-fore having a take-away late in the evening. He smokes 20 cigarettes a day and drinks around 30 units of alcohol a week. There is no family history of cardiac or GI disease.

Examination

Simon is overweight, with a body mass index of 29 kg/m². The rest of the exami-nation is normal. There are no signs of pallor or lymphadenopathy which sug-gest a cancer or reproducible chest wall tenderness which implies the pain is musculoskeletal.

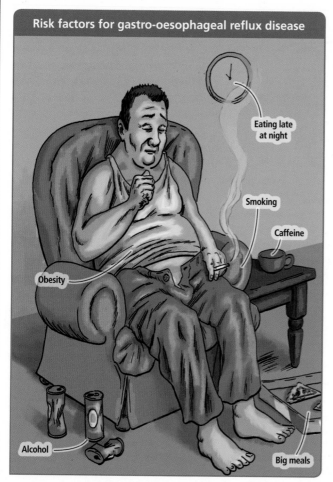

Risk factors for gastro-oesophageal reflux disease

Eating late at night

Smoking

Caffeine

Obesity

Alcohol

Big meals

Figure 3.1 Lifestyle risk factors for gastro-oesophageal reflux disease (GORD). The patient is holding his chest in discomfort, a typical sign in GORD.

Case 1 *continued*

Interpretation of findings

Clinical examination is usually normal in patients with GORD, so these examination findings support a diagnosis of GORD. Together with his lifestyle (diet, smoking and drinking alcohol, etc.), being overweight will exacerbate Simon's symptoms.

Investigations

In view of his fairly young age and lack of alarm symptoms, there is no need for further investigation. Referral for upper

GI endoscopy is considered when there are progressive or persistent symptoms despite appropriate treatment. There is often a poor correlation between the severity of symptoms and the findings at endoscopy, that is, many people with severe reflux have a normal-looking oesophagus.

Diagnosis

Simon's GP makes a diagnosis of GORD and considers that a hiatus hernia is

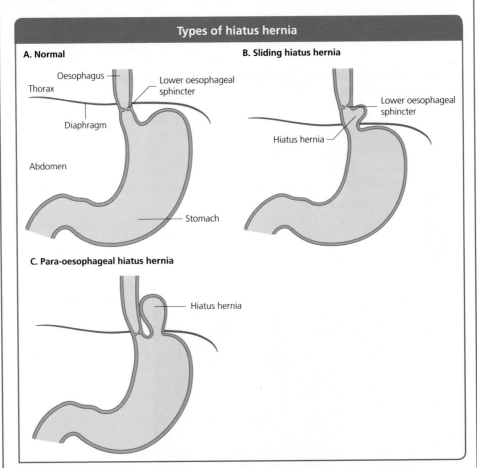

Types of hiatus hernia

Figure 3.2 Types of hiatus hernia. (a) Normal stomach position below the diaphragm. (b) Most hiatus hernias are 'sliding'. Part of the gastric cardia and lower oesophageal sphincter moves above the diaphragm through a widened oesophageal hiatus. (c) The less-common para-oesophageal (rolling) hiatus hernia occurs when part of the stomach protrudes alongside the oesophagus due to a defect in the phreno-oesophageal membrane.

Case 1 *continued*

present as this is commonly present in patients with reflux (**Figure 3.2**). He discusses lifestyle changes to help improve the symptoms, such as losing weight, not eating late at night, reducing caffeine and alcohol intake and stopping smoking. Simon is prescribed a proton pump inhibitor as this medication reduces gastric acid production. On review 8 weeks later he has intentionally lost 3 kg in weight and his symptoms are greatly improved. His GP congratulates him on his weight loss and encourages him to persist with the other lifestyle changes.

Case 2 Difficulty in swallowing

Presentation

Tom Evans is a 68-year-old man who presents to his GP with difficulty swallowing and a weight loss of 4 kg over the previous month.

Initial interpretation

The many causes of dysphagia are classified by site (pharyngeal or oesophageal) and as benign or malignant (**Table 3.3**), but there is occasionally a central neurological cause. Mr Evans' symptoms must be considered further in terms of:

- Duration
- Whether they are progressive or intermittent
- The level at which the symptoms occur, i.e. in the throat, upper or lower chest.
- Whether the problem is with swallowing solids and/or liquids
- An unintentional weight loss of 4 kg in a month is significant and is a cause for concern as it sometimes means a cancer is present.

History

Mr Evans reports a 15-year history of chronic heartburn controlled with over-the-counter medications. He says that swallowing has become increasingly

Causes of oesophageal dysphagia	
Malignant	
Adenocarcinoma	
Squamous cell carcinoma	
Extrinsic compression secondary to lung malignancy or mediastinal lymphadenopathy	
Benign	
Peptic stricture	
Radiation-induced stricture	
Oesophagitis	Reflux related
	Infective, e.g. candidiasis, herpes simplex virus infection, American trypanosomiasis (Chagas' disease)
	Medication-induced, e.g. bisphosphonates
	Caustic ingestion
	Eosinophilic
Oesophageal dysmotility	Nutcracker oesophagus
	Diffuse oesophageal spasm
	Secondary to systemic disorders, e.g. scleroderma
	Achalasia
Schatzki ring or oesophageal web	
Oesophageal diverticulum	
Extrinsic compression secondary to goitre, cardiac atria or enlargement of osteophytes	

Table 3.3 Malignant and benign causes of oesophageal dysphagia

Case 2 *continued*

Diagnosis of oesophageal cancer

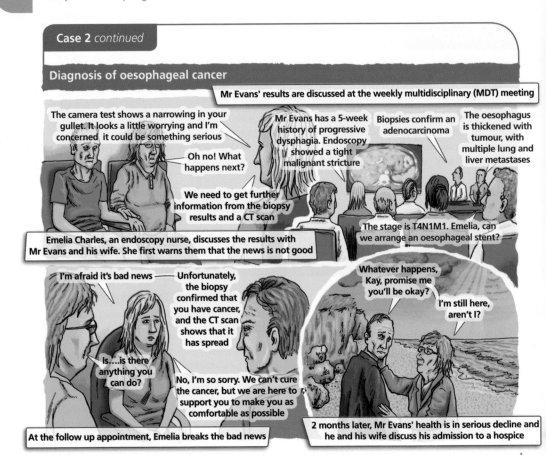

Mr Evans' results are discussed at the weekly multidisciplinary (MDT) meeting

The camera test shows a narrowing in your gullet. It looks a little worrying and I'm concerned it could be something serious

Oh no! What happens next?

Mr Evans has a 5-week history of progressive dysphagia. Endoscopy showed a tight malignant stricture

Biopsies confirm an adenocarcinoma

The oesophagus is thickened with tumour, with multiple lung and liver metastases

We need to get further information from the biopsy results and a CT scan

The stage is T4N1M1. Emelia, can we arrange an oesophageal stent?

Emelia Charles, an endoscopy nurse, discusses the results with Mr Evans and his wife. She first warns them that the news is not good

I'm afraid it's bad news

Unfortunately, the biopsy confirmed that you have cancer, and the CT scan shows that it has spread

Is....is there anything you can do?

No, I'm so sorry. We can't cure the cancer, but we are here to support you to make you as comfortable as possible

Whatever happens, Kay, promise me you'll be okay?

I'm still here, aren't I?

At the follow up appointment, Emelia breaks the bad news

2 months later, Mr Evans' health is in serious decline and he and his wife discuss his admission to a hospice

difficult over the last 5 weeks, with food feeling as if it is sticking in the region of his lower chest. He initially noticed problems with meat, but this gradually progressed over the 5 weeks and he is now able to tolerate only liquids. He is a non-smoker.

Interpretation of history

Chronic intermittent symptoms suggest a benign condition such as oesophageal dysmotility, whereas a progressive history suggests a stricture (narrowing), which is malignant or benign.

Mr Evans' recent history of progressive dysphagia from solids to liquids over a short period of time together with weight loss is very concerning and raises the alarm that he could have an oesophageal cancer.

Examination

Mr Evans looks pale and cachectic (visible muscle wasting and weight loss). Abdominal, respiratory and cardiovascular examinations are normal, and there are no palpable lymph nodes.

Interpretation of findings

The combination of progressive dysphagia and weight loss alerts the GP to a sinister cause, particularly in an older patient. Chronic gastro-oesophageal reflux is a risk factor for Barrett's oesophagus, a premalignant change that in turn increases the risk of oesophageal cancer. Clinical examination is usually normal in patients with any condition of the oesophagus.

Case 2 *continued*

Investigations

Mr Evans is referred for an urgent upper GI endoscopy. This shows a circumferential and ulcerated stricture in the lower oesophagus, through which the gastroscope cannot be passed as the lumen is too narrow (**Figure 3.3**). Biopsies are taken. CT of the chest and abdomen shows spread to the local lymph nodes and extensive liver and lung metastases.

Diagnosis

Mr Evans' results are discussed at a weekly multidisciplinary (MDT) meeting. After a review of the biopsies and imaging, metastatic oesophageal adenocarcinoma is diagnosed. In view of the advanced disease, the MDT recommends a palliative oesophageal stent to help the swallowing. The diagnosis of cancer and the management plan from the MDT is discussed with

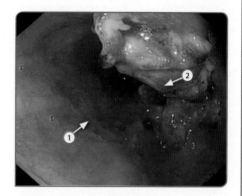

Figure 3.3 Endoscopic image of an oesophageal carcinoma with stricturing of the lumen. (1) Barrett's oesophagus. (2) Ulcerated mass causing narrowing of the oesophageal lumen

Mr Evans and his wife in the outpatient clinic. Although both are upset, they were already aware that this was the likely diagnosis as this was stated at the time of the endoscopy.

Gastro-oesophageal reflux disease

GORD is very common. It is caused by reflux of the acidic contents of the stomach and bile through the gastro-oesophageal junction into the oesophagus.

Epidemiology

Up to one third of the population in developed countries experience symptoms of GORD at least once a week. Men and women are equally affected.

Aetiology

Several mechanisms prevent reflux of acid and bile into the oesophagus:

- The lower oesophageal sphincter, which is formed by the distal 4 cm of oesophageal smooth muscle

- An external sphincter, formed by the crura of the diaphragm
- Peristalsis, which clears the oesophagus of any refluxed contents

Impairment of any of these will predispose towards GORD.

A hiatus hernia is a herniation of part of the stomach through the diaphragm and into the chest. A hiatus hernia is present in approximately one third of the population over the age of 50 years. It predisposes to reflux due to impaired ability of the crura to act as an external sphincter (**Figure 3.2**).

Other risk factors for GORD are listed in **Table 3.4**.

Risk factors for GORD	
Mechanical (raised intra-abdominal pressure)	Pregnancy
	Obesity
	Sports such as weight lifting
	Stooping
Drugs and diet	Caffeine
	Chocolate
	Spicy foods
	Calcium channel antagonists
	Anticholinergic agents
	Nitrates
	Alcohol
	Smoking
Other	Systemic sclerosis
	Asthma

Table 3.4 Risk factors for gastro-oesophageal reflux disease (GORD)

Patients with a hiatus hernia often experience no symptoms. The hernia is found incidentally during endoscopy and radiological investigation. Conversely, many patients have symptoms of GORD in the absence of a hiatus hernia.

Clinical features

Symptoms include one or more of the following:

- Heartburn
- Waterbrash – excess saliva produced as a response to acid in the lower oesophagus
- Regurgitation of food or fluid
- Nocturnal cough or wheeze – from possible bronchospasm caused by aspiration of acid on lying flat
- Chest pain – which is caused by oesophageal spasm and is sometimes difficult to differentiate from cardiac chest pain
- Hiccoughs or belching
- Odynophagia or dysphagia – which is often a sign of complications of GORD such as oesophagitis or a stricture (**Figure 3.4**)

None of these symptoms are particularly sensitive or specific for GORD and they are frequently reported even in the absence of documented signs of gastro-oesophageal reflux on invasive tests.

Clinical examination is often normal, although patients are often overweight or display other risk factors for symptoms (**Figure 3.1**). Acid regurgitation occasionally causes pharyngitis, laryngitis, or dental erosions.

Diagnostic approach

In most patients the symptoms are mild and further investigation is unnecessary. In the absence of alarm symptoms, lifestyle advice is given, appropriate treatment started and the patient reviewed after a month or so on treatment to ensure the symptoms are controlled.

Symptoms of gastro-oesophageal reflux characteristically respond well to proton pump inhibitors and these are therefore used as a diagnostic test. Patients often report that their symptoms reoccur shortly after stopping treatment.

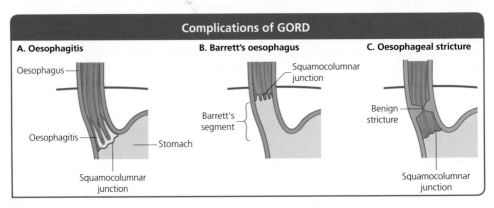

Complications of GORD

A. Oesophagitis
Oesophagus
Oesophagitis
Stomach
Squamocolumnar junction

B. Barrett's oesophagus
Squamocolumnar junction
Barrett's segment

C. Oesophageal stricture
Benign stricture
Squamocolumnar junction

Figure 3.4 Complications of gastro-oesophageal reflux disease (GORD).

Investigations

Further investigation is warranted if symptoms are persistent despite medication, or any alarm features are present (**Table 3.2**).

Blood tests

A normal full blood count and ferritin concentrations exclude iron deficiency anaemia.

Endoscopy

Upper GI endoscopy is the first-line investigation used to exclude more serious underlying pathology. There is often a poor correlation between the endoscopic changes and severity of symptoms, with the results of endoscopy frequently being normal. A hiatus hernia or changes caused by gastro-oesophageal reflux, such as oesophagitis or a benign oesophageal stricture, is often seen. Barrett's oesophagus is sometimes also identified.

pH studies and manometry

The pH is monitored for 24 hours to quantify the amount of acid refluxing into the oesophagus if there is diagnostic uncertainty and to ensure that surgical treatment to reduce reflux will be helpful. A thin tube is passed through the nose into the distal oesophagus, where it remains for 24 hours to investigate how eating, physical activity and sleep influence acid production. The frequency and severity of acid reflux, and its correlation with the patient's symptoms, is recorded in an events diary. Oesophageal manometry is usually performed at the same time as pH studies, with the same tube, to assess the lower oesophageal sphincter pressure and oesophageal contractions.

Management

GORD is normally managed with a step-up or step-down approach to achieve adequate symptom control (**Table 3.5**). A step-up approach starts with lifestyle advice and antacids. This is escalated by replacing the antacids with H_2-receptor antagonists, which in turn are switched to proton pump inhibitors if the symptoms are not alleviated. A 'step-down' approach starts with the most effective treatment medical treatment (i.e. proton

Management of GORD		
Management option		**Mechanism of action**
Lifestyle measures	Weight loss	Lowers intra-abdominal pressure
	Avoid eating late at night	Eating promotes gastric acid production; lying down increases reflux of gastric contents into oesophagus
	Smoking cessation Avoid excess alcohol	Smoking, alcohol and other drugs increase reflux by causing relaxation of LOS
Medication	Antacids	Neutralise pH
	Alginates	Form a protective cover (or 'raft') in oesophagus as a barrier to acid
	H_2 receptor antagonist (e.g. ranitidine)	Decrease acid by inhibiting gastric parietal cells
	Proton pump inhibitor (e.g. omeprazole)	Irreversibly block H^+–K^+ ATP pump on parietal cells
	Prokinetic (e.g. domperidone)	Moves contents of oesophagus and stomach forwards by promoting peristalsis
Surgical	Nissen fundoplication	Gastric fundus is wrapped around the lower oesophagus to reinforce it and prevent reflux
LOS, lower oesophageal sphincter		

Table 3.5 Management of gastro-oesophageal reflux disease (GORD). Patients are advised about lifestyle measures, and medication is stepped up or down depending upon response.

pump inhibitors), the dose being reduced as the symptoms improve.

Occasionally surgery is undertaken if patients do not want to continue or do not tolerate long term acid suppressants, which may result in complications such as dysphagia, inability to belch or vomit, and excess flatulence.

Prognosis

Although persistent symptoms of GORD affect quality of life, there is no increase in mortality.

Barrett's oesophagus

Barrett's oesophagus is a premalignant condition of the oesophageal lining that is associated with a 40-fold increased lifetime risk of oesophageal adenocarcinoma (**Figure 3.3**).

Epidemiology

The true prevalence is unknown as endoscopy is required for diagnosis. However, studies have estimated it to be approximately 1.5% of the UK population.

Aetiology

Prolonged irritation of the lower oesophagus by gastric acid causes a transformation (metaplasia) from squamous epithelium to columnar-type intestinal epithelium (**Figure 3.5**). This intestinal metaplastic change is called Barrett's oesophagus. Dysplastic change occasionally occurs within Barrett's and this dysplasia predisposes to malignant transformation. For this reason, individuals diagnosed with this condition are offered surveillance endoscopies to identify dysplastic or premalignant change as early as possible.

The main risk factor for the development of Barrett's oesophagus is GORD. Risk also

Management of Barrett's oesophagus	
Classification	Treatment
No dysplasia	Upper GI endoscopy with acetic acid spray and quadrantic biopsies every 2 cm on initial detection, then repeated:
	Every 2–3 years if ≥3 cm in length
	Every 3–5 years if < 3cm in length and intestinal metaplasia present
Low-grade dysplasia	Surveillance upper GI endoscopy every 6 months
High-grade dysplasia or intramucosal cancer	Discussion by multidisciplinary team and repeat endoscopy in a specialist centre
	Options are: ■ Radiofrequency ablation (see page 154) if no visible lesion ■ Endoscopic resection if visible lesion ■ Oesophagectomy (endoscopic techniques preferred due to decreased risk of morbidity and mortality)

Table 3.6 Endoscopic surveillance and management of Barrett's oesophagus

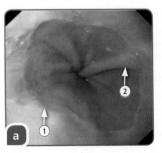
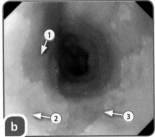

Figure 3.5 Endoscopic image of Barrett's oesophagus. (a) Normal appearance of the lower oesophagus. ① Squamocolumnar junction. ② Top of gastric folds. (b) Barrett's oesophagus. ① Barrett's oesophagus (redder columnar epithelium). ② Pale squamous epithelium. ③ Squamocolumnar junction.

increases with age due to a longer exposure of gastric acid, obesity which is associated with higher rates of GORD and the male sex for an unknown reason (3:1 male:female).

Clinical features

Patients are typically asymptomatic and therefore many are not diagnosed. Gastro-oesophageal reflux or other GI symptoms usually prompt the initial endoscopy. Clinical examination is usually normal.

Diagnostic approach

The diagnosis of Barrett's oesophagus is made endoscopically and confirmed histologically with biopsies.

Investigations

At endoscopy, Barrett's oesophagus is identified by replacement of the paler squamous epithelium with pinker columnar epithelium that is visible above the gastro-oesophageal junction (**Figure 3.5**). The diagnosis is confirmed by biopsy.

Management

Long-term high-dose proton pump inhibitors are given to prevent acid reflux.

Patients diagnosed with Barrett's oesophagus are offered endoscopic surveillance to detect signs of the dysplasia that sometimes complicates it. Management options are outlined in **Table 3.6**.

Prognosis

This depends on the presence and grade of dysplasia. Up to 40% of patients undergoing oesophageal resection for high-grade dysplasia are found to have early adenocarcinoma. At present, there is no proven benefit to screening the general population for Barrett's oesophagus.

Oesophagitis

Oesophagitis is inflammation of the oesophagus and is acute or chronic. The most common cause is gastro-oesophageal reflux.

Epidemiology

The causes and features for the different causes of oesophagitis are given in **Table 3.7**.

Aetiology

Reflux of acidic gastric contents through the lower gastro-oesophageal sphincter into the oesophagus is the most common cause of oesophageal inflammation as it irritates the mucosa. Acid reflux into the oesophagus is more common with a hiatus hernia and if certain lifestyle factors are present (**Table 3.4**).

Oesophagitis is sometimes due to the ingestion of medications or caustic agents, infiltration with eosinophils usually related to food or other allergies, infection, the presence of a nasogastric tube because of trauma and radiotherapy to the oesophagus or nearby structures.

Clinical features

Oesophagitis is sometimes asymptomatic. However, it is most commonly associated with:

- Heartburn
- Odynophagia
- Dysphagia – this results from strictures secondary to chronic oesophagitis or conditions such as eosinophilic oesophagitis, which causes intermittent dysphagia and presents with food bolus obstruction
- Chest pain
- Nausea
- Dry cough – which is caused by acid reflux
- Fevers – which usually occur soon after caustic ingestion

Physical examination is usually normal.

Diagnostic approach

A careful history will often help determine the underlying cause. The patient should be asked about:

Types of oesophagitis	
Type	Features
Reflux	More common with a hiatus hernia and lifestyle factors (see page 168)
Infective	Usually Candida but also herpes simplex and cytomegalovirus
	More common in immunosuppressive states or with drugs, e.g. HIV/AIDS, cancer chemotherapy and steroid treatment
Eosinophilic	Oesophageal mucosa becomes infiltrated with eosinophils
	More common in those with food and other allergies
Drugs	Ingestion of tablets that are corrosive if they stick in the oesophagus, including non-steroidal anti-inflammatories, bisphosphonates, potassium salts, tetracycline and doxycycline
Caustic	Accidental or deliberate ingestion of fluids that are acidic or alkaline, e.g. bleach
Radiotherapy	Commonly occurs when treating cancers of the oesophagus, lung, breast and the chest wall
Mechanical	Nasogastric tubes, particularly when in situ for a long time, cause irritation of the oesophagus

Table 3.7 Types of oesophagitis

- Medication that has been taken
- Response to acid-suppressant medication
- Allergies
- Other medical history, including immunosuppressive conditions such as cancer and its treatments
- A psychiatric history if caustic ingestion is suspected, although this occasionally happens accidentally

Investigations

Investigation is not required for patients with symptoms typical of gastro-oesophageal reflux because they are usually treated successfully without an endoscopy. Other underlying aetiologies are considered in those with risk factors or an atypical history. Many of these patients are diagnosed and managed successfully without invasive investigations; this is the case with, for example, a person taking a bisphosphonate who has central chest pain or a person who has pain on swallowing in the presence of oral candidiasis after recent chemotherapy.

Investigation is necessary if an opportunistic infection or eosinophilic oesophagitis is suspected. It is also indicated if typical symptoms of GORD have not responded to adequate treatment to see if there is another cause for oesophagitis and to exclude malignancy.

Blood tests

The results are usually normal. However, the eosinophil count (part of the full blood count) is sometimes elevated with eosinophilic oesophagitis.

Endoscopy

Upper GI endoscopy is the preferred investigation (**Figure 3.6**) because oesophagitis is identified and the mucosa closely inspected. Biopsies are taken of strictures or any abnormal areas to exclude underlying malignancy.

The endoscopic findings of eosinophilic oesophagitis vary and it sometimes looks normal. Diagnosis is made by an increased eosinophil count in biopsies – this is seen in GORD within the distal oesophagus and so biopsies are taken from the proximal oesophagus.

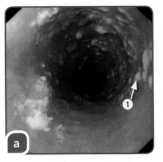
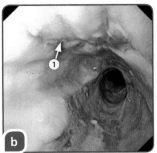

Figure 3.6 Common types of oesophagitis. (a) Candidiasis – white plaques seen throughout the oesophagus ①. (b) Reflux oesophagitis in the lower oesophagus – red streaks are seen extending up the oesophagus ①.

Imaging

A barium swallow is less sensitive and helpful only if a structural or motility disorder is suspected.

Management

Each cause of oesophagitis has a specific treatment (**Table 3.8**). As reflux oesophagitis is so common, most patients with compatible symptoms are initially given an empirical trial of acid suppression with a proton pump inhibitor.

Oesophageal strictures develop with reflux, caustic, eosinophilic and radiotherapy-related oesophagitis. Endoscopic dilatation is undertaken in patients with progressive dysphagia who are unable to tolerate an oral diet despite appropriate medical therapy. Counselling is required as there is an increased risk of perforation with oesophageal dilatation – up to 2% for benign strictures (compared with 0.1% with a diagnostic gastroscopy).

Management of oesophagitis	
Type	Treatment
Reflux	Lifestyle modifications
	Antacids
	H₂ receptor antagonists
	Proton pump inhibitors
	Fundoplication (surgery)
Infective:	
Candida	Oral fluconazole
Herpes simplex	Oral aciclovir
Cytomegalovirus	Intravenous ganciclovir
Eosinophilic	Swallow inhaled steroids
Drugs	Avoid or stop the agent
Caustic	Discuss with poisons advice service, management varies with fluid swallowed
Radiotherapy	Temporarily or permanently stop radiotherapy or alter regimen
Mechanical	Remove tube if severe and consider other feeding, e.g. via a percutaneous endoscopic gastrostomy (PEG) tube

Table 3.8 Types of oesophagitis and their management

Oesophageal neoplasia

Oesophageal carcinoma usually presents with dysphagia. The two main types of carcinoma are adenocarcinoma, which affects the lower oesophagus, and squamous cell carcinoma, which more commonly affects the middle and upper oesophagus.

Epidemiology

Oesophageal carcinoma is the eighth most common cancer worldwide and affects more than twice as many men as women. The incidence varies throughout the world; it is lowest in Western Africa and highest in Eastern Asia. Most diagnoses are made in people aged over 60 years old. In developed countries the incidence of adenocarcinoma is rising, but that of squamous cell carcinoma is stable.

Aetiology

There are a number of different risk factors for both types of oesophageal cancer (**Table 3.9**).

Clinical features

Presentation is often late in the disease process and symptoms that are present are:

- Progressive dysphagia – which occurs due to growth of the tumour into the oesophageal lumen. Initially, there is a problem swallowing solids, but this progresses to difficulty with liquids
- Weight loss – which occurs over weeks to months and is caused by reduced oral intake
- Odynophagia – pain on swallowing when tumours are ulcerated

Risk factors for oesophageal carcinoma	
Carcinoma type	**Risk factors**
Squamous cell carcinoma	Cigarette smoking
	Excess alcohol consumption
	Achalasia (particularly if it is longstanding and untreated)
	Caustic strictures
	Family history (without identifiable pattern of inheritance)
	Dietary – vitamin or mineral deficiencies (global deficiencies – no specific culprit is known)
	Plummer–Vinson syndrome*
	Familial tylosis (palmar hyperkeratosis), a rare autosomal dominant condition
Adenocarcinoma	Gastro-oesophageal reflux disease (see page 167)
	Barrett's oesophagus (see page 170)

*Also called Patterson–Brown–Kelly syndrome.

Table 3.9 Risk factors for oesophageal carcinoma

- Haematemesis – which occasionally occurs due to oozing of blood from the tumour
- Hoarse voice – due to local invasion of tumour into the recurrent laryngeal nerve, which causes vocal cord paralysis
- Recurrent chest infections – due to tumour invasion into the trachea or bronchus, causing a connection (fistula) to form between the oesophagus and the lungs

Patients often appear cachectic with signs of muscle wasting. Physical examination is usually normal unless there is extensive metastatic disease; in this setting cervical lymphadenopathy or hepatomegaly is often evident.

> **Dysphagia is occasionally due to acute or chronic progressive neurological disorders,** e.g. Parkinson's disease or motor neurone disease as well as conditions affecting the oesophagus or pharynx.

Diagnostic approach

Diagnosis is made using a combination of blood tests, upper GI endoscopy and radiological imaging.

Investigations

If malignancy is suspected, initial blood tests (a full blood count, ferritin, liver function tests) are performed and an urgent referral made for upper GI endoscopy. Radiology is required for staging if the diagnosis is confirmed.

Blood tests
Low haemoglobin, mean cell volume (MCV) and ferritin levels occur with iron deficiency anaemia, secondary to chronic blood loss.

Endoscopy
Upper GI endoscopy is the investigation of choice and shows oesophageal nodularity, ulceration and stricturing. Subtle changes are enhanced using dyes – acetic acid for Barrett's oesophagus and Lugol's iodine for squamous mucosa. Endoscopic measurements record the position and length of the tumour, which helps guide further treatment. Biopsies differentiate between adenocarcinoma and squamous cell carcinoma.

Imaging
Mucosal abnormalities and strictures are identified on a barium swallow used to investigate dysphagia. CT and positron emission tomography assess for local and distant spread. Endoscopic ultrasound provides accurate information on the depth of invasion into the oesophageal wall (T-stage).

Management

Management is individualised after discussion with the MDT and considering the carcinoma type, co-morbidity and stage of disease using the TNM classification. A combination of treatments is often chosen.

Endoscopic treatment

Endoscopic mucosal or submucosal resection is possible for early cancers. Laser can be used to obliterate tumour, as a palliative treatment for dysphagia.

Chemotherapy/radiotherapy

Chemotherapy and radiotherapy are used alone or in combination (chemo-radiotherapy) as curative or palliative treatments. Chemo-radiotherapy is the treatment of choice for localised squamous cell carcinoma. Palliative radiotherapy is used to treat dysphagia, pain or bleeding from advanced carcinoma.

Surgery

The section of oesophagus containing the carcinoma is removed and the stomach is moved into the thoracic cavity to connect it to the remaining oesophagus. The proximal part of the stomach is often removed if the tumour is in the lower oesophagus.

Palliative treatment

Self-expanding metal or biodegradable stents are inserted into the oesophagus at endoscopy to relieve symptoms of dysphagia (**Figure 3.7**). Covered stents (metal stents containing a plastic coating) are used to treat complications such as tracheo-oesophageal fistulae, to cover the hole. Dietary advice is required to avoid stent occlusion secondary to solid boluses of food such as lumps of meat or bread.

Prognosis

Oesophageal cancer often presents late and has an overall 5-year survival of approximately 15%. Detection of early cancers through surveillance endoscopy in patients with Barrett's oesophagus significantly improves survival rates by detecting dysplasia and cancer at an earlier, often asymptomatic stage.

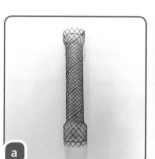
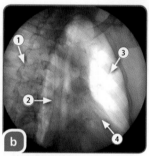

Figure 3.7 (a) Oesophageal stent. (b) Radiograph showing an oesophageal stent. ① Spine, ② metal stent, ③ lung, ④ heart.

Motility disorders

The most common disorder of oesophageal motility is a defective lower oesophageal sphincter, which leads to gastro-oesophageal reflux. Achalasia and other forms of 'spastic' dysmotility (**Figure 3.8**) also occur.

Achalasia

This is characterised by the absence of peristaltic waves in the distal oesophagus and a lower oesophageal sphincter that does not relax on swallowing. It is caused by degeneration of the enteric nerves, although the cause of this is unknown. Males and females

are equally affected. It occurs at any age including young adult life, but is most common in the third to fifth decades; achalasia very rarely occurs in children.

Clinical features

Dysphagia with respect to both liquids and solids is the main symptom. It is often longstanding and slowly progressive. Other symptoms are:

- Regurgitation of undigested food and liquids with a risk of aspiration/chest infections

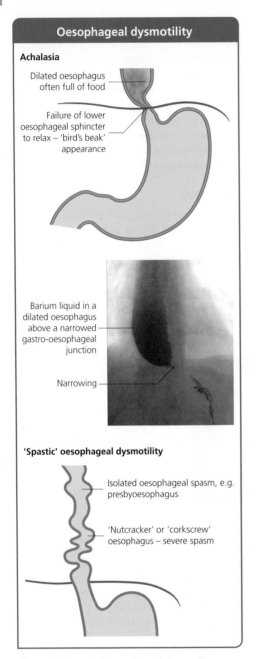

Oesophageal dysmotility

Achalasia

Dilated oesophagus often full of food

Failure of lower oesophageal sphincter to relax – 'bird's beak' appearance

Barium liquid in a dilated oesophagus above a narrowed gastro-oesophageal junction

Narrowing

'Spastic' oesophageal dysmotility

Isolated oesophageal spasm, e.g. presbyoesophagus

'Nutcracker' or 'corkscrew' oesophagus – severe spasm

Figure 3.8 Forms of oesophageal dysmotility.

- Retrosternal chest pain, which sometimes precedes symptoms of dysphagia
- Weight loss

Clinical examination is usually normal.

Diagnostic approach
It is sometimes difficult to diagnose the exact cause of dysphagia from the symptoms alone. Investigations are always performed to determine the underlying cause.

Investigations

Endoscopy
Upper GI endoscopy is required to exclude malignancy. The results are often normal in early achalasia. Later, endoscopy usually shows a dilated oesophagus full of old food above a tight lower oesophageal sphincter that only occasionally relaxes.

Other tests
Barium swallow shows a tapering at the gastro-oesophageal junction (which gives a 'bird's beak' appearance), oesophageal dilatation and lack of peristalsis (**Figure 3.8**).

Oesophageal manometry records pressures throughout the length of oesophagus. The diagnostic features of achalasia are the absence of distal oesophageal peristaltic waves and an elevated pressure at the lower oesophageal sphincter with incomplete relaxation after swallowing.

Management
Drugs are of no benefit because they cannot overcome the dysfunction in the oesophagus. Management options are:

- Endoscopy with botulinum toxin injection, into the lower oesophageal sphincter which is effective in up to 75% of patients, although the benefit wears off after several months
- Balloon dilatation of the lower oesophageal sphincter, which is effective in 90% of patients; however, most develop reflux, and there is a 2% risk of perforation
- Cardiomyotomy, a surgical procedure in which a lengthwise cut is made in the outer muscular layer of the oesophagus. This is effective in 90% of patients and is usually carried out laparoscopically

- Peroral endoscopic myotomy (POEM), an advanced endoscopic technique involving a cut through the wall of the oesophagus, with division of the underlying circular muscle. This is effective in 90% of patients

The risk of oesophageal carcinoma is increased up to 100-fold in longstanding, untreated achalasia.

> 'Pseudo-achalasia' has identical symptoms to motility disorders and has the same abnormalities on barium meal, but it is due to a cancer of the gastric cardia.

'Spastic' oesophageal dysmotility

High-amplitude, non-peristaltic waves are seen in this condition. It is precipitated by gastro-oesophageal reflux and is rarely associated with systemic conditions such as scleroderma. It is more common in the elderly, many of whom have some dysmotility with no symptoms ('presbyoesophagus').

Clinical features

There is not usually any weight loss. Features include:

- Dysphagia for both liquids and solids, which is often intermittent

- Chest pain, which often occurs at rest. This often has the characteristics of reflux or is sometimes central and crushing (i.e. 'cardiac' like, similar to angina)
- Coexisting symptoms of irritable bowel syndrome

Clinical examination is normal.

Investigations

Endoscopy
Upper GI endoscopy is performed to exclude strictures and is very often normal. However, abnormal peristaltic waves are sometimes seen.

Other tests
Barium swallow is more helpful than endoscopy and shows 'spasms' that are diffuse ('corkscrew oesophagus'). Oesophageal manometry sometimes shows high-amplitude waves but, like barium swallow, the results are often normal as dysmotility is intermittent.

Management

A proton pump inhibitor will help some individuals. A 'spasm' pain is treated with sublingual nitrate, which causes smooth muscle relaxation, or calcium channel antagonists, for example nifedipine. Low-dosage tricyclic antidepressants and botulinum toxin injection during endoscopy are other options.

Pharyngo-oesophageal disorders

Neuromuscular, structural and functional abnormalities occur near the pharyngo-oesophageal junction (**Table 3.10**). These present primarily with difficulty swallowing.

> Patients with high dysphagia (i.e. at the level of the throat) are initially assessed by a barium swallow or ENT examination. Oesophagogastroduodenoscopy (OGD) does not produce optimal views of this region, and the presence of a pouch increases the risk of perforation when intubating the oesophagus.

Neuromuscular abnormalities

Many neuromuscular disorders cause pharyngeal weakness (**Table 3.10**). This results in problems with swallowing and predisposes to aspiration of contents into the airway, leading to a cough or pneumonia. A change in voice is often present. These disorders usually have other systemic neurological features which help in identifying why there is pharyngeal weakness. For the majority of patients, there is no specific

Neuromuscular causes of pharyngeal weakness	
Site	Causes
Central nervous system	Cerebrovascular accident ('stroke')
	Parkinson's disease
	Multiple sclerosis
	Dementia
	Brain tumours
	Cerebral palsy
Peripheral nerve	Guillain–Barré syndrome
	Motor neurone disease (amyotrophic lateral sclerosis)
Neuromuscular junction	Myasthenia gravis
Muscle (primary muscle disorders)	Muscular dystrophy, e.g. Duchenne's, oculopharyngeal
	Myotonic dystrophy
	Polymyositis
	Dermatomyositis

Table 3.10 Neuromuscular causes of pharyngeal weakness

treatment for the underlying condition and so the treatment is supportive – modifying the diet, e.g. thickening fluids under the direction of a speech and language therapist together with a dietician. A percutaneous endoscopic gastrostomy is sometimes necessary to maintain hydration and nutritional intake if the swallow is very unsafe leading to a high risk of aspiration.

Functional abnormalities (globus pharyngeus)

Globus pharyngeus is a functional disorder resulting from spasm of the cricopharyngeal muscle. The cause of this spasm is not always apparent. It is more common in patients with anxiety but also occurs as a response to gastro-oesophageal reflux or abnormal upper oesophageal sphincter function.

Clinical features

Features include:

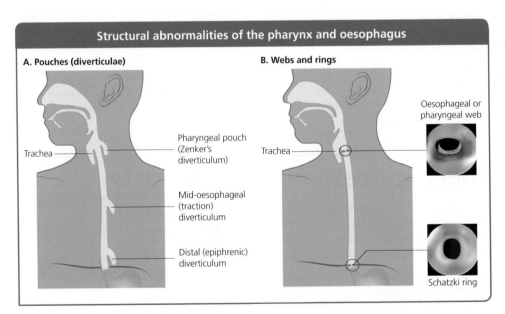

Figure 3.9 Structural abnormalities of the pharynx and oesophagus.

- A 'lump at the back of the throat'
- High dysphagia – at the level of the larynx – which is usually intermittent
- Recurrent throat clearing or cough
- Coexisting symptoms of other functional problems, e.g. irritable bowel syndrome

Diagnostic approach

Globus pharyngeus is frequently diagnosed on the basis of symptoms alone. However, upper GI endoscopy or a barium swallow is often carried out to exclude other causes, including malignancy. Upper GI endoscopy is normal. A barium swallow occasionally shows cricopharyngeal spasm but is usually normal.

Management

Reassurance and explanation are key. If a trial of proton pump inhibitor to reduce reflux is helpful, it is continued.

Dietary modification including drinking plenty of fluid with meals is useful. If there is an underlying mood disorder this will need appropriate management.

Structural abnormalities

Pouches and diverticulae

Pharyngeal pouch (Zenker's diverticulum)

A pharyngeal pouch (Figure 3.9a) is a herniation of the mucosa of the oesophagus between the cricopharyngeus and inferior pharyngeal constrictor muscles of the pharynx, above the upper oesophageal sphincter. Its cause is unknown. It usually presents with intermittent high dysphagia and regurgitation, with an increased risk of aspiration. It is

more common in elderly patients and is usually diagnosed by barium swallow. If the condition is troublesome, patients are referred to an ENT specialist to consider surgery. Diverticulae in the more distal oesophagus rarely cause any problems.

Webs and rings

The most commonly encountered webs and rings are illustrated in **Figure 3.9b**.

Oesophageal webs

These are semi-circular thickenings of the oesophagus. They sometimes cause dysphagia but are difficult to see at endoscopy as they are often inadvertently ruptured when the tube enters the oesophagus but are seen on barium swallow. They usually occur in the post-cricoid area. There is a very rare condition called Plummer–Vinson syndrome which is characterised by iron deficiency anaemia, dysphagia and oesophageal webs. It is associated with an increased risk of squamous cell cancer of the proximal oesophagus and pharynx.

'Schatzki' rings

These are circumferential, fibrotic, oesophageal thickenings most commonly seen in the mid or distal oesophagus at endoscopy or on imaging. They often cause longstanding, mild dysphagia and also food bolus obstruction with lumps of food. If symptomatic, they are dilated using a balloon at oesophagogastroduodenoscopy.

> **Globus pharyngeus was formerly called globus hystericus** because it was thought to be a psychogenic disorder.

Answers to starter questions

1. Hiatus hernias are very common; they are present in a third of people over 50 years of age. They occur when the stomach protrudes through the diaphragm at the point that the oesophagus enters the abdominal cavity. Some are congenital, but most develop over time and are more common with increasing age and obesity. They sometimes occur when coughing or straining, for example when carrying heavy objects.

2. Although heartburn is often dismissed as being a nuisance, gastro-oesophageal reflux disease is potentially serious. By inducing intestinal metaplasia (Barrett's oesophagus), chronic acid reflux can be considered as the initial trigger to developing oesophageal adenocarcinoma.

3. The incidence of adenocarcinoma of the oesophagus is rising very rapidly in the West. This is likely to be due to increasing rates of gastro-oesophageal reflux associated with poor diet and obesity. A healthy balanced diet, weight loss, avoidance of late-night eating before bed, reduction in alcohol intake and smoking cessation are all recommended to treat gastro-oesophageal reflux. However, there is no evidence these measures will prevent oesophageal adenocarcinoma.

Chapter 4
Gastric disease

Starter questions

Reading this chapter will enable you to answer the following questions. Answers are on page 198.

1. How does *Helicobacter pylori* infection cause a range of different upper GI conditions?
2. Why do patients with gastric ulcers need a follow up endoscopy, whereas those with duodenal ulcers do not?
3. How can nonsteroidal anti-inflammatory drugs be taken more safely in patients who need them?
4. Why is there such a variation in the rates of gastric cancer around the world?

Introduction

Gastric disease involves any part of the stomach from the gastro-oesophageal sphincter to the pylorus. Gastric symptoms are very common, many people will experience episodes of nausea and vomiting, upper abdominal pain and bloating which occur particularly after eating.

The most common diseases of the stomach are gastritis, peptic ulcers and functional dyspepsia (with this condition there is no structural or biochemical abnormality and there are often other symptoms, for example irritable bowel syndrome). These conditions are usually triggered by factors such as diet, alcohol, stress, non-steroidal anti-inflammatory agents (NSAIDs) or *Helicobacter pylori* infection. Gastric cancer is relatively uncommon in the Western World compared to East Asia and often presents in an advanced state with metastases. Motility abnormalities of the stomach are rare but cause many symptoms; gastric emptying is either delayed (gastroparesis) or accelerated (e.g. dumping syndrome).

Case 3 Abdominal pain after eating

Presentation

Jocelyn King is a 43-year-old woman with a 6-month history of intermittent upper abdominal discomfort.

Initial interpretation

Abdominal pain is a common symptom with a wide differential diagnosis that includes peptic ulcer disease, gallstones and pancreatitis. Furthermore, the pain may originate outside the gastrointestinal (GI) tract, including the cardiac, respiratory, musculoskeletal, urological and gynaecological systems. Therefore a thorough history must be taken to further characterise Jocelyn's pain in terms of its nature, onset, aggravating and relieving factors, etc., to provide diagnostic clues.

History

Jocelyn says she has been experiencing almost daily upper abdominal pain with a feeling of fullness and bloating. It is worse after eating, particularly with large meals, and at night. She sometimes feels nauseous but has not vomited. She reports no dysphagia or weight loss. In response to questioning she confirms she has no symptoms suggesting GI bleeding (e.g. haematemesis or melaena).

Over the last few months she has been taking ibuprofen for back pain. She is a smoker and drinks approximately 21 units of alcohol per week. There is no family history of ischaemic heart disease or gastric malignancy. She received treatment for *H. pylori* 3 years ago when she previously had upper abdominal pain. This bacterium is present in the stomach of many people but rarely leads to conditions such as peptic ulcers, and is only treated when dyspepsia is confirmed.

Jocelyn has tried over-the-counter antacids, which seem to help.

Gastric symptoms are very common but often mild and treated with over-the-counter medication obtained by the patient from a supermarket or pharmacy, without needing to visit a doctor for a prescription.

Examination

On examination Jocelyn is found to be overweight with a body mass index of 28 kg/m². There is no conjunctival pallor or palpable lymph nodes in the neck or supraclavicular region. She has mild epigastric tenderness but no palpable mass or enlarged organs (organomegaly). The rest of the examination is normal.

Interpretation of findings

Jocelyn's symptoms are in keeping with dyspepsia (indigestion).

She is demonstrating a group of symptoms that are common in the general population and are caused by:

- underlying peptic ulcer disease with *H. pylori* infection
- taking NSAIDs such as ibuprofen
- functional (non-ulcer) dyspepsia

It is important to check for any alarm features that suggest a more serious underlying disease such as gastric cancer, for example dysphagia, unintentional weight loss, persistent nausea and vomiting, GI bleeding, an epigastric mass or iron deficiency anaemia. Urgent further investigation is required if an 'alarm' feature is present (see Table 3.2).

Investigations

The results of Jocelyn's blood tests, including a full blood count and coeliac serology, are normal.

Case 3 *continued*

Management of dyspepsia

Jocelyn discusses her symptoms with her GP, Dr Seymour. He checks that she has no alarm symptoms, and suggests lifestyle changes that might help

Jocelyn also talks about her frustration with her symptoms and their effect on her confidence

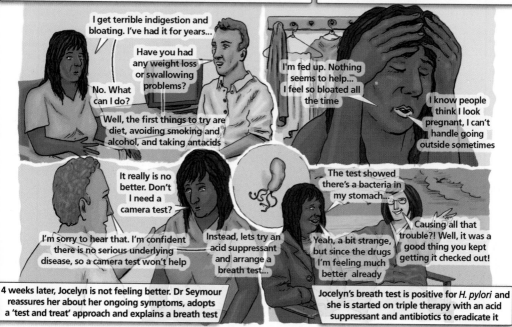

4 weeks later, Jocelyn is not feeling better. Dr Seymour reassures her about her ongoing symptoms, adopts a 'test and treat' approach and explains a breath test

Jocelyn's breath test is positive for *H. pylori* and she is started on triple therapy with an acid suppressant and antibiotics to eradicate it

Most patients, particularly those under 55 years old, require no further investigation because the symptoms of dyspepsia are usually managed effectively with lifestyle changes and medication, and gastric cancer would be a very unlikely diagnosis. In view of Jocelyn's age and lack of alarm features, an upper GI endoscopy is not indicated.

Jocelyn is offered general lifestyle advice, such as losing weight, avoiding smoking and excess alcohol, and avoiding spicy foods. She is told to stop taking NSAIDs. If these measures are ineffective, a 'test-and-treat' approach for *H. pylori* is used. In fact, Jocelyn has previously had treatment for this infection. This is effective in the majority of patients but in some the bacteria do persist and recurrent infection does sometimes occur. If a patient has already received eradication therapy, a carbon urea breath test is the most appropriate investigation to see if *H. pylori* is present (**Figure 4.1**).

Diagnosis

Jocelyn's breath test is positive, indicating *H. pylori* infection. Therefore in addition to the advice on lifestyle and cessation of NSAIDs she is given a course of eradication therapy (see **Table 4.4**). She is reviewed by her general practitioner (GP) 1 month later, when she reports that her symptoms have greatly improved.

Case 3 *continued*

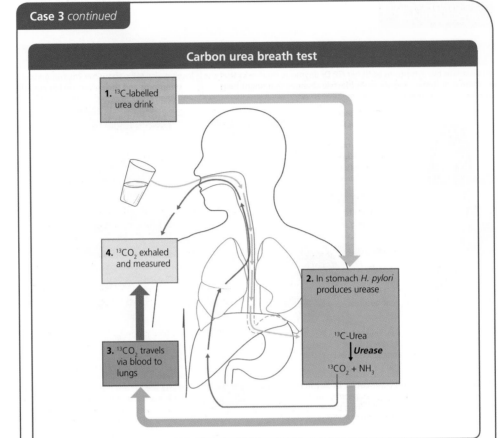

Carbon urea breath test

1. ^{13}C-labelled urea drink

2. In stomach *H. pylori* produces urease

^{13}C-Urea

↓ *Urease*

$^{13}CO_2 + NH_3$

3. $^{13}CO_2$ travels via blood to lungs

4. $^{13}CO_2$ exhaled and measured

Figure 4.1 Carbon urea breath test. Either ^{13}C- or ^{14}C-labelled urea is administered orally after an overnight fast. If *Helicobacter pylori* is present ^{13}C- or ^{14}C-labelled carbon dioxide is detectable by a breath meter.

Case 4 Nausea and vomiting

Presentation

Jack Brown, a 51-year-old man, has been seen by his GP for symptoms of nausea over the previous 6 weeks. He has a past medical history of type 2 diabetes that is well controlled by oral antidiabetic drugs. His GP has referred him to the gastroenterology clinic for consideration of an upper GI endoscopy.

Initial interpretation

Jack's nausea must be categorised further in terms of its onset, precipitating or relieving factors, whether the symptoms are continuous or intermittent and any associated vomiting. This information is often in the GP referral letter. Nausea is a common symptom with many potential causes, only some of which relate to the GI tract (**Table 4.1**).

Case 4 *continued*

Causes of nausea and vomiting	
Causes	**Examples**
Gastrointestinal	Dyspepsia
	Pancreatitis, cholecystitis
	Hepatitis
	Gastric outlet and small bowel obstruction
	Gastroparesis
Central nervous system	Migrainous headache
	Intracerebral lesions and raised intracranial pressure
	Labyrinth and vestibular disorders, e.g. Ménière's disease
Metabolic and endocrine	Pregnancy
	Diabetes, e.g. ketoacidosis
	Addison's disease
	Hypercalcaemia and hyponatraemia
	Renal failure
Infectious	Viral and bacterial gastroenteritis
	Systemic infections
Drugs	NSAIDs, opiates
	Chemotherapy agents
	Digoxin
Other	Eating disorders
	Functional disorders
	Alcohol

NSAID, non-steroidal anti-inflammatory drug.

Table 4.1 Causes of nausea and vomiting

Jack's history is relevant because diabetes causes complications such as delayed gastric emptying (gastroparesis), and antidiabetic drugs cause GI side effects.

> **Gastrointestinal symptoms are common side effects of most medications** and are always considered in the differential diagnosis. Side effects such as dyspepsia, nausea, vomiting, abdominal cramps, diarrhoea and constipation usually occur without any visible abnormality and resolve shortly after the drug is stopped.

Jack has not lost weight, which makes a malignant cause less likely. However, a detailed clinical history must be obtained to assess for other features signalling cancer, such as persistent vomiting or early satiety as well as any precipitants for his symptoms.

Further history

Jack describes how his symptoms began after he developed shingles (varicella zoster) affecting his right chest wall, after which he developed a sharp burning pain. His GP started an antiepileptic medication as a treatment for neuropathic pain.

Jack has a normal appetite with no symptoms of abdominal pain, heartburn or vomiting. There is no history of headache or other extra-intestinal features. His diabetes has been well controlled with the same medications since his diagnosis 2 years previously. He is teetotal.

Examination

Jack appears slightly overweight. There is no evidence of dehydration, e.g. dry mucous membranes, drowsiness, hypotension or tachycardia, which occasionally occurs when vomiting is severe or prolonged. There are several small scars over his right chest wall but the abdominal, cardiovascular and respiratory examinations are otherwise normal. There are no palpable lymph nodes.

Interpretation of findings

Clinical examination is often normal in patients with nausea and vomiting unless they are secondary to a systemic condition such as infection. The clinical history is key to establishing the potential causes. The main differential diagnoses for Jack's presentation include side effects of the medications prescribed for neuropathic pain and GI complication of diabetes. The relatively short history of well-controlled diabetes makes the latter less likely.

Case 4 *continued*

Investigations

Basic blood tests will exclude metabolic causes of nausea. A low ferritin concentration indicates whether there are underlying pathologies causing chronic blood loss. Glycated haemoglobin (HbA1c) is measured to assess diabetic control; this would be increased if blood sugar had been high in recent weeks, however it is found to be normal.

Jack's full blood count, ferritin, urea and electrolyte, liver function test, bone profile and thyroid function test results are all found to be normal.

Diagnosis

Because there are no alarm symptoms, blood tests are normal and Jack's symptoms have occurred in relationship to a change in medication, an upper GI endoscopy is not necessary. Jack's good diabetic control with normal HbA1c results suggest that it is very unlikely that his symptoms are GI complications of diabetes. The relationship between the onset of his symptoms to the diagnosis of shingles and change in treatment strongly suggest that his problems are side effects of antiepileptic medication.

During assessment in the gastroenterology clinic the consultant advises discontinuation of the antiepileptic medication prescribed for the neuropathic pain. Jack is reviewed in the clinic 2 months later and reports that his symptoms have completely resolved. He is discharged back to GP care, without the need for invasive investigation.

Peptic ulcer disease

There are two types of peptic ulcer, named according to their location, i.e. gastric and duodenal ulcers. They occur when there is a breach in the mucosal surface of the stomach or duodenum due to an imbalance between acid secretion and mucosal defences. Nearly all peptic ulcers are associated with *Helicobacter pylori* infection or NSAID use.

Epidemiology

Approximately 70% of peptic ulcers occur in the duodenum. Gastric ulcers are less common and are usually seen in the elderly. Duodenal ulcers are twice as common in men as women and affect 15% of the population at some point during life (**Table 4.2**).

> **The prevalence of *H. pylori* has been decreasing in developed countries due to improved sanitation.** However, in some developing countries, up to 90% of the population are infected.

Aetiology

The most common cause of peptic ulcer disease worldwide is *H. pylori* infection: over 90% of duodenal ulcers and 70% of gastric ulcers are associated with this species. *Helicobacter pylori* is a spirally shaped Gram-negative, urease-producing bacterium that colonises more than 50% of the population worldwide. Infection is transmitted by the oro-oral route or by the gastro-oral or faeco-oral route (contact with infected vomit or stools, respectively).

Helicobacter pylori has several adaptive features that allow it to colonise the gastric mucosa:

- Flagella to burrow into the mucus lining of the stomach and into the epithelial layer where the pH is more neutral which is a better environment for the organism's survival
- Adhesins on its surface ensure it adheres to the gastric mucosa

- Production of the enzyme urease, which neutralises the stomach acid

> Although infection with *H. pylori* is usually asymptomatic it carries a lifetime risk of 10–20% for peptic ulceration and 1% for gastric cancer.

Infection of the gastric antrum, which is where most of the gastrin-producing G cells are located, leads to increased gastrin production and in turn increased gastric acid secretion. This often results in increased acid within the lumen of the duodenum, predisposing to duodenal ulcers (**Figure 4.2**).

NSAIDs are also a common cause of peptic ulcers. They inhibit the enzyme cyclo-oxygenase, which results in reduced prostaglandin production and therefore damage to the mucosal surface. This is not a local effect; it is a systemic effect and therefore occurs even if the drug is given by non-oral routes, for example intravenously.

The *Helicobacter*- or NSAID-induced impairment of the mucus–bicarbonate barrier and reduced prostaglandin-mediated mucosal protection are also thought to play a role in ulcer development. Other, rarer, causes of peptic ulcer include:

- Other drugs (e.g. aspirin, bisphosphonates, theophyllines)
- Gastric adenocarcinoma
- Lymphoma
- Zollinger–Ellison syndrome, which occurs with excess gastrin production from a neuroendocrine tumour (see page 191)
- Physiological stress, e.g. burns or head trauma
- Multiple endocrine neoplasia type 1
- Crohn's disease

> Although *H. pylori* is classified as a carcinogen by the World Health Organization, there is no evidence to support screening the whole community.

Clinical features

Infection with *H. pylori* is often asymptomatic but if it is not it leads to gastritis or peptic ulceration. The clinical features of gastric and duodenal ulcers are compared in **Table 4.2**. Examination is often normal or reveals epigastric tenderness.

Comparison of gastric and duodenal ulcers		
	Gastric	Duodenal
Clinical features	Epigastric pain soon after eating	Nocturnal or hunger pain
	Relieved by antacids	Relieved by eating
	± Vomiting	Vomiting unusual
	Poor appetite, weight loss	No weight loss
Demographics	Mostly elderly	Mostly <40 years
	Men:women 1:1	Men:women 2:1
Endoscopy	For diagnosis; repeat to assess healing	For diagnosis
Biopsy and testing	CLO test to detect *H. pylori*	CLO test to detect *H. pylori*
	Biopsy of ulcer to detect underlying malignancy	
Treatment	Eradication of *H. pylori* if present	Eradication of *H. pylori* if present
	Acid suppression	Acid suppression
CLO, *Campylobacter*-like organism.		

Table 4.2 Comparison of gastric and duodenal ulcers

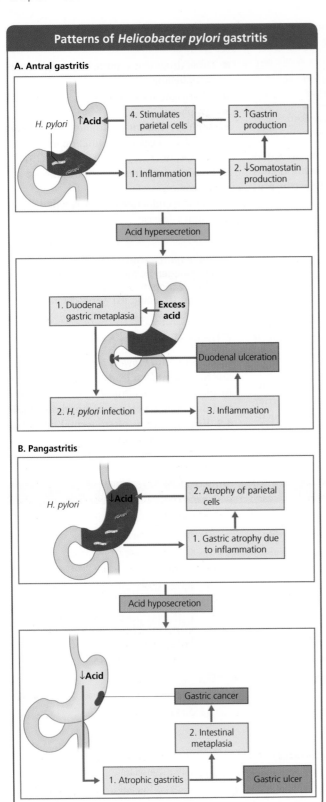

Figure 4.2 Patterns of *Helicobacter pylori* infection. (a) Antral gastritis resulting in duodenal ulceration. (b) Pangastritis resulting in gastric ulcers or cancer.

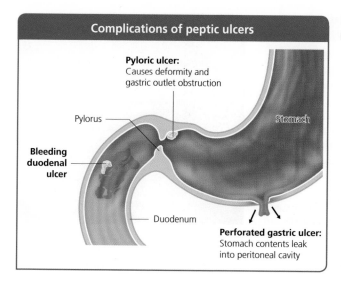

Figure 4.3 Complications of peptic ulcers.

Complications include (**Figure 4.3**):

- **Gastrointestinal bleeding** – this occurs when an ulcer erodes into a blood vessel. It is the most common complication and is sometimes life threatening (see Chapter 10)
- **Perforation** – erosion through the wall of the stomach or duodenum is a surgical emergency and presents with pain and signs of peritonitis
- **Pyloric stenosis and gastric outlet obstruction** – this is caused by duodenal ulcers or ulcers in the very distal stomach, i.e. the antrum when they scar during healing. It causes vomiting of undigested food from the stomach

Diagnostic approach

The diagnosis is usually suggested by the clinical history. The differential diagnosis includes gastro-oesophageal reflux disease, functional (non-ulcer) dyspepsia, gallstone disease and gastric cancer, all of which produce similar symptoms. Endoscopy is the investigation of choice for confirming the diagnosis. Underlying *H. pylori* infection is sought (see below) and eradicated if found. False negatives for the faecal antigen, carbon urea and rapid urease tests are seen if a patient is taking a proton pump inhibitor, so this medication is stopped for 2 weeks before the test is performed.

Investigations

There are several methods of diagnosing *H. pylori* infection, as listed in **Table 4.3**. Serology is often used in primary care but is only of value if the patient has never had treatment previously. Endoscopy does not need to be performed just to diagnose *H. pylori* infection or to check how effective previous treatment has been. The carbon urea breath test is the most reliable.

Blood tests

Iron deficiency anaemia is often present because of chronic bleeding from the ulcer.

> *Helicobacter pylori* **serology is helpful only as an initial test** because antibodies remain in the blood for many years after successful eradication of the infection.

Endoscopy and biopsy

Diagnosis of peptic ulcers is confirmed by gastroscopy (**Figure 4.4**). Ulcers are visible as convex disruptions in the mucosal surface. Biopsies are taken to distinguish between benign and malignant ulcers and a rapid urease or '*Campylobacter*-like organism' ('CLO') test is done to identify *H. pylori* infection (**Figure 4.5**).

Methods of detecting *H. pylori*

Investigation	Description
Urea breath test	Detects *Helicobacter* breakdown of urea into CO_2 and ammonia – see Figure 4.1
Serology	Detects IgG antibodies, confirming past or present exposure (rather than definitively identifying infection)
Faecal antigen test	Detects *H. pylori* antigen, confirming current infection (test also used to confirm eradication)
CLO* test (also called rapid urease test)	Confirms *Helicobacter* urease activity in biopsy specimen placed on pre-prepared slide (see Figure 4.5)
Histology	*Helicobacter pylori* visualised in gastric biopsies on haematoxylin and eosin stains
Culture	Identifies *Helicobacter* antibiotic sensitivities if there is resistance to first- and second-line antibiotics (see Table 4.4)

*Campylobacter-like organism.

Table 4.3 Methods of detecting *Helicobacter pylori*

A repeat endoscopy is scheduled 6–8 weeks after diagnosis of a gastric ulcer to ensure healing and exclude cancer.

Management

Proton pump inhibitors form the mainstay of treatment, together with eradication of *H. pylori* if it is detected. Advice is given on lifestyle measures, such as smoking cessation, limiting alcohol consumption and avoiding precipitating drugs such as NSAIDs or bisphosphonates.

Medication

H. pylori eradication usually involves triple therapy with a proton pump inhibitor and two antibiotics. The concomitant use of two antibiotics increases the success rate of treatment and reduces the development of antibiotic resistance. Antibiotic choice depends on factors such as penicillin allergy (amoxicillin must be avoided), concurrent warfarin therapy (clarithromycin must be avoided because it raises INR) and local guidance based on patterns of antibiotic resistance. Re-testing

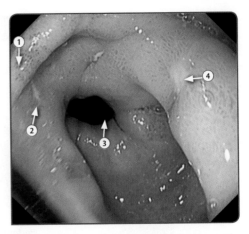

Figure 4.4 Endoscopic image of gastric ulcers and gastritis. ① Red mucosa caused by gastritis. ② Erosion. ③ Pylorus. ④ Superficial gastric ulcer.

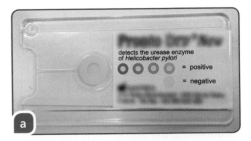

detects the urease enzyme of *Helicobacter pylori*
○ ○ ○ ○ = positive
= negative

a

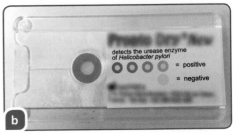

detects the urease enzyme of *Helicobacter pylori*
○ ○ ○ ○ = positive
= negative

b

Figure 4.5 *Campylobacter*-like organism (CLO) test. A biopsy specimen is placed on a gel containing urea and a pH indicator: infection causes urea to be broken down to ammonia, which raises pH and causes a colour change. (a) Negative CLO test. (b) Positive CLO test indicating the presence of *H. pylori*.

for *H. pylori* is performed in patients with ongoing symptoms: if infection persists a second-line regime is prescribed. Examples of 7-day *H. pylori* eradication regimes are given in **Table 4.4**.

Proton pump inhibitors are usually given orally. A 72-hour intravenous infusion is used after endoscopy if there is a high risk of the

7-day *H. pylori* eradication regimes		
	Antibacterial	Acid suppressant
First line	Amoxicillin + clarithromycin *OR* metronidazole + clarithromycin *OR* amoxicillin + metronidazole	Proton pump inhibitor (PPI), e.g. omeprazole
Second line	Amoxicillin + quinolone or tetracycline *OR* metronidazole + levofloxacin *OR* metronidazole + tetracycline + bismuth	

Table 4.4 7-day *Helicobacter pylori* eradication regimes: a combination of one PPI plus ≥2 antibiotics is prescribed. A second-line regime is chosen if the first-line regime fails.

ulcer bleeding, for example if there is a visible artery or active bleeding. It makes the stomach less acidic and therefore stabilises any clot on the ulcer.

H$_2$ receptor antagonists are also effective but are rarely used unless patients experience side effects with proton pump inhibitors as the ulcer takes longer to heal.

> **To remember the 7-day *H. pylori* eradication regimen (triple therapy)**, think 3-2-1: three drugs, twice a day, for 1 week.

Endoscopic treatment

Endoscopic techniques to help achieve haemostasis are used if there are signs of bleeding. These include injection of adrenaline (epinephrine), use of thermal devices or mechanical methods such as clips (see page 153).

Surgery

Surgery is very rarely required but is used to treat complications such as:

- Haemorrhage that cannot be controlled at endoscopy: the vessel is under-run
- Perforation: the defect is treated by oversewing or surgical resection
- Gastric outlet obstruction

> **Surgery for peptic ulcers is now seldom required because of advances in medical and endoscopic treatments.** It occasionally has a role, e.g. after the ulcer has perforated. You will encounter older patients who underwent this surgery a long time ago.

Prognosis

Triple therapy eradicates *H. pylori* in more than 90% of patients. As treatment is effective, re-testing is only done in those who have persistent or recurrent symptoms and in patients in whom a significant complication such as a peptic ulcer bleed has occurred. The carbon urea breath test is the most reliable method to confirm eradication after treatment; the faecal antigen test is also reliable.

Duodenal ulcers are usually benign and, in the absence of complications, heal completely with appropriate treatment.

> **Around 4% of gastric ulcers are malignant.** Therefore, endoscopy is repeated 6–8 weeks after treatment to assess healing and take further biopsies.

Zollinger–Ellison syndrome

This condition is rare. A neuroendocrine tumour in the pancreas or duodenum secretes large amounts of the hormone gastrin which increases the amount of gastric acid produced in the stomach. Patients present with recurrent multiple peptic ulcers and diarrhoea. Zollinger–Ellison syndrome is suspected if a patient has multiple or persistent ulcers with no apparent cause or has received only limited benefit from treatment with PPIs.

Serum gastrin is markedly increased in Zollinger–Ellison syndrome. However false-positive results do sometimes occur in patients taking acid suppressants such as proton pump inhibitors: the feedback mechanism causes a rise in serum gastrin when the pH rises in the stomach. Because of this effect, acid-suppressing treatment should always be stopped for several days before measuring gastrin.

In Zollinger–Ellison syndrome, somatostatin receptor scintigraphy ('octreoscan') helps to locate the tumour because it usually has this receptor on its surface.

Surgical resection of the tumour is the treatment of choice and patients subsequently receive lifelong high-dose proton pump inhibitors. Injections of a somatostatin analogue, e.g. octreotide, are used to help manage the symptoms of diarrhoea and flushing.

Gastritis

Gastritis is inflammation of the stomach lining and is acute or chronic. Acute causes of gastritis are usually secondary to ingestion of medications such as NSAIDs or alcohol. The diagnosis of gastritis is made histologically by endoscopy. Gastritis is identified during investigation of symptoms such as dyspepsia or as a coincidental finding at endoscopy during the investigation of other GI symptoms.

Aetiology

Inflammation of the stomach lining has infectious and non-infectious causes, as summarised in **Table 4.5**. *Helicobacter pylori* is one of the most common causes worldwide.

Clinical features

Gastritis is usually asymptomatic but occasionally presents with epigastric pain, vomiting, haematemesis and weight loss. Clinical examination is normal unless the underlying cause is part of a systemic disease, for example Crohn's disease.

Diagnostic approach

A detailed clinical history is necessary to identify potential causes, including alcohol consumption and over-the-counter medications.

Investigations

If gastritis is suspected, blood tests and non-invasive investigations for *H. pylori* are undertaken in symptomatic patients. These include *H. pylori* serology, faecal antigen and the urea breath test (**Table 4.3**).

Blood tests

Patients are sometimes anaemic as a result of iron or vitamin B_{12} deficiency. If the cause is Crohn's disease they may have raised inflammatory markers.

Endoscopy

Upper GI endoscopy determines the extent of gastritis (antrum, body or whole stomach) and shows erythema, erosions, ulceration or haemorrhage (**Figure 4.4**). Mucosal biopsies are taken to determine the aetiology, and a rapid urease test identifies *H. pylori* infection.

Management

The approach to management depends on identification of the underlying cause (see **Table 4.5**).

Medications

NSAID-induced gastritis is treated by discontinuation of the medication and proton pump inhibitor therapy if symptomatic. Combined with antibiotics, it is also a component of the treatment of *H. pylori* infection (see **Table 4.4**). Vitamin B_{12} injections are required if autoimmune gastritis has caused a deficiency, to avoid complications such as anaemia and peripheral neuropathy. Vitamin B_{12} deficiency occurs due to reduced production of intrinsic factor.

Prognosis

Gastritis is caused by benign aetiologies that do not usually affect life expectancy unless they are a component of a life-shortening systemic disease or therapy, e.g. infections related to immunosuppressive states such as HIV or chemotherapy for cancer.

Causes and treatment of gastritis		
	Cause	Treatment
Infectious		
Bacterial	*Helicobacter pylori*	*H. pylori* eradication (see **Table 4.4**)
	Mycobacteria, actinomycosis, syphilis	Antibiotic
Viral	Herpes viruses (e.g. cytomegalovirus, herpes simplex virus), measles	Antiviral
Fungal	Candidiasis, histoplasmosis	Antifungal
Parasites	Cryptosporidiosis, strongyloidiasis, ascariasis	Antihelmintic/supportive treatment
Non-infectious		
Reactive	NSAIDs, alcohol, cocaine	Discontinue Proton pump inhibitor
	Bile acid reflux	Sucralfate
	Radiation induced (radiotherapy)	No specific treatment
	Ischaemic	Treat underlying causes
Granulomatous	Crohn's disease	See page 211
	Sarcoidosis	Glucocorticosteroids
Other causes	Autoimmune	Vitamin B_{12} replacement
	Atrophic	Vitamin B_{12} or iron replacement
	Collagenous	No known treatment
	Lymphocytic	Eradicate *H. pylori* if present
	Eosinophilic	Glucocorticosteroids
NSAID, non-steroidal anti-inflammatory drug.		

Table 4.5 Aetiology of gastritis, with a summary of treatment

Functional dyspepsia

Functional (non-ulcer) dyspepsia is defined as the presence of symptoms of chronic indigestion with no demonstrable organic abnormality in the upper GI tract.

Epidemiology

Functional dyspepsia occurs at any age. In patients presenting to primary care with upper GI symptoms, it is as common as reflux (i.e. GORD) and more common than ulcer disease.

Aetiology

The condition is poorly understood but is thought to have several dietary and psychological precipitants such as spicy foods, alcohol, anxiety and depression. There is a large overlap with other functional conditions such as irritable bowel syndrome (**Figure 4.6**); patients often have typical features of IBS which if present supports a diagnosis of functional dyspepsia. *Helicobacter pylori* infection is also slightly more common in patients with functional dyspepsia than in the general population.

Clinical features

Patients present with bloating, nausea, early satiety, belching and other dyspeptic symptoms. Symptoms are often similar to those

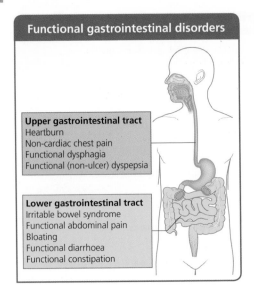

Functional gastrointestinal disorders

Upper gastrointestinal tract
Heartburn
Non-cardiac chest pain
Functional dysphagia
Functional (non-ulcer) dyspepsia

Lower gastrointestinal tract
Irritable bowel syndrome
Functional abdominal pain
Bloating
Functional diarrhoea
Functional constipation

Figure 4.6 Functional gastrointestinal disorders.

significantly (and with the targeted exclusion of other diagnoses, e.g. gallstones which are visible on an abdominal ultrasound) functional dyspepsia is the likely diagnosis.

Investigations

These are undertaken to exclude other significant pathology that give similar symptoms such as liver or biliary tree disease, peptic ulcers or gastric cancer:

- Full blood count and liver function tests are normal in patients with functional dyspepsia
- *H. pylori* testing is positive or negative
- Symptoms are atypical or severe in a minority of patients, so an endoscopy must be carried out to exclude other diagnoses such as ulcers or cancer. The result will be normal.

seen in gastro-oesophageal reflux disease and peptic ulcer disease. It is common for patients to have coexisting irritable bowel syndrome, but no weight loss or 'alarm' upper GI symptoms suggestive of more serious disease and malignancy (see **Table 3.2**) are present.

Diagnostic approach

It is often difficult to be certain whether the patient has gastro-oesophageal reflux, an ulcer or functional dyspepsia from the history. In the absence of any symptoms suggesting an upper GI tract malignancy, the patient is offered a trial of acid suppression and *H. pylori* treatment. If this does not help

Management

The patient is informed about lifestyle and dietary changes that will benefit them. Regular meals, avoiding identifiable food precipitants, smoking cessation and reduced alcohol consumption help reduce the symptoms. Some patients are helped by antispasmodics (e.g. hyoscine), prokinetics (e.g. domperidone), or low-dosage tricyclic antidepressants (e.g. amitriptyline).

If *H. pylori* is detected, eradication treatment is given. However this provides long-term benefit in very few of these patients because *H. pylori* appears to play only a minor role in this setting.

Gastric neoplasia

Gastric neoplasia refers to the abnormal growth of cells in the stomach, resulting in a malignant or benign tumour. Ninety-five percent of gastric tumours are adenocarcinomas but other types also occur, including lymphomas, GI stromal tumours and benign neoplasms (**Table 4.6**).

Epidemiology

Gastric cancer has huge geographical variation. It is the fourth most common cancer worldwide, being particularly common in Asia, but only the 15th most common cancer in the UK. It is primarily found in people over 65 years old and has a male-to-female ratio of 3:1. It is more common in smokers.

Features of gastric neoplasms	
Type	**Features**
Malignant	
Adenocarcinoma (95% of gastric cancers)	Initially: barely visible at endoscopy
	Later: polypoidal, ulcerative or diffusely infiltrating (linitis plastica)
Primary gastric lymphoma	Usually B-cell non-Hodgkin's, most of which are high grade
	Fewer are low-grade MALT lymphomas occurring as an immunological response to chronic *H. pylori* infection
Gastrointestinal stromal tumour	Develop in submucosa or muscularis mucosae
	Express c-KIT oncogene (tyrosine kinase receptor)
	Variable malignant potential
Benign	
Hyperplastic or cystic fundal polyp(s)	Asymptomatic but very common endoscopy finding
	More common in patients taking long-term proton pump inhibitors
Adenoma	Uncommon and premalignant
MALT, mucosa-associated lymphoid tissue.	

Table 4.6 Features of gastric neoplasms

Aetiology

In patients with pangastritis and *H. pylori* infection (see **Figure 4.2**), there is an initial atrophic gastritis and then intestinal metaplasia before dysplasia and cancer develop. In Asia, where gastric cancer is more prevalent, the local diet (containing a higher level of N-nitrosamines than the Western diet) and genetic factors contribute.

Clinical features

The initial symptoms of gastric cancer are often vague and many patients do not consult a doctor. By the time they do present, the cancer is often advanced with metastases. Patients may have one or more of the following typical symptoms:

- Weight loss
- Anorexia and lethargy
- Abdominal pain or dyspepsia
- Early satiety
- Nausea and vomiting
- Haematemesis or melaena

Benign lesions are asymptomatic but occasionally are seen at the time of endoscopy, where close inspection and biopsy help determine their nature.

Diagnostic approach

The suspicion of gastric cancer arises when a patient presents with the clinical features listed above. To confirm this suspicion, endoscopy and scans are required; these are also used to stage the tumour if one is found.

Investigations

Blood tests

The results often show iron deficiency, which is caused by bleeding from the tumour. Abnormal liver function tests suggest liver metastases and the likelihood of incurable disease. There is no tumour marker for gastric cancer.

Endoscopy

Upper GI endoscopy is the preferred investigation (**Figure 4.7**). Histological confirmation is obtained from biopsies.

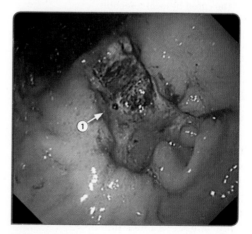

Figure 4.7 Endoscopic appearance of gastric cancer. ① Large malignant gastric ulcer with rolled irregular edges.

Imaging

CT scans diagnose the cancer or help in staging if the chest and abdomen are imaged to determine lymph node involvement and metastatic spread. Endoscopic ultrasound is also used for staging.

Laparoscopy

Diagnostic laparoscopy is used in selected patients in whom the cancer appears to be localised, to determine surgical resectability.

Management (Table 4.7)

When an adenocarcinoma is confined to the gastric wall, it can be removed by endoscopic or surgical resection (which is often laparoscopic) (see Figure 2.38). In more locally advanced disease, combined chemo-radiotherapy is occasionally used to reduce the size of the tumour prior to surgery or used as palliative treatment if there are metastases which cannot be cured.

Prognosis

Only 15% of patients are alive at 5 years after diagnosis.

> **In Asia, where gastric cancer is particularly common, some countries have screening programmes.** Early stomach cancer is picked up by endoscopy before it causes symptoms and at a stage where it is more likely to be cured by local resection.

Treatment of gastric neoplasms	
Type	Treatment
Malignant	
Adenocarcinoma (95% of malignant gastric lesions)	Early stage: curative endoscopic or surgical resection
	Palliation and downstaging: chemotherapy (e.g. epirubicin, cisplatin, 5-fluorouracil and capecitabine)
Lymphoma	Surgery or combined chemo-radiotherapy, depending on extent and type
	MALT lymphomas: *H. pylori* eradication (cures 80%; the rest are treated as for other lymphomas)
Gastrointestinal stromal tumour	Imatinib (monoclonal antibody against tyrosine kinase inhibitor) is generally effective (see Table 4.6)
	Curative endoscopic or surgical resection for localised disease
Benign	
Hyperplastic or cystic fundal polyps	No action required
Adenomas	Endoscopic or surgical removal

MALT, mucosa-associated lymphoid tissue.

Table 4.7 Treatment of gastric neoplasms

Motility disorders

Motility refers to the peristaltic movement of muscles within the oesophagus, stomach and small intestine. When there is a change in muscle contractions there is either a delay in gastric emptying or a rapid emptying of gastric content. Motility problems are also present in some people with functional dyspepsia.

Gastroparesis

In this condition there is a delay in gastric emptying from the stomach into the small intestine. It is more common in individuals with diabetes but is sometimes idiopathic and occurs in those taking opioid analgesia.

Aetiology

The change in motility seen in gastroparesis is usually neurological in origin; there is abnormal contraction in the stomach or the pylorus opens at incorrect times, preventing food from leaving the stomach. This must be distinguished from mechanical causes in which the pylorus is narrowed because of cancer, an ulcer or a congenital cause (presenting with projectile vomiting in newborn children).

Clinical features

These include:

- Nausea and vomiting, which often occurs with undigested food a while after eating
- Early satiety and bloating
- Weight loss if the condition is severe or chronic

Investigations

If gastroparesis is suspected from the history, further investigation is carried out. Endoscopy is the usual initial investigation to exclude a mechanical cause. Even though the patient has fasted, endoscopy sometimes shows a distended stomach containing food. A gastric emptying study or barium meal study confirms delayed emptying and is diagnostic.

Management

Minor symptoms often respond to dietary modification. Patients are told to eat more frequent, smaller meals that are lower in fat and fibre. If the patient is diabetic, optimising blood sugar control sometimes improves the gastric symptoms. Trials of prokinetic agents, for example domperidone, are variably helpful.

In severe symptoms, injection of botulinum toxin into the pylorus at endoscopy occasionally helps and feeding through a jejunostomy is sometimes necessary. Gastric stimulation via the surgical insertion of a gastric pacemaker is a possible treatment but the benefits are variable.

Dumping syndrome

This occurs when gastric contents, which are normally stored in the stomach and released periodically through the pylorus, pass too quickly into the small intestine. This causes osmotic fluid shifts and has an effect on nutrient digestion and absorption. Dumping is described as 'early' (during or shortly after meals) or 'late' (up to 3 hours after food) and many patients experience both. It usually occurs as a consequence of gastric surgery (see Figure 2.38).

Clinical features

These include:

- Nausea, vomiting, cramping epigastric pain, diarrhoea, fatigue and dizziness (early dumping)
- Hypoglycaemia, weakness, sweating and dizziness (late dumping)

Diagnostic approach

Dumping syndrome is considered in any patient with compatible symptoms who has had a previous gastrectomy. Tests are often performed to exclude other causes of these symptoms, such as a peptic ulcer, intestinal obstruction and gallstones.

Investigations

Blood tests and endoscopy findings are normal, apart from any evidence of previous surgery. Barium meal and radio-isotope scans confirm accelerated gastric emptying.

Management

The main approach is dietary. Measures that help include eating smaller, more frequent meals with an increased intake of soluble fibre, fats, complex carbohydrates and proteins. Patients are also told to limit their fluid intake with food, reduce the intake of simple sugars and change, for example, solid food such as meat to minced products.

Answers to starter questions

1. Different patterns of *H. pylori* infection predispose to different diseases. Infection of the antrum causes increased gastrin production and acid levels, which leads to duodenitis and duodenal ulcers. Infection of the gastric body (i.e. the main, central region of the stomach) leads to reduced acid production with resultant gastric atrophy, gastric ulcers and malignancy. Only a small minority of patients with *H. pylori* infection develop cancer – this is thought to depend on the *H. pylori* subtype and different host–infection interactions.

2. All patients with a gastric ulcer diagnosed at oesophagogastroduodenoscopy should have a repeat endoscopy after receiving treatment with a proton pump inhibitor for 6–8 weeks (and *H. pylori* eradication if appropriate). This is because up to 5% of gastric ulcers are an ulcerated malignancy whereas duodenal cancer is extremely rare and virtually never seen in clinical practice. Patients should have repeat endoscopies with biopsies until the ulcer has healed in order to detect malignancy as early as possible.

3. Nonsteroidal anti-inflammatory drugs (NSAIDs) cause a number of different GI side effects including peptic ulcers, bleeding from any site, hepatitis and colitis. They should therefore be used sparingly, and patients should be advised to monitor for dyspepsia and other GI symptoms. Co-prescription with a PPI has been shown to reduce the frequency of NSAID-induced upper GI damage.

4. Gastric cancer is thought to be more prevalent in South East Asia due to higher rates of *H. pylori* infection, particularly with certain bacterial subtypes. Other influences likely include genetic factors leading to a greater susceptibility to carcinogenesis, and a diet high in N-nitrosamines, e.g. beer, processed fish, and meat and cheese products preserved with nitrites.

Chapter 5
Small intestine and malabsorption disorders

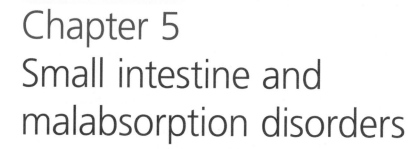

Starter questions

Reading this chapter will enable you to answer the following questions. Answers are on page 215.

1. How is suspected malabsorption investigated?
2. Is coeliac disease curable?
3. How do the pathological features of Crohn's disease explain its different clinical presentations?
4. Why is cancer of the small bowel so uncommon?

Introduction

The small intestine is crucial for health as it is the primary site where nutrients are digested and absorbed. Significant dysfunction results in marked weight loss and malabsorption, with diarrhoea, steatorrhoea and deficiencies of several minerals and vitamins. The clinical presentation is, however, often more subtle. In contrast, small bowel obstruction is a surgical emergency.

The most common diseases of the small bowel are due to infection, inflammation, autoimmune-mediated damage and, more rarely, cancer. Worldwide, infectious aetiologies are common, leading to significant morbidity and mortality. Crohn's disease is a chronic inflammatory disorder that affects any region of the intestine, especially the terminal ileum and is particularly common in North America and some parts of Europe. Coeliac disease is an autoimmune condition triggered by dietary gluten and is relatively common in developed countries; however, only a minority of patients are diagnosed because symptoms, if they are present, are often only minor or non-specific.

Case 5 Weight loss and anaemia

Presentation

Chloe Evans is a 24-year-old woman who presents to her general practitioner (GP) with a 4-month history of increasing lethargy, weight loss of 6 kg and diarrhoea. She has hypothyroidism that is adequately controlled with levothyroxine.

Initial interpretation

Diarrhoea can be caused by:

- Small or large bowel disease
- Pancreatic disorders
- Endocrine conditions such as hyperthyroidism
- Exogenous factors including drugs, excess alcohol and diet
- Infections

Diarrhoea must be assessed in terms of its onset, frequency (including nocturnal symptoms), consistency and colour. Stool consistency can broadly be described as liquid, semi-formed or formed, but the Bristol stool chart allows a more accurate description (see Figure 2.4). Pale, offensive or oily stool is due to the presence of excess fat and suggests malabsorption in the small intestine. The chronic nature of Chloe's symptoms makes an infective aetiology less likely.

Lethargy is a common and non-specific symptom. It can occur secondary to anaemia and haematinic deficiencies or one of several underlying metabolic disorders. Chloe's history of hypothyroidism means that thyroid function tests should be undertaken.

An unintentional weight loss of 6 kg over 4 months is a worrying sign and usually indicates the presence of a significant medical condition. In Chloe's context, it supports an underlying gastrointestinal (GI) pathology. A history of rectal bleeding

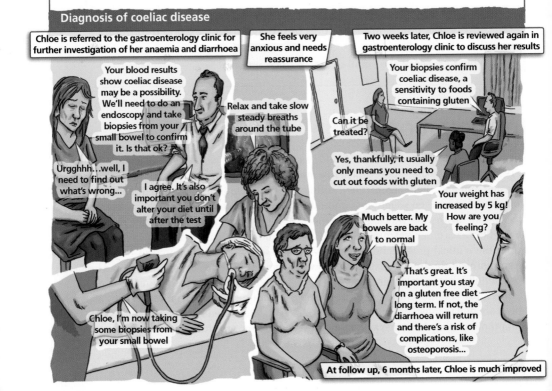

Diagnosis of coeliac disease

Chloe is referred to the gastroenterology clinic for further investigation of her anaemia and diarrhoea

She feels very anxious and needs reassurance

Two weeks later, Chloe is reviewed again in gastroenterology clinic to discuss her results

Your blood results show coeliac disease may be a possibility. We'll need to do an endoscopy and take biopsies from your small bowel to confirm it. Is that ok?

Relax and take slow steady breaths around the tube

Your biopsies confirm coeliac disease, a sensitivity to foods containing gluten

Urgghhh...well, I need to find out what's wrong...

I agree. It's also important you don't alter your diet until after the test

Can it be treated?

Yes, thankfully, it usually only means you need to cut out foods with gluten

Your weight has increased by 5 kg! How are you feeling?

Much better. My bowels are back to normal

Chloe, I'm now taking some biopsies from your small bowel

That's great. It's important you stay on a gluten free diet long term. If not, the diarrhoea will return and there's a risk of complications, like osteoporosis...

At follow up, 6 months later, Chloe is much improved

Case 5 *continued*

suggests a colonic cause such as inflammatory bowel disease or malignancy.

> **Talking about diarrhoea is often embarrassing for patients but make sure you ask about stool frequency.** This includes nocturnal symptoms. Example questions include 'How many times a day do you open your bowels?' and 'Do you ever wake at night to open your bowels?'

Further history

Chloe also describes abdominal bloating and distension that is worse after eating bread and pasta. She has a normal appetite with no upper GI symptoms, abdominal or joint pains. She passes pale, semi-formed stool six times during the day. She also wakes up twice during the night to defaecate. There is no history of blood or mucus being passed from the rectum. She has recently noticed an itchy rash over her trunk and the extensor surfaces of her arms and legs.

Chloe's mother has experienced similar GI symptoms and has recently been diagnosed with osteoporosis at the age of 50.

Examination

Chloe appears thin and her body mass index (BMI) is 15 kg/m², meaning she is underweight. She has pale conjunctivae and angular stomatitis (**Figure 5.1**). The remainder of her abdominal examination is normal and there are no palpable lymph nodes. Small blisters are noted on her thighs. Rectal examination reveals no masses.

There are no abnormal findings on examination of the cardiovascular and respiratory systems.

Interpretation of findings

Together, the pale and loose stool, bloating and significant weight loss suggest

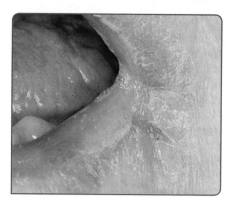

Figure 5.1 Angular stomatitis (cheilitis) is cracking or inflammation at the corners of the mouth that is secondary to iron deficiency anaemia.

Features of small bowel disease	
Category	Features
Symptoms	Steatorrhoea (pale stool)
	Weight loss
	Diarrhoea
	Abdominal bloating or distension
	Abdominal pain (colicky)
Physical signs	Thin body or evidence of weight loss
	Angular stomatitis or glossitis
	Koilonychia
	Aphthoid mouth ulcers
	Distended abdomen
Signs revealed by laboratory tests	Haematinic deficiency
	Anaemia
	Raised CRP or ESR
	Low albumin
	Low magnesium or calcium

CRP, C-reactive protein; ESR, erythrocyte sedimentation rate.

Table 5.1 Features of small bowel disease

a small bowel disease that is causing malabsorption (**Table 5.1**). Abdominal palpation is often normal in small bowel disease. Disease of the large bowel is less likely to be the cause because there is no sign of rectal bleeding.

Case 5 *continued*

Chloe's pale conjunctivae and angular stomatitis suggest iron deficiency anaemia, which is often seen in conditions causing malabsorption. The family history raises the possibility of a hereditary component to the condition.

The main differential diagnoses to consider are coeliac disease and small bowel Crohn's disease. Because of the dietary triggers identified, coeliac disease is most likely.

Investigations

Blood tests for coeliac serology (anti-tTG antibodies and IgA levels) are requested, as well as inflammatory markers [C-reactive protein (CRP) and erythrocyte sedimentation rate (ESR)] that are increased in Crohn's disease. Ferritin, folate, vitamin D and vitamin B_{12} levels are also assessed as these are often low in small bowel disorders due to malabsorption. Three stool samples are taken to exclude infective causes and measure faecal calprotectin (released by white cells in the intestinal wall).

The results of Chloe's blood tests are given in **Table 5.2**. No cysts, ova or parasites are detected in the stool samples, and the faecal calprotectin level is low (20 µg/g, normal being levels <100 µg/g), suggesting the cause is not an inflammatory disease.

Chloe's test results show a mixed pattern of haematinic deficiency (low ferritin and folate, with normal vitamin B12) so her GP refers her to the hospital gastroenterology department for further assessment in accordance with **Table 5.3**. This includes outpatient upper GI tract endoscopy with duodenal biopsies. Chloe is advised to remain on a normal diet while awaiting the endoscopy and is prescribed oral iron and folic acid supplements because her low ferritin and folate levels show these are both deficient which has made her anaemic.

Chloe's blood test results	
Test	Result (normal range)
Haemoglobin (Hb)	90 g/L (115–165 g/L in women)
Mean corpuscular volume (MCV)	70 fL (80–96 fL)
Mean cell haemoglobin	24 pg (28–32 pg)
Platelets	165 x 10^9/L (150–400 x 10^9/L)
Ferritin	5 µg/L (15–300 µg/L)
Vitamin B_{12}	324 ng/L (160–760 ng/L)
Folate	1.2 µg/L (2–11 µg/L)
Vitamin D	32 ng/mL (20–50 ng/mL)
Anti-tissue transglutaminase (anti-tTG) antibodies	125 U/mL (<15 U/mL)
IgA	1.2 g/L (0.8–3.0 g/L)
Erythrocyte sedimentation rate (ESR)	8 mm/h (0–15 mm/h)
C-reactive protein (CRP)	2 mg/L (<5 mg/L)

Table 5.2 Chloe's blood test results

On upper GI endoscopy, the duodenal mucosa has a flattened appearance. Duodenal biopsies are taken; they show a flattened villous architecture and a higher than normal number of intraepithelial lymphocytes.

Diagnosis

The biopsy confirms a diagnosis of coeliac disease. In the outpatient clinic, Chloe is reviewed by a gastroenterologist and by a specialist dietician, who gives her advice on a gluten-free diet. The rash is diagnosed as dermatitis herpetiformis, which occurs in 2–5% of people with coeliac disease (**Figure 5.2**). A baseline dual-energy X-ray absorptiometry (DEXA) bone scan

Case 5 *continued*

Investigation of haematinic deficiency

Deficiency	Investigations
Iron	Premenopausal women: anti-tTG antibodies*
	Men and postmenopausal women: upper and lower GI endoscopy (or alternative) ± small bowel studies; urine dipstick for haematuria
Vitamin B₁₂	Intrinsic factor
	Anti-tTG antibodies
Folate	Anti-tTG antibodies
Mixed	Anti-tTG antibodies
	Upper GI endoscopy; lower GI tract or small bowel investigations
	Faecal elastase if diarrhoeal symptoms

tTG, tissue transglutaminase.

*In premenopausal women, menstrual blood loss is by far the commonest cause of iron deficiency.

Table 5.3 Investigation of deficiency of haematinics (nutrients required for red blood cell formation)

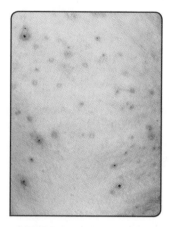

Figure 5.2 Dermatitis herpetiformis is an intensely itchy blistering rash typically seen on the extensor surfaces of the limbs and trunk. It is strongly associated with coeliac disease.

shows that her bone density is within the normal range. Osteoporosis often occurs in untreated coeliac disease due to the malabsorption of calcium and vitamin D, but Chloe has not developed this problem.

The hyposplenism, present in about a third of patents with coeliac disease, increases the risk of infection, particularly with encapsulated bacteria. Chloe is therefore told to be vaccinated against pneumococcus, meningitis C and *Haemophilus influenzae* type B which provide lifelong immunity. She is also advised to have the annual flu vaccine.

When Chloe returns to the clinic for her 6-month follow-up, her BMI and anti-tTG antibodies have both returned to normal levels.

Malabsorption

Malabsorption is the failure of absorption of one or more nutrients from the GI tract. It is caused by disease processes that disrupt digestion, mucosal function or motility. The site of absorption of the various nutrients is summarised in Figure 1.50 and Table 1.27.

Epidemiology

This varies considerably depending on the aetiology. Infective causes are more prevalent in developing countries (**Table 5.4**), whereas inflammatory bowel disease is more common in developed countries.

Infective causes of malabsorption		
Causative pathogen	Distinguishing features	Evidence of infection
Tropical sprue	Recent enteric infection Tropical area (Asia, South America)	Partial villous atrophy on duodenal biopsy
Giardiasis (*Giardia lamblia*)	Travel history Watery diarrhoea, anorexia, abdominal pain	Stool culture for cysts Parasites or villous atrophy seen on duodenal biopsy
Whipple's disease (*Tropheryma whipplei*)	Arthropathy, skin pigmentation Lymphadenopathy, fever	Macrophages on periodic acid-–Schiff staining on duodenal biopsy
Intestinal tuberculosis (*Mycobacterium tuberculosis*)	Weight loss, anorexia, abdominal pain, right iliac fossa mass HIV infection, area endemic for TB	Small bowel imaging Laparoscopy and biopsy Tuberculin test, chest radiograph
Cholera (*Vibrio cholerae*)	Profuse watery diarrhoea ('rice-water stool') Dehydration, acute renal impairment, electrolyte imbalance	Identification of the bacteria in a stool sample
HIV enteropathy	HIV infection, profuse diarrhoea	Absence of identifiable GI pathogen in confirmed HIV
Other parasitic infection (hookworm, roundworm)	Worldwide prevalence, particularly deprived rural areas	Ova detected on stool microscopy

Table 5.4 Common infective causes of malabsorption

Aetiology

The main non-infective causes of malabsorption are:

- Coeliac disease
- Crohn's disease
- Lactase deficiency
- Bacterial overgrowth
- Bile salt malabsorption
- Short bowel syndrome
- Radiation enteropathy
- Pancreatic insufficiency

Clinical features

The clinical features help target investigations that will make the diagnosis (**Table 5.5**). They vary depending on the underlying cause and its severity. Mild disease is usually asymptomatic, but more severe malabsorption presents with diarrhoea and weight loss. Steatorrhoea (pale, malodorous, voluminous stools that are difficult to flush away) is typical of fat malabsorption. However, it is not as common as diarrhoea. Non-specific symptoms such as bloating and abdominal discomfort often occur.

Further clues from the history sometimes suggest the underlying aetiology:

- A family history suggests a diagnosis of coeliac or Crohn's disease
- Lactose intolerance (also called 'lactase deficiency') affects over 90% of Asians and black African populations but has a prevalence of less than 10% in Northern Europe
- Alcohol excess suggests underlying chronic pancreatitis
- A history of travel points towards an infective cause particularly if the travelling was in the developing world
- A previous history of surgery or radiotherapy is also significant because both cause diarrhoea when part of the GI tract is removed or damaged

Physical examination is often completely normal or sometimes includes features of haematinic deficiency, such as conjunctival pallor or glossitis (**Figure 5.3**). Patients sometimes appear underweight. Specific nutritional deficiencies are occasionally seen (**Table 5.6**).

Non-infective causes of malabsorption		
Cause	Clinical features*	Investigation
Coeliac disease	Often asymptomatic Family history Other autoimmune conditions Relation to foods containing gluten	Raised anti-tTG antibodies Villous atrophy on duodenal biopsy
Crohn's disease	Family history Extraintestinal features	Raised inflammatory markers Raised faecal calprotectin Small bowel radiology Colonoscopy
Lactase deficiency	Relation to dairy products African/Asian ethnicity	Lactose intolerance test
Bacterial overgrowth	Previous surgery, small bowel diverticulosis Immunosuppression, diabetes mellitus	Glucose hydrogen breath test
Bile salt malabsorption	Postprandial diarrhoea Past cholecystectomy, Crohn's disease, ileal resection	Abnormal SeHCAT scan
Short bowel syndrome	Previous extensive surgical resection	Electrolyte imbalance
Radiation enteropathy	Previous radiotherapy	Small bowel imaging
Pancreatic insufficiency	Steatorrhoea Alcohol excess	Low faecal elastase

tTG, tissue transglutaminase.
*In addition to malabsorption

Table 5.5 Clinical features and investigation of non-infective causes of malabsorption

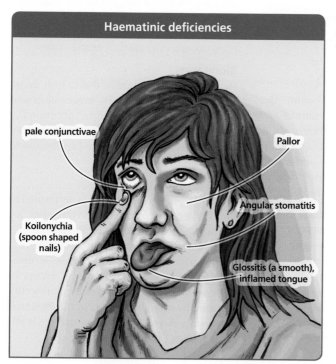

Haematinic deficiencies

pale conjunctivae

Pallor

Angular stomatitis

Koilonychia
(spoon shaped
nails)

Glossitis (a smooth),
inflamed tongue

Figure 5.3 Haematinic deficiencies produce several signs on clinical examination.

Nutritional consequences of malabsorption	
Deficiency	**Clinical features**
Iron	Pallor, glossitis, angular stomatitis
Folate	Pallor, glossitis
Vitamin B$_{12}$	Neuropathy, psychological effects
Protein	Oedema, muscle wasting
Fat-soluble vitamins:	
Vitamin A	Night blindness, dry eyes
Vitamin D	Osteomalacia (adults), rickets (children)
Vitamin K	Prolonged prothrombin time, easy bruising
Vitamin E	Ataxia, neuropathy
Calcium	Tetany or weakness
Magnesium	Weakness, fatigue
Trace elements, e.g. selenium, zinc	Fatigue, hair and nail changes, rash

Table 5.6 Nutritional consequences of malabsorption

> **Always consider malabsorption in a patient who presents with weight loss, diarrhoea and nutrient deficiencies.**

Diagnostic approach

Initial investigations (full blood count, electrolyte and bone profile, haematinic and vitamin levels) often show deficiencies of one or more of the nutrients listed in **Table 5.6**. More specific tests are then performed, which are guided by the initial investigation results and clinical features (**Table 5.5**):

■ Further blood tests (inflammatory markers, thyroid function, anti-tTG antibodies, immunoglobulin A [IgA] concentrations)
■ Stool microscopy – infection is considered particularly where risk factors exist (see **Table 5.4**)
■ Faecal elastase is measured where there is history of chronic pancreatitis

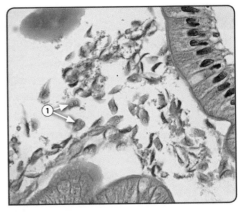

Figure 5.4 Duodenal biopsy showing *Giardia lamblia* trophozoites ①.

or significant alcohol ingestion which damages the pancreas.
■ The faecal calprotectin level is increased where there is inflammation of the intestinal lining
■ Upper GI endoscopy with duodenal biopsies (**Figure 5.4**)
■ Further imaging and/or breath tests

Investigations

The order and priority of investigations depends on which conditions are suspected from the history. A combination of investigations is usually required to diagnose the underlying cause and assess the consequences.

Blood tests

Patients are often anaemic due to iron, folate or B$_{12}$ deficiency. Calcium, magnesium and albumin concentrations are occasionally low. A prolonged prothrombin time is caused by vitamin K deficiency. Raised antibodies to tTG suggest coeliac disease.

Stool tests

Stool microscopy and culture is performed to look for bacteria, ova, cysts and parasites, for example *Giardia lamblia*. Repeated samples are taken as excretion is often intermittent.

The pancreatic enzyme elastase is measurable in the faeces; a low level occurs in pancreatic insufficiency. Faecal calprotectin, released by white blood cells in the intestinal mucosa, is increased in inflammatory conditions such as Crohn's disease.

Non-pathogenic microorganisms are present throughout the GI tract and have immune and metabolic functions, e.g. regulating fat storage and producing vitamins B and K and short-chain fatty acids. The small intestine is relatively sterile compared with the large intestine, but it experiences bacterial overgrowth if there are changes in structure (e.g. after surgery) or metabolism (e.g. diabetes mellitus) that promote bacterial colonisation.

Endoscopy

Upper GI endoscopy with duodenal biopsies is the initial investigation of choice to diagnose coeliac disease. Capsule endoscopy visualises the mucosa of the more distal small intestine which lies beyond the reach of the endoscope.

Imaging

Small bowel radiology such as a magnetic resonance enterogram (see page 121) identifies underlying structural abnormalities including stricturing Crohn's disease or jejunal diverticulosis.

Hydrogen breath tests

These tests screen for underlying lactose intolerance or bacterial overgrowth in the small intestine (see page 115).

SeHCAT scan

Retention of less than 15% of the administered dosage of tauroselcholic [^{75}selenium] acid after 1 week signifies excess bile salt loss, demonstrating bile salt malabsorption (see page 127).

Management

The approach to management is divided into:

- Identification and treatment of the underlying cause (see **Tables 5.4** and **5.5**)
- Correction of nutritional and haematinic deficiencies, for example iron, vitamin B$_{12}$ and vitamin D. This is achieved through enriched foods and if these are insufficient, the use of oral, intramuscular or intravenous supplements

Prognosis

Once identified, most small bowel causes of malabsorption are treated with dietary modifications or medications, without any long-term impact on survival.

Coeliac disease

Coeliac disease is a lifelong sensitivity to the protein gluten. It is an autoimmune disorder rather than a food intolerance or allergy (**Table 5.7**). It leads to disruption of the structure and function of the small intestine mucosa, resulting in malabsorption. Coeliac disease sometimes interferes significantly with quality of life but is simple to treat by adopting a life-long gluten-free diet.

Types of disorder causing symptoms after food ingestion		
Type of reaction	Mechanism	Symptoms
Autoimmune, e.g. coeliac disease	T-cell-mediated immune response	Asymptomatic, GI symptoms (see page 208)
Intolerance, e.g. lactose or fructose	Non-immune, due to specific enzyme deficit or reaction to salicylates or other chemicals in food	Abdominal pain, bloating, diarrhoea
Allergy, e.g. peanuts	Immunoglobulin E-mediated immune reaction	Systemic upset, rash, oedema, bronchospasm

Table 5.7 A comparison of types of disorder causing symptoms after ingestion of food

Epidemiology

Up to 1% of the population in Europe and North America are affected. It presents at any age and there is a slight (2:1) female preponderance. There is a 10% risk of having coeliac disease if a first-degree relative is also affected.

Aetiology

Gluten is a protein present in wheat, barley and rye. In coeliac disease, ingestion of gluten leads to an abnormal T-cell-mediated immune response.

Gliadin, one of the two main protein groups in gluten, is absorbed into the mucosa of the small intestine and is then modified in the lamina propria by the enzyme tissue transglutaminase (tTG). Individuals with coeliac disease have T cells that recognise this modified gliadin and secrete lymphokines which lead to persistent inflammation and damage to the endothelial villi, particularly in the duodenum and jejunum. These lymphokines also stimulate plasma B cells to produce anti-tTG antibodies (including types of immunoglobulin A), which attack the tTG. These anti-tTG antibodies are measured to obtain a diagnosis.

> Some individuals with coeliac disease also seem to be sensitive to oats, but this is probably because of cross-contamination during cereal growth or harvesting or in food manufacturing.

Clinical features

In patients with coeliac disease there are often no abnormal findings on physical examination. Coeliac disease is sometimes asymptomatic or presents with one or more of a wide range of features:

- Fatigue, caused by the symptoms or a nutrient deficiency
- Gastrointestinal symptoms that are wide ranging and include bloating, diarrhoea, steatorrhoea, abdominal pain and even constipation
- Weight loss that is either gradual or occurs over many months or years

- Nutrient deficiencies with specific consequences (**Table 5.6**)
- Failure to thrive (infants) and delayed puberty and short stature (children) because of malnutrition and nutrient malabsorption during critical developmental periods
- Dermatitis herpetiformis

A few patients have associated conditions including inflammatory bowel disease, microscopic colitis, Down's syndrome and Turner's syndrome. Autoimmune disorders such as type 1 diabetes mellitus, Addison's disease, thyroid disorders, autoimmune hepatitis, primary biliary cholangitis and Sjögren's syndrome are sometimes also present. It is not known whether these conditions have the same predisposition to coeliac disease or are in any way related to the gluten-induced damage to the small intestine.

> **Always check coeliac serology in patients with GI symptoms even if these are not obviously related to eating food containing gluten.** Coeliac disease affects 1% of the population and presents with a wide range of symptoms.

Complications

Complications occur secondary to untreated or poorly controlled coeliac disease, and all resolve or become much less common when the condition is treated. They include:

- Malabsorption of vitamins and minerals
- Osteoporosis and osteomalacia as a result of vitamin D malabsorption
- Lactose intolerance due to the destruction of villi and a decreased amount of the enzyme lactase
- Hyposplenism (a small, underactive spleen) (the mechanism is unclear)
- Reduced fertility, probably due to nutrient deficiencies
- With pregnancy, low-birthweight and premature birth, due to nutrient deficiencies
- Neurological conditions – peripheral neuropathy, epilepsy, depression and

bipolar disease; vitamin and other nutrient deficiencies contribute to these
- T-cell lymphomas and adenocarcinomas of the small intestine

Diagnostic approach

Because it affects so many people and has a wide range of presentations, coeliac disease is considered in all patients presenting with GI symptoms or nutrient deficiencies. Suspicion is further raised if the history reveals there is a coexisting autoimmune condition or a family history of coeliac disease. The diagnosis is then made using a combination of blood tests and histology following biopsy of the small intestine.

Investigations

If coeliac disease is suspected, the usual sequence for investigation is:

- Initially, blood tests for anti-tTG antibodies – the patient is referred to a gastroenterologist if the level is raised or there is strong suspicion of the diagnosis
- Upper GI endoscopy to obtain duodenal biopsies
- Further blood tests and a DEXA scan to assess for associated complications

Blood tests
Testing for raised IgA autoantibodies against tTG is highly sensitive and specific for untreated coeliac disease. False-negative results occur if the individual is on a gluten-free diet, because their tTG antibody level returns to normal. A false negative result also occurs if the patient has IgA deficiency, a genetic disorder that is usually asymptomatic. IgA deficiency occurs in 2.5% of individuals with coeliac disease but only 0.5% of the general population; the reason for this is unknown.

Duodenal biopsy
The duodenal lining often looks flattened at endoscopy. Biopsies show villous atrophy with compensatory crypt hyperplasia and lymphocytes in the epithelium of the small intestine (**Figure 5.5**). Because these resolve with gluten avoidance, it is essential that initial biopsies are obtained on an unrestricted diet.

Other tests
After the diagnosis has been made, blood tests are performed to look for deficiencies

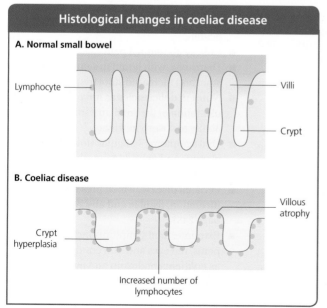

A. Normal small bowel
Lymphocyte — Villi
— Crypt

B. Coeliac disease
Crypt hyperplasia — Villous atrophy
Increased number of lymphocytes

Figure 5.5 Histological changes in coeliac disease: villous atrophy, crypt hyperplasia and increased numbers of intraepithelial lymphocytes.

of haematinics, vitamins and minerals. A DEXA scan is performed to assess bone density for osteoporosis.

Management

A permanent gluten-free diet resolves the symptoms of malabsorption and reduces the long-term consequences. A dietitian will advise on a balanced and appropriate intake, which sometimes includes supplements for nutrient deficiencies. The complications associated with coeliac disease should be treated.

Prognosis

The sensitivity to gluten continues throughout life in those with coeliac disease. In the absence of complications, adopting a gluten-free diet results in normal life expectancy.

Small bowel Crohn's disease

Crohn's disease is an inflammatory bowel disease that involves any part of the GI tract from the mouth to the anus. It affects the small intestine alone or in combination with the large intestine (see page 236). The most common site is the distal small intestine (terminal ileum).

Although its exact cause is unknown, effective medical therapies have been developed to treat the inflammation and obtain remission. Nevertheless, the majority of patients will require surgery at some point in their lives.

Epidemiology

The prevalence of Crohn's disease varies significantly worldwide from 0.6 per 100,000 in parts of Greece to 322 per 100,000 in sections of Italy, with considerable regional variation. There is an equal sex distribution, and patients characteristically present in late adolescence and early adulthood.

Aetiology

A genetic predisposition and environmental precipitants such as current smoking and previous infection contribute to the sustained disturbed immune response that causes Crohn's disease in predisposed individuals. The response is an inappropriate immune attack against bacteria in the GI tract, resulting in chronic inflammation.

No specific pathogens have been confirmed to be causative, although several have been suggested, for example *Mycobacterium avium*.

The increased risk observed in family members supports a genetic predisposition; for example 5% of children who have a parent with Crohn's disease develop the condition. Genome studies have identified several genes in which mutations increase susceptibility to Crohn's; however, these mutations are present in only a minority of patients. One such gene is *NOD2*, which produces a protein involved in the recognition of bacterial peptidoglycans.

Clinical features

Patients are usually chronically unwell and present with a combination of symptoms. However, they occasionally present more acutely. Symptoms include:

■ Weight loss, which occurs gradually or acutely
■ Colicky abdominal pain
■ Diarrhoea, with liquid to semi-formed stool and increased stool frequency
■ Nutrient deficiencies as inflammation and ulceration of the small intestine affect its ability to absorb nutrients
■ Oral symptoms – angular stomatitis, glossitis and aphthoid mouth ulcers (**Figures 5.1** and **5.6**)
■ Perianal disease, which presents with ulceration, fistulae and abscesses (see page 245)
■ Extraintestinal symptoms including joint pains, red eyes and skin conditions such as erythema nodosum and pyoderma gangrenosum

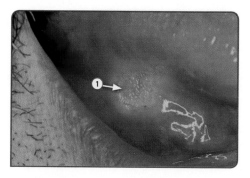

Figure 5.6 Aphthoid mouth ulcer ①. These are recurrent, painful ulcers seen on the mucosal surface of the mouth.

Complications

Crohn's disease causes a chronic transmural inflammation. This can lead to several complications (**Figure 5.7**):

- Stricture – narrowing of the bowel resulting from chronic inflammation

and formation of scar tissue. This causes postprandial pain and features of bowel obstruction such as abdominal distension and vomiting
- Fistula – a communication between the small intestine and the skin or adjacent organs including the large intestine, bladder or vagina. It results from deep transmural ulceration affecting the full thickness of the bowel wall. The patient reports the passage of stool into the connecting organ
- Abscess – a collection of pus within the abdominal cavity or perianal region. This is caused in the same way as a fistula. It often presents with signs of infection such as fever or pain

Diagnostic approach

The clinical history, including risk factors such as family history and smoking, sometimes suggests the diagnosis.

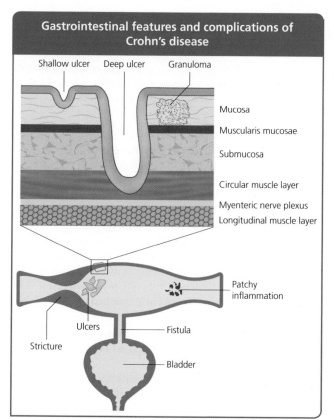

Gastrointestinal features and complications of Crohn's disease

Shallow ulcer   Deep ulcer   Granuloma

Mucosa
Muscularis mucosae
Submucosa

Circular muscle layer
Myenteric nerve plexus
Longitudinal muscle layer

Patchy inflammation

Ulcers
Stricture
Fistula
Bladder

Figure 5.7 Gastrointestinal features and complications of Crohn's disease. Granulomas and ulcers are seen at endoscopy and on histology of the small intestine.

Investigations

A combination of investigations is required to diagnose Crohn's disease and assess what regions of the GI tract are involved as well as how active the inflammation is. Although non-invasive blood, stool and radiological investigations support a diagnosis, a definitive diagnosis is only made from histology. The tissue sample is obtained at endoscopy or after operative resection of the small intestine.

Blood tests

Raised CRP, ESR, white cell and platelet levels indicate inflammation. A low vitamin B_{12} level occurs with 'terminal' ileal disease, i.e. disease involving the very distal part of the ileum where the vitamin is absorbed from the GI tract.

Stool tests

The level of calprotectin is increased in inflammatory bowel conditions such as Crohn's disease. Coexisting infection is excluded by microscopy and measuring glutamate dehydrogenase, which indicates the presence of *Clostridium difficile* (see page 114).

Imaging and endoscopy

The gold standard radiological investigation of the small intestine is magnetic resonance or CT enterography. This demonstrates the extent and activity of disease as well as any large bowel or extraluminal complications. A barium follow-through is an alternative but less effective way of visualising the small intestine.

A labelled white cell scan is a non-invasive test that evaluates the presence and extent of inflammation. A gamma camera detects a radioactive isotope which has been tagged to the patients' neutrophils and then reinjected into their blood stream.

Oesophagogastroduodenoscopy is used to visualise the lumen and epithelium of the duodenum. Colonoscopy allows the terminal ileum to be assessed for ulceration. Capsule endoscopy allows imaging of the entire small intestine to assess for inflammation and ulcers (**Figure 5.8**). However, it is used with caution in patients with possible strictures due to an increased risk of retention, where the capsule gets stuck in the narrowed lumen.

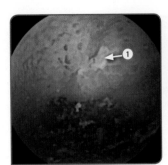

Figure 5.8 Small bowel ulcer ① in a patient with Crohn's disease identified at capsule endoscopy.

Histology of the small intestine reveals transmural, patchy chronic inflammation and ulcers with granulomas, which are a collection of macrophages (**Figure 5.7**).

Management

Crohn's is an incurable condition, but the disease and its complications are managed using a variety of medical and surgical treatments. In the absence of complications, medical therapies are usually the first-line approach.

> **Crohn's disease cannot be cured even by surgically removing all affected tissue.** After ileocaecal resection, colonoscopy shows recurrence in most patients after only 1 year, and 20% will have symptoms related to this. The most effective strategy to reduce recurrence post-surgery is smoking cessation – smokers have over twice the risk of a further operation during the next 10 years.

Medication

Corticosteroids, e.g. prednisolone, are used as a short-term treatment (no more than a few months) to decrease inflammation and therefore induce remission (see page 139). Oral budesonide treats distal ileal and right-sided colonic Crohn's disease as it is released in these regions to act topically – it has fewer systemic side effects than prednisolone. Corticosteroids are always prescribed with calcium supplements to reduce the risk of osteoporosis.

Because of their side effects, which include glucose intolerance and osteoporosis, corticosteroids are not used as maintenance treatment. Medications used in the longer term to treat inflammation include:

- Immunomodulators such as azathioprine, 6-mercaptopurine and methotrexate
- Biological agents, which are antibodies, e.g. against tumour necrosis factor-α or $\alpha4\beta7$ integrin

Despite these treatments, only 10% of patients have prolonged remission, and at least 50% require surgery within the first 10 years of the disease.

Surgery

The lifetime need for surgery is as high as 80%. Surgery is indicated when medical therapy is not effective or tolerated, and also when there are complications such as intestinal obstruction.

Stricturoplasty is the widening of a narrowed segment of intestine. A lengthways cut is made along one side of the intestine and the two cut ends pulled together along the width of the intestine. The ends are then sutured together. This technique is preferred for short strictures as it minimises the amount of small intestine that is removed.

Vitamin B_{12} deficiency and bile salt acid malabsorption commonly occur if ileocaecal resection has been carried out.

> **You can live without an oesophagus, stomach or colon if these are removed surgically but you cannot survive without having at least some of your small bowel present.** If a large amount is removed intravenous fluid and nutrition is required.

Complications

Complications of Crohn's disease (e.g. stricture, fistula and abscess) usually require a combination of medical and surgical treatments, as described above.

Prognosis

Crohn's disease is a lifelong disease of varying severity with periods of relapse and remission. Its course is positively influenced by modifying risk factors. Smoking cessation reduces the risk of relapse by approximately two thirds.

Small bowel neoplasia

Both benign and malignant tumours arise in the small intestine (**Table 5.8**). Even though the small intestine forms approximately 90% of the surface area and 75% of the length of the GI tract, cancer in this area accounts for only 2% of GI malignancies. It is not known why they are so uncommon – the worldwide incidence is fewer than 1 per 100,000 people. It is more common in men and people over 60 years of age.

The most common malignancies are metastases from melanomas, the breast and lung. Most primary cancers are adenocarcinomas, followed by neuroendocrine tumours (NETS) of the small intestine. Risk factors for adenocarcinoma include a diet high in animal fat, protein and red meats, and untreated coeliac disease. Both benign and malignant small bowel tumours occur more frequently in association with genetic or other disorders (**Table 5.8**).

> **Secondary tumours are at least twice as common as primary malignancies in the small intestine.** It is not known why cancer is much rarer in the small intestine than other sites in the GI tract – each year, only one new case is diagnosed for every 32 patients with colorectal cancer.

Clinical features

Presentation is usually non-specific with abdominal pain, weight loss, diarrhoea or iron deficiency anaemia. Less frequently, patients present acutely with abdominal obstruction or perforation and bleeding (as melaena). Blockage of the ampulla of Vater results in pancreatitis. This produces epigastric and back pain, and jaundice.

Small bowel tumour types		
Tumour type	Cell of origin	Associated conditions (if none, indicated by –)
Benign		
Hamartoma	Excess of normal tissue	Peutz–Jeghers syndrome
Adenoma	Mucosal glands	FAP, HNPCC, MAP
Leiomyoma	Smooth muscle	–
Lipoma	Mature fat cells	–
Haemangioma	Vasculature	–
Fibroma	Fibroblasts	–
Neurofibroma	Neurones	–
Malignant		
Adenocarcinoma	Mucosal glands	Coeliac disease, FAP, HNPCC, MAP, Crohn's disease, Peutz–Jeghers syndrome
Lymphoma		
B cell	Lymphocytes	Cystic fibrosis, FAP, HNPCC, MAP, Crohn's disease, Peutz–Jeghers syndrome
T cell	Lymphocytes	Coeliac disease
Neuroendocrine tumours (NETs)	Enterochromaffin-like cells	–
Sarcomas		
Leiomyosarcoma	Smooth muscle	Neurofibromatosis
Gastrointestinal stromal tumour	Mesenchymal cells	–
Angiosarcoma	Vascular endothelial cells	–
Fibrosarcoma	Fibroblasts	–
Kaposi's sarcoma	Spindle cells	AIDS
Metastases from another site		
Melanoma	Melanocytes	–
Other primary site (e.g. breast, lung cancers)	Any	–

AIDS, acquired immune deficiency syndrome; FAP, familial adenomatous polyposis; HNPCC, hereditary non-polyposis colorectal cancer; MAP, *MUTYH*-associated polyposis.

Table 5.8 Types of small bowel tumour, their cell of origin and associated conditions

Most NETs of the small intestine are non-functioning (i.e. do not release peptide or hormones). 'Carcinoid syndrome' occurs when vasoactive compounds including serotonin and tachykinins are released into the bloodstream by a NET. These cause 'dry' flushing (i.e. without sweating) of the skin (particularly the face), diarrhoea and abdominal pain.

Tumours are usually diagnosed by radiology and endoscopy. NETS are diagnosed by testing for chromogranin A (secreted by tumours and detected in blood samples) and 5-hydroxyindoleacetic acid (the main metabolite of serotonin, excreted by the kidneys and measured by a 24-hour collection of urine).

Management

Patients with malignant tumours have a CT scan to stage how extensive it is and whether there are metastases to lymph nodes, the liver, etc. This will determine the most appropriate treatment.

Medication

Chemotherapy is used to treat adenocarcinomas, sarcomas and lymphoma. Oral tyrosine kinase inhibitors are used to treat GI stromal tumours. Somatostatin analogues, such as octreotide, are used to treat the symptoms of carcinoid syndrome and slow tumour progression if the tumour is inoperable.

Surgery

Benign tumours such as adenomas are sometimes removed at endoscopy. Alternatively, benign and malignant tumours are removed by laparoscopic or open surgery. An ileostomy is sometimes required in patients with more advanced disease to prevent or treat bowel obstruction.

Lifelong fluid and nutritional supplementation is usually required if less than 2 m of small intestine remains after surgery as this is an insufficient length for normal functioning. Extensive resection, particularly if the large intestine has also been removed, frequently results in intestinal failure requiring long-term parenteral nutrition. Rarely, intestinal transplantation is considered.

Prognosis

This varies with the type of tumour, stage of disease and histological grade. Adenocarcinoma has an overall 5-year survival of 35%, increasing to 50% for sarcomas.

Answers to starter questions

1. Several simple tests are initially performed to investigate suspected malabsorption. Blood tests that suggest malabsorption include: anaemia or haematinic deficiency, abnormalities of electrolytes, magnesium, calcium, or albumin. More specific investigations are then done to determine the cause, including blood tests for anti-TTG antibodies, stool microscopy and faecal elastase. Upper GI endoscopy and duodenal biopsies allow small bowel mucosal abnormalities to be identified. Further investigation comprising small bowel and pancreatic imaging, breath tests and a SeHCAT scan is performed when there is a suspicion of other diagnoses including Crohn's disease, pancreatic insufficiency, pancreatic insufficiency, bacterial overgrowth in the small intestine, lactose intolerance or bile salt malabsorption.

2. Coeliac disease is a life-long condition without a true cure. However, a permanent gluten free diet is a very effective treatment. This means avoiding all products containing wheat, barley and rye. Dietetic advice is essential to ensure gluten avoidance and a balanced intake. Patients are helped by the fact that supermarkets now routinely stock gluten-free foods including pasta and breads. Charities such as Coeliac UK provide regularly updated lists of suitable products that patients can safely eat.

3. Crohn's disease is associated with transmural inflammation, which can lead to the development of strictures. Muscle hypertrophy and collagen deposition lead to narrowed segments of small bowel, resulting in abdominal pain and sometimes obstruction, presenting with abdominal pain, distension, vomiting and reduced bowel frequency. Aphthous ulcers can progress to transmural fissures and inflammation with abscess formation, leading to adherence of the bowel to adjacent structures and fistula formation.

4. Considering the small bowel makes up 75% of the length and over 90% of the surface area of the GI tract, tumours are remarkably rare; they comprise only

Answers *continued*

2% of GI malignancies. In contrast, colorectal cancer is the third most common cancer worldwide. The reason why small bowel cancers are rare is not known; theories include the quick transit in and relative sterility of the small intestine, and the protective effects of secreted IgA within it. The increased incidence in chronic inflammatory disease (e.g. Crohns disease) suggest inflammation may be involved.

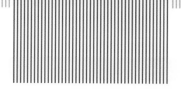

Chapter 6
Colorectal disorders

Starter questions

Reading this chapter will enable you to answer the following questions. Answers are on page 247.

1. Why do polyps develop in the large intestine?
2. Can colorectal cancer be prevented?
3. Does food cause irritable bowel syndrome?
4. Why do diverticulae form in the gastrointestinal tract, and why does their global incidence vary?

Introduction

The primary function of the large intestine is to absorb water from the liquid contents of the small intestine:

- to reduce fluid loss from the body
- to form more solid stool

The main symptoms of large intestinal disorders arise when this process is affected, which causes changes in defaecation such as diarrhoea or constipation. Pain, bloating and bleeding (either visible blood loss or occult loss, leading to iron deficiency) are other symptoms that commonly occur.

Self-limiting diarrhoeal illnesses caused by infection occur periodically in most people. Chronic conditions, such as irritable bowel syndrome and diverticulosis, are also very common. The large intestine is the third most common site of cancer worldwide; early detection and treatment often greatly improve its prognosis.

Inflammation of the large intestine (colitis) occurs due to several different disorders, as summarised in **Table 6.1**.

Types of colitis		
Type	**Features**	**Treatment**
Infective	Usually self-limiting diarrhoea	See page 223

Inflammatory bowel disease:
  Ulcerative colitis
  Crohn's disease
	Chronic intermittent diarrhoea ± blood	See page 229

Microscopic	Watery diarrhoea	See page 238

Ischaemic
 	
  Acute
  Chronic
	
	Severe abdominal pain and leucocytosis
	Abdominal pain after eating, weight loss and bloody diarrhoea
		
		Treatment of risk factors, e.g. atrial fibrillation, diabetes

Diversion (colitis in a defunctioned colon, i.e. when a stoma has been formed in a proximal part of the intestine)	Presents with a bloody discharge	Steroid, 5-ASA or short-chain fatty acid enemas
Radiation induced (proctopathy)	Bloody diarrhoea May present with symptoms many years after radiotherapy	Sucralfate enemas Metronidazole Topical formalin Argon photocoagulation Hyperbaric oxygen
NSAID induced	Symptoms identical to ulcerative colitis	Stop NSAID therapy

5-ASA, 5-aminosalicylic acid; NSAID, non-steroidal anti-inflammatory drug.

Table 6.1 Types of colitis and their distinguishing features

Case 6 Bloody diarrhoea

Presentation

Josh Edwards is a 27-year-old man who presents to his general practitioner (GP) with a 2-month history of abdominal pain and bloody diarrhoea.

Initial interpretation

Diarrhoea is caused by disease of the small or large intestine and is described in terms of stool frequency and consistency (see **Figure 2.4**). Information about the onset, severity, timing and aggravating and relieving factors is also required. It is important to ask about any nocturnal (night time) symptoms, which indicate more severe disease and is uncommon in conditions such as irritable bowel syndrome.

The presence of blood is more suggestive of pathology in the large intestine than the small intestine. The colour and volume of the blood and whether it is surrounding or mixed with the stool suggests an origin of blood loss from within the large intestine.

The duration of the symptoms helps to point to the underlying diagnosis. Sudden-onset symptoms, which resolve on their own without treatment is suggestive of an infective cause. More long-standing symptoms raise the possibility of underlying disease of the large intestine, such as inflammatory bowel disease. It is important to establish if there are any sinister features suggestive of colorectal malignancy, such as significant weight loss, as a delay in diagnosis sometimes affects prognosis. Although colorectal malignancy often presents with similar symptoms, it is uncommon in people under the age of 50 years old and without a family history, such as Josh.

Case 6 *continued*

History

Josh has been opening his bowels seven or eight times during the day. He is also waking two or three times per night to open his bowels. The stool is liquid and he has noticed fresh red blood mixed with the stool each time. He is also passing mucus and has been experiencing cramps in the lower abdomen.

Over the last 2 months, Josh has started to feel generally lethargic and fatigued. Three months ago he stopped smoking as part of a healthy lifestyle change.

He has recently been taking over-the-counter ibuprofen for pains in his joints, particularly his lower back. There is no history of recent foreign travel. Josh reports that his father underwent an emergency colectomy 30 years ago, but is unsure of further details.

Examination

Josh looks unwell. He has a tachycardia of 105 beats per minute. His sclerae are slightly reddened although his conjunctivae are pale. An ulcerated area is noted on his lower legs (**Figure 6.1**). There is tenderness in the left iliac fossa but no guarding (see page 88, Chapter 2).

Rectal examination reveals fresh blood on the glove but no palpable masses. There are no abnormal findings on perianal examination or on examination of the respiratory and cardiovascular systems.

Interpretation of findings

The tachycardia and abdominal tenderness indicate that he is not well and requires an urgent outpatient assessment or admission to hospital.

A small intestine cause is unlikely because bleeding and mucus are present. Josh's symptoms are suggestive of colitis (**Table 6.1**). For patients in this age group presenting with these symptoms, the most likely diagnosis is an inflammatory bowel disease. However, stool tests are required to exclude coexisting infection.

Investigations

Josh's blood and stool test results are outlined in **Table 6.2**. Three stool samples testing for *Clostridium difficile* glutamate dehydrogenase and microscopy, culture and sensitivity are negative.

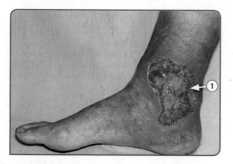

Figure 6.1 An ulcer overlying the right ankle ① that has been caused by pyoderma gangrenosum.

Josh's blood results	
Test	Result (normal range)
Haemoglobin (Hb)	103 g/L (130–180 g/L in men)
Mean corpuscular volume (MCV)	72 fL (80–96 fL)
Mean corpuscular haemoglobin (MCH)	25 pg (28–32 pg)
Platelets	415 × 10⁹/L (150–400 × 10⁹/L)
Erythrocyte sedimentation rate (ESR)	78 mm/h (0–15 mm/h)
C-reactive protein (CRP)	115 mg/L (<5 mg/L)
Albumin	28 g/L (37–49 g/L)
Faecal calprotectin	660 µg/g (<100 µg/g)

Table 6.2 Case 6: Josh's blood results

Case 6 *continued*

The GP refers Josh to the gastroenterology department for urgent investigation due to the severity of his symptoms and because he looks unwell. A flexible sigmoidoscopy is arranged, which shows continuous superficial inflammation and ulceration extending from the rectum up to the splenic flexure. Biopsies show superficial neutrophilic infiltration with loss of crypt architecture and crypt abscesses. No granulomas are identified.

Diagnosis

These results are in keeping with a diagnosis of inflammatory bowel disease. The continuous nature of the inflammation and absence of granulomas on biopsy makes ulcerative colitis most likely. The findings are explained to Josh when he is reviewed in the outpatient department by a consultant gastroenterologist and nurse specialist in inflammatory bowel disease.

Josh is prescribed a 7-week course of oral steroids with a gradually reducing dose, to suppress the inflammation of the large intestine. He is also given calcium and vitamin D supplements to minimise bone loss, occurring as a side effect of steroid treatment. Oral and rectal 5-aminosalicylic acid medications are given long-term to suppress inflammation of the large intestine. Oral iron supplements treat the microcytic (low MCV), hypochromic (low MCH) anaemia occurring due to an iron deficiency. He is advised to stop taking non-steroidal anti-inflammatory drugs (NSAIDs) as they commonly exacerbate colitis. Paracetamol is recommended as an alternative painkiller. Josh is told that his joint pains are likely to be due to the ulcerative colitis and usually disappear as the inflammation of the large intestine improves.

The specialist nurse recognises that Josh had stopped smoking a few months before

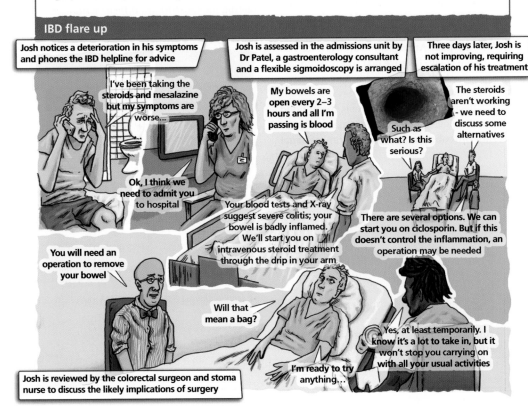

IBD flare up

Josh notices a deterioration in his symptoms and phones the IBD helpline for advice

Josh is assessed in the admissions unit by Dr Patel, a gastroenterology consultant and a flexible sigmoidoscopy is arranged

Three days later, Josh is not improving, requiring escalation of his treatment

I've been taking the steroids and mesalazine but my symptoms are worse...

My bowels are open every 2–3 hours and all I'm passing is blood

Such as what? Is this serious?

The steroids aren't working - we need to discuss some alternatives

Ok, I think we need to admit you to hospital

Your blood tests and X-ray suggest severe colitis; your bowel is badly inflamed. We'll start you on intravenous steroid treatment through the drip in your arm

There are several options. We can start you on ciclosporin. But if this doesn't control the inflammation, an operation may be needed

You will need an operation to remove your bowel

Will that mean a bag?

Yes, at least temporarily. I know it's a lot to take in, but it won't stop you carrying on with all your usual activities

I'm ready to try anything...

Josh is reviewed by the colorectal surgeon and stoma nurse to discuss the likely implications of surgery

the symptoms started. She explains that although smoking sometimes improves the symptoms of ulcerative colitis, the other health benefits of stopping smoking far outweigh this.

Before his planned review in the outpatient clinic 4 weeks later, Josh's symptoms deteriorate and he has worsening diarrhoea and rectal bleeding. He rings the specialist nurse, who suggests admission to hospital.

Case 7 Intermittent abdominal pain

Presentation

Sarah Morgan is a 21-year-old woman who makes an appointment with her GP to discuss lower abdominal pain and bloating that she has experienced for the last 4 years.

Initial interpretation

Sarah is young and has had these symptoms for some time before seeking medical advice, making the risk of anything sinister such as cancer unlikely. Information about the onset, severity, site and any relieving or aggravating factors of the pain is needed to help determine the potential cause. These symptoms could originate from a gynaecological or bowel source, but bloating is more suggestive of an underlying gastrointestinal (GI) disorder.

History

Sarah has cramp-like pains in the left iliac fossa. Each bout of pain lasts for up to an hour. The pain sometimes occurs several times in one day but then does not occur again for a week or more. The pain is improved by defaecation.

The abdominal bloating usually occurs when the pain is present and often gets worse through the day. When it is particularly obvious, colleagues have told Sarah that she looks pregnant.

The pain has no obvious link to Sarah's menstrual cycle. She has a regular 28-day cycle and no menorrhagia (heavy periods).

Interpretation of history

As the pain is alleviated by defaecation and has no specific relationship to menstruation, it appears to be originating from the GI tract rather than from a gynaecological disorder. Abdominal distension has a range of causes (see page 90) but in Sarah's case it probably has a gastrointestinal origin as it is intermittent and coexists with the pain.

A further history will help to determine a likely cause. It is important to ask about other bowel symptoms, which are suggestive of a gastrointestinal origin such as constipation or diarrhoea. The presence of 'alarm' symptoms would raise the possibility of an underlying malignancy.

Further history

Sarah's bowel habit has varied over the last few years. Since early childhood, she has tended towards bouts of constipation. She passes small amounts of hard stool and often goes several days before opening her bowels. Her bloating and pain are worse when she is constipated. Less frequently, she has slightly looser stool, sometimes with mucus, and opens her bowels two or three times first thing in the morning. There has been no rectal

Case 7 *continued*

bleeding, no weight loss and no symptoms during the night.

Sarah says her symptoms are worse when she is stressed and wonders if foods containing wheat and certain vegetables make her more bloated. There is no family history of inflammatory bowel disease, coeliac disease or bowel cancer.

Examination

Sarah looks well. Her body mass index is 21 kg/m². There are no palpable abdominal masses although there is slight tenderness on deep palpation of the left iliac fossa. The rectal examination is normal, as are examinations of the cardiovascular and respiratory systems.

Interpretation of findings

From her symptoms, the most likely diagnosis is irritable bowel syndrome. Physical examination in individuals with irritable bowel syndrome is often normal, although there is sometimes mild abdominal tenderness. Some patients also have a degree of distension, which is resonant to percussion. Faecal loading of the large intestine is sometimes palpable if constipation predominates.

Any other abnormality would bring a diagnosis of irritable bowel syndrome into doubt. Blood tests are required to exclude other conditions such as coeliac and thyroid disease.

Investigations

The results of Sarah's blood and stool tests are outlined in **Table 6.3**. Renal, liver, glucose and immunoglobulin A concentrations are also normal.

The level of faecal calprotectin in the stool is useful in younger patients with diarrhoeal symptoms. Calprotectin is a biochemical marker of inflammation. It helps

Sarah's blood results	
Test	Result (normal range)
Haemoglobin (Hb)	130 g/L (115–165 g/L in women)
Mean corpuscular volume (MCV)	87 fL (80–96 fL)
Erythrocyte sedimentation rate (ESR)	5 mm/h (0–15 mm/h)
C-reactive protein (CRP)	3 mg/L (<5 mg/L)
Thyroid-stimulating hormone (TSH)	3.4 mIU/L (0.5–5 mU/L)
Free T4	12 pmol/L (10–20 pmol/L)
Anti-tissue transglutaminase	2 U/mL (< 15 U/mL)
Ferritin	180 µg/L (15–300 µg/L)
Vitamin B$_{12}$	550 ng/L (160–760 ng/L)
Folate	10 µg/L (2–11 µg/L)
Faecal calprotectin	17 µg/g (<100 µg/g)

Table 6.3 Case 7: Sarah's blood results

to distinguish between irritable bowel syndrome where the level is normal and inflammatory or infective conditions when it is raised.

Diagnosis

The history, physical examination, normal blood tests and low faecal calprotectin level are consistent with a diagnosis of irritable bowel syndrome (see **Table 6.5**).

Management

Sarah is reviewed by her GP, who reassures her by explaining the diagnosis and its basis. He explains that endoscopic or radiological tests are not required as these would be normal.

Sarah is prescribed an oral stool softener and peppermint capsules, which improve her constipation, abdominal pain and bloating. She is advised to keep a food

Case 7 *continued*

diary to identify precipitants. Sarah and her GP discuss the possibility of psychological treatments, for example hypnosis, if her symptoms do not improve. This therapy is helpful in some people who do not respond to other treatments.

Irritable bowel syndrome is usually managed effectively in primary care. The only patients who require referral for fur-ther assessment are those with atypical or alarm features (including a family history of colorectal cancer), unexplained rectal bleeding, an onset at an older age, for example over 50 years, or abnormalities on the physical examination (e.g. rectal or abdominal mass) or initial blood tests (e.g. iron deficiency anaemia).

Infective diarrhoea

Infective (also called infectious) diarrhoea is diarrhoea due to some types of infection of the GI tract. It is the most common cause of diarrhoea worldwide. Although it is usually self-limiting, it is a major cause of morbidity and mortality, particularly in the developing world.

Most infections that result in diarrhoea are caused by viruses, bacteria or protozoa. Transmission is usually via the faecal–oral route.

Epidemiology

Despite improvements in public health and economic wealth in the developed world, the incidence of infective diarrhoea is still high with 3 billion cases occurring worldwide annually, and 17 million in the UK. More than 300 people die of infective diarrhoea in the UK each year.

Traveller's diarrhoea is a type of infective diarrhoea that occurs when a person travels from a developed to a resource-limited (developing) destination and affects more than 15 million travellers annually.

Aetiology

Numerous bacterial, viral and parasitic pathogens cause infective diarrhoea (**Table 6.4**). However, in 60% of patients with symptoms, no aetiological agent is isolated during testing. Spread is commonly faecal–oral either through the ingestion of contaminated food or fluids, or by direct person-to-person contact.

> **Vomiting is a prominent early symptom of norovirus infection.** This results in aerosol spread and explains why norovirus is highly contagious in community and hospital outbreaks.

Patients who are immunocompromised or elderly are often more susceptible. Gastric acid kills some of the bacteria responsible for infective diarrhoea. Therefore, individuals with reduced gastric acid secretion such as those on proton pump inhibitor medication are more susceptible to diarrhoea from organisms such as *C. difficile*, *Salmonella*, *Campylobacter*, *E. coli* and cholera-associated diarrhoea.

Acute or recurrent *C. difficile* diarrhoea infection is caused by Gram-positive, spore-forming bacilli. The majority of patients who develop symptomatic infection have recently received antibiotic treatment. Broad-spectrum antibiotics such as penicillin and cephalosporins disrupt the normal gut flora, allowing the number of *C. difficile* bacteria to increase to a high level.

Common causes of infective diarrhoea			
Pathogen	Source or mode of infection	Incubation period	Related conditions and features
Bacteria Bloody diarrhoea:			
Campylobacter	Undercooked poultry	2–5 days	Rarely associated with a reactive arthritis or Guillain–Barré syndrome (rapid-onset muscle weakness)
Shigella	Person-to-person spread	12–24 h	Can cause haemolytic–uraemic syndrome
Escherichia coli	Undercooked meat, unpasteurised milk	1–3 days	Haemolytic–uraemic syndrome occurs in 15% of cases
Non-bloody diarrhoea:			
Salmonella*	Milk, beef, eggs	12–48 h	Entry of Salmonella into lymphatic system and release of toxins cause typhoid fever
Vibrio cholerae	Travel to endemic area	1–2 days	Life-threatening watery diarrhoea
Clostridium difficile	Person-to-person spread (greater risk with antibiotics)	1–7 days	Can cause pseudomembranous colitis
Viruses Rotavirus	Person-to-person spread (children predominantly affected)	2 days	–
Norovirus	Person-to-person spread; outbreaks in densely housed populations, e.g. hospitals and cruise ships	12–48 hours	–
Parasites Giardia lamblia	Contaminated soil, food or water	1–3 weeks	Chronic diarrhoea, malabsorption
Entamoeba histolytica*	Cysts ingested from infected soil, food or water	2–4 weeks	Can cause liver abscesses and rarely fulminant colitis (blood present)

*In some patients the diarrhoea is bloody

Table 6.4 Common causes of infective diarrhoea

Over 500 different organisms live in the normal human intestine and form the gut microbiota. They have several important roles including the prevention of infection and in aiding digestion. The number, species and location of bacteria are altered by interventions including surgery, antibiotics and radiotherapy. This sometimes leads to symptoms such as diarrhoea and bloating.

Clinical features

Infective diarrhoea presents as:

- Acute watery diarrhoea
- Bloody diarrhoea (dysentery)
- Persistent diarrhoea – where diarrhoea has continued for more than 2 weeks

Patients often feel unwell with non-specific symptoms of fever, anorexia, malaise, vomiting and colicky abdominal pain. A history of recent foreign travel or the ingestion of unusual or suspect food provides information about the potential organisms causing the infection. Ascertaining recent antibiotic use is also important because it is associated with an increased risk of *C. difficile* infection.

Physical examination is usually normal, although if the symptoms of diarrhoea are severe, patients often show signs of dehydration with dry mucous membranes and reduced skin turgor.

Complications

An acute kidney injury and electrolyte disturbance (e.g. low potassium) sometimes occur as a result of fluid loss. Toxic megacolon (acute colonic distension) and perforation rarely results from severe infection.

Diagnostic approach

A diagnosis of infective diarrhoea is usually based solely on the clinical history. Most cases resolve rapidly without the need for specific treatment or investigation. However, further investigation is needed in patients with severe symptoms and those who are immunosuppressed due to medications (e.g. biologics) or diseases (e.g. HIV), where additional treatment such as antibiotics are sometimes required.

Investigations

Blood tests

Biochemistry tests show elevated urea and creatinine levels indicating renal impairment due to dehydration, if symptoms are severe. Potassium and sodium electrolyte levels often fall due to fluid loss. An elevated C-reactive protein (CRP), erythrocyte sedimentation rate (ESR) and white cell count (leucocytosis) occur with infection. However, these are not specific findings and are also present in conditions such as inflammatory bowel disease.

Escherichia coli subtype 0157 results in haemolytic–uraemic syndrome in approximately 15% of cases. This complication consists of the destruction of red blood cells in small blood vessels (microangiopathic haemolytic anaemia), a low platelet count (thrombocytopenia) and acute renal failure. It carries a mortality of 3–5%.

Stool tests

Although frequently negative, stool microscopy is performed to look for ova, cysts and parasites, such as *Giardia lamblia* and *Entamoeba histolytica* (**Table 6.4**), and cultured to identify potential causative organisms.

Clostridium difficile diarrhoea is diagnosed by the presence of glutamate dehydrogenase and subsequent identification of *C. difficile* toxin.

Imaging

Abdominal imaging, such as a plain radiograph or CT, is often of limited value. However, it is used to detect the presence of complications such as toxic megacolon.

Sigmoidoscopy

If diarrhoea persists, a flexible sigmoidoscopy and biopsy is considered to exclude other underlying conditions. In patients with *C. difficile* infection, characteristic plaques of inflammatory exudate called pseudomembranes are sometimes seen (**Figure 6.2**).

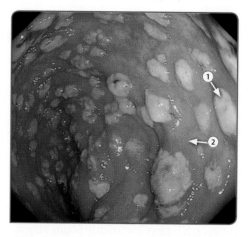

Figure 6.2 Pseudomembranes ① associated with *Clostridium difficile* diarrhoea. Normal colonic mucosa can be seen between the plaques ②.

Management

The mainstay of treatment is adequate rehydration and correction of underlying electrolyte imbalance such as a low potassium or sodium. Oral fluids and oral rehydration solutions are usually sufficient. However, if there is severe fluid loss or profound vomiting, intravenous rehydration is almost always required. Cases of infective diarrhoea due to some species, such as *Campylobacter* and *E. coli*, must be reported to public health authorities to try and establish a source and trace any related cases.

Medication

Antibiotics are rarely required because symptoms are usually short-lived and resolve without treatment and because they are ineffective against viral causes of diarrhoea. However, they are occasionally used if symptoms are persistent or in immunosuppressed individuals if a specific organism is identified.

Oral metronidazole is the first-line treatment of mild to moderate *Clostridium difficile* diarrhoea infection. It is as effective as treatment with vancomycin, but cheaper. Oral vancomycin is used for severe infection due to its faster response rate and the failure of metronidazole to treat some cases.

The use of anti-diarrhoeal agents, such as loperamide and codeine phosphate, should be avoided because they slow expulsion of the organisms from the GI tract, delaying recovery and increasing the risk of complications such as toxic megacolon.

> **Recurrent *C. difficile* infection is often difficult to treat.** Faecal transplant is one way of re-establishing the normal healthy gut microbiota, with cure rates of up to 94%. It involves transplanting the faeces of a healthy donor into the recipient via an enema, nasogastric tube or at colonoscopy.

Surgery

This is rarely required except for complications such as toxic megacolon or perforation.

Prognosis

Most cases are self-limiting with no long-term sequelae. Persistent diarrhoea sometimes occurs with post-infective irritable bowel syndrome, secondary hypolactasia (reduced lactase enzyme activity), persistent infection (e.g. with *Giardia lamblia*) or co-existing undiagnosed conditions such as inflammatory bowel disease.

Irritable bowel syndrome

Irritable bowel syndrome is a chronic functional disorder of the intestine characterised by the presence of abdominal symptoms in the absence of any structural, biochemical or pathological abnormality.

Epidemiology

Irritable bowel syndrome is very common. It affects up to 20% of adults in developed countries and is found worldwide. It can occur at any age but is more common in young adults. Women and girls are more frequently affected, particularly with constipation-predominant symptoms.

The majority of people with irritable bowel syndrome do not seek medical advice because their symptoms are often mild or they recognise its occurrence with specific factors such as stress. However its prevalence makes it one of the most common reasons for consultation with a GP.

Aetiology

There is no single unifying hypothesis for the cause of irritable bowel syndrome. Several different mechanisms contribute to and exacerbate it (**Figure 6.3**).

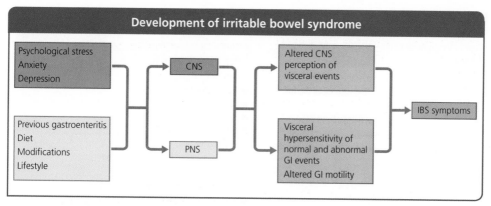

Figure 6.3 Development of irritable bowel syndrome. There are multiple psychological and GI factors and mechanisms involved; ultimately the same symptoms can develop via several different pathways. CNS, central nervous system; GI, gastrointestinal; PNS, peripheral nervous system.

Clinical features

Abdominal pain is a characteristic feature of irritable bowel syndrome, which forms part of the Rome diagnostic criteria. Other components are a change in the stool frequency and consistency. Irritable bowel syndrome is divided into three subgroups depending on bowel function:

- Constipation predominant
- Diarrhoea predominant
- Alternating constipation and diarrhoea

Other abdominal symptoms are commonly found:

- Bloating – sensation that the abdomen is full or distended
- Distension – swelling of the abdomen
- Mucus passed per rectum – patients sometimes refer to this as slime
- A sensation of incomplete evacuation of stool
- Borborygmi – excessive stomach noises or rumbling
- Excess flatus
- Upper GI symptoms such as nausea, early satiety and heartburn

Non-GI symptoms with no structural cause such as chronic fatigue, backache, fibromyalgia, headache, urinary frequency, dyspareunia (painful sexual intercourse) and tinnitus also occur.

The ABCD of irritable bowel syndrome:

- Abdominal pain
- Bloating
- Constipation
- Diarrhoea

Diagnostic approach

Irritable bowel syndrome is diagnosed by identifying compatible symptoms in the absence of any alarm features that would prompt further investigation (**Table 6.5**). Physical examination is usually normal but sometimes shows abdominal distension, non-specific tenderness or faecal loading.

Invasive investigations are not mandatory. They often increase the patients' anxiety and reduce their confidence in the diagnosis. Examination of the large intestine should be performed in patients with new symptoms over 50 years of age and those who have alarm symptoms, provided there are no contraindications. There is a greater diagnostic yield in those with persistent diarrhoeal symptoms, due to an increased incidence of conditions such as microscopic colitis.

Investigations

There is no single investigation that will diagnose irritable bowel syndrome, but

Diagnosing irritable bowel syndrome	
Features suggestive of IBS – the 'Rome IV' diagnostic criteria	Features not supporting a diagnosis of IBS and requiring further assessment
Abdominal pain occurring on average at least 1 day/week over the last 3 months, associated with ≥2 of the following: ■ Related to defaecation ■ Associated with a change in frequency of stool ■ Associated with a change in consistency of stool Symptoms must also have started at least 6 months ago	Symptoms ■ Rectal bleeding ■ Steatorrhoea ■ Weight loss ■ Nocturnal occurrence ■ Onset >50 years old ■ Family history of IBD or bowel cancer Examination ■ Palpable mass in abdomen (but not stool) ■ Abnormality on rectal examination Investigations ■ Any abnormality on blood tests, endoscopy, pathology or radiology ■ Raised faecal calprotectin

IBD, inflammatory bowel disease; IBS, irritable bowel syndrome.

Table 6.5 Diagnosing irritable bowel syndrome

some tests are required to exclude other conditions.

Blood tests
A full blood count, CRP, liver function tests, haematinics, thyroid function tests and coeliac serology are performed to exclude other conditions causing similar symptoms. Alternative diagnoses are considered if any of these results are abnormal.

> Check that blood test results are normal in irritable bowel syndrome. Remember that 20% of women under the age of 50 years have low ferritin as a result of normal or high menstrual blood loss.

Stool tests
Ascertaining the level of faecal calprotectin is helpful in patients under 50 years of age who have diarrhoea-predominant symptoms. It sometimes identifies other underlying pathology such as inflammatory bowel disease. The level is normal in patients with irritable bowel syndrome.

Imaging
Endoscopic or radiological investigation is only necessary in patients over the age of 50 years old, those with atypical or alarm symptoms, abnormal blood or stool test results.

Management
The patient's concerns and beliefs must be addressed. Strong reassurance is provided, with an explanation that irritable bowel syndrome is a benign, chronically relapsing and remitting disorder that sometimes significantly impairs quality of life but does not reduce life expectancy. As irritable bowel syndrome has no single cause, different therapeutic approaches help in different individuals.

Diet
Many patients link their symptoms to what they eat. Although the trigger can be from any food group, the most common are wheat, dairy, caffeine, sweeteners, alcohol and spicy foods. It is worth asking the patient to keep a record of what is eaten and when symptoms occur: this often helps identify trigger foods.

A dietician can provide advice based on review of a food diary and guide an 'exclusion' diet to ensure that adequate nutrients are still consumed. Fibre supplementation may help with constipation, although it sometimes exacerbates symptoms or causes bloating. A low 'FODMAP' diet (see Table 2.38) helps up to 70% of IBS patients, especially those with bloating: for a trial period this diet restricts then gradually reintroduces fermentable oligo-, di- and mono-saccharides and polyols (e.g. fructose, lactose, fructans, galactans and sorbitol) to identify the problem foods.

> A 'FODMAP' diet can be very effective in treating irritable bowel syndrome but for best results should be supervised by a dietitian because it initially excludes many fruit and vegetables as well as dairy products.

Medication

Drug treatment is principally focused on the symptoms:

- **Antispasmodics** (e.g. mebeverine, peppermint oil) and anti-cholinergics (e.g. hyoscine) these are well tolerated but are only marginally more effective than placebo drugs
- **Laxatives** include osmotic agents, stool softeners and stimulants, and are used either as required or on a regular basis (see page 136)
- **Antidiarrhoeals** (e.g. loperamide) are used in variable doses according to a patient's symptoms; unlike codeine

phosphate, which is also sometimes used for diarrhoea, loperamide can be safely used long term
- **Tricyclic antidepressants** (e.g. amitriptyline) are effective in low doses even in the absence of mood disturbance, due to their effect on the gut–brain axis and gut neurotransmitters. Common side-effects are constipation and drowsiness
- **Selective serotonin uptake inhibitors** (e.g. citalopram) have some benefit in the treatment of irritable bowel syndrome; they are mainly used when there is concurrent depression or anxiety
- **Probiotics** have some benefit, particularly in patients with bloating
- **Newer agents** such as prucalopride (selective serotonin 5-HT$_4$ agonist) and linaclotide (guanylate cyclase 2C agonist) target specific receptors in the GI tract and are used in the treatment of constipation-predominant symptoms

Psychological interventions

Cognitive–behavioural therapy, psychotherapy and hypnotherapy are often of benefit but are not always widely available (see page 149).

Prognosis

Although irritable bowel syndrome causes excess morbidity, life expectancy is normal.

Inflammatory bowel disease: ulcerative colitis and Crohn's disease

Inflammatory bowel disease is particularly prevalent in developed countries: it affects approximately 1 in 250 people in the UK, for example. In developing countries it is less common. Although the reasons for this are uncertain, it is probably due to unknown environmental factors. The two main types affecting the large intestine are ulcerative colitis and Crohn's disease.

Ulcerative colitis and Crohn's disease are both autoimmune conditions characterised by inflammation of the intestine

with periods of remission and relapse. They share a number of overlapping clinical, radiological and histological features but there are also differences between them (**Table 6.6**), for example whereas ulcerative colitis is confined to the large intestine, Crohn's disease affects any part of the GI tract from mouth to anus (**Figure 6.4**). In around 5% of patients the diagnostic distinction is less clear and the condition is termed inflammatory bowel disease type unclassified.

Features of ulcerative colitis and Crohn's disease		
Feature	Ulcerative colitis	Crohn's disease
Gender	M = F	M = F
Genetic factors	HLA-DR103 is strongly associated with severe disease	NOD2 (CARD15)
Clinical presentation	Bloody diarrhoea	Variable – abdominal pain, weight loss, diarrhoea Perianal disease
Distribution	Confined to large intestine	Affects any part of GI tract Predominantly ileocaecal
Endoscopic findings	Continuous inflammation with ulceration	Patchy non-continuous 'Skip lesions' Cobblestone appearance
Histology	Limited to the mucosal layer Acute and chronic inflammatory cells Crypt abscesses	Transmural Non-caseating granulomas Goblet cells

GI, gastrointestinal.

Table 6.6 Distinguishing features of inflammatory bowel disease

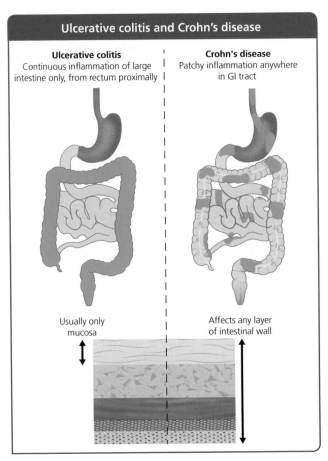

Ulcerative colitis and Crohn's disease

Ulcerative colitis
Continuous inflammation of large intestine only, from rectum proximally

Crohn's disease
Patchy inflammation anywhere in GI tract

Usually only mucosa

Affects any layer of intestinal wall

Figure 6.4 The location of inflammation differs in ulcerative colitis and Crohn's disease.

> **Irritable bowel syndrome and inflammatory bowel disease are two separate disorders**. Don't let their abbreviations – IBS and IBD – cause confusion.

Ulcerative colitis

Ulcerative colitis is a chronic condition causing inflammation of the large intestine.

Epidemiology

The incidence (number of new cases) is approximately 10 per 100,000 population per year and the prevalence (total number of cases) 240 per 100,000, in the UK. Symptoms can develop at any age, but there is one peak between 15 and 35 years and a second peak in the sixth and seventh decades.

Aetiology

The aetiology of ulcerative colitis remains unclear. However, it is thought that an environmental trigger causes an abnormal inflammatory response in genetically susceptible individuals. The inflammatory mediators that are released, for example tumour necrosis factor and interleukins 12 and 23, cause tissue damage. Studies in twins have suggested a genetic predisposition, although the evidence for this is weaker for ulcerative colitis than it is for Crohn's disease.

Environmental factors that have been implicated are:

- Smoking – ulcerative colitis is predominantly a disease of lifelong non-smokers and recent ex-smokers
- Drugs – NSAIDs exacerbate inflammatory bowel disease
- Stress – this sometimes plays a role in relapses or exacerbations
- Hygiene – reduced exposure to gut microorganisms may explain the increased prevalence in developed countries
- Diet – excess refined sugar, low fibre and red meat is weakly associated
- Appendectomy – this appears to have a protective effect in ulcerative colitis

Immunological factors are also thought to play an important role. Gut microbiota are required for the development of gut-associated lymphoid tissue (e.g. Peyer's patches located in the ileum), which store immune cells involved in managing pathogens within the intestine. Defects in the mechanisms in which a patient's intestine recognises and clears bacteria is thought to lead to the development of inflammatory bowel disease.

It is likely that a combination of the factors outlined above interact, resulting in gut tissue damage and inflammation.

> **It is often difficult to distinguish an infective from an inflammatory cause of acute diarrhoea**. If stool microscopy and culture are negative and symptoms persist, further investigations such as sigmoidoscopy are indicated to detect the inflammation and ulceration that occur in inflammatory bowel disease.

Clinical features

These vary depending on the site, extent and severity of the disease and may include:

- Bloody diarrhoea
- Faecal urgency – the sudden need to open the bowels
- Mucus per rectum
- Tenesmus – a recurrent sensation of needing to evacuate the bowels
- Colicky abdominal pain

Untreated inflammation always involves the rectum (proctitis). However, it sometimes extends to involve the sigmoid and descending colon (left-sided colitis) up to the hepatic flexure (extensive colitis), or to involve the whole colon (pancolitis) (**Figure 6.5**). The inflammation is confluent and confined to the mucosa, sparing the deeper layers of the bowel wall. Extraintestinal manifestations of inflammatory bowel disease are outlined in **Figure 6.6**. They are often related to the underlying disease activity and improve as inflammation of the intestine is treated.

Clinical features and signs are used to identify patients with severe colitis (**Table 6.7**).

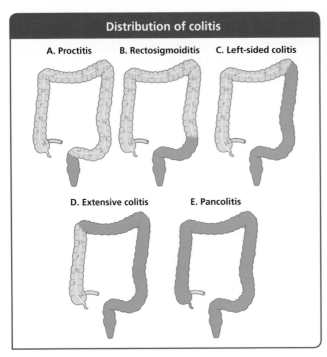

Figure 6.5 Distribution of colitis.

Features of acute severe colitis	
Category	Feature
Symptoms	Stool frequency >8 times a day with blood
	Abdominal pain
Signs	Tachycardia >100/min
	Fever >37.5°C
	Abdominal tenderness
Investigations	Haemoglobin <100 g/L
	Albumin <30 g/L
	ESR >35 mm/h
	CRP >20 mg/L
	Large intestine dilated to >6 cm diameter on abdominal radiograph

CRP, C-reactive protein; ESR, erythrocyte sedimentation rate.

Table 6.7 Clinical and laboratory features of acute severe ulcerative colitis

Diagnostic approach

A combination of blood tests, radiology, endoscopic examination and histology is required for both diagnosis and assessment of disease activity.

Investigations

Blood tests

Elevated white cell counts, ESR and CRP levels indicate inflammation. Anaemia commonly occurs due to iron deficiency resulting from blood loss and anaemia of chronic disease.

Cholestatic liver function tests with raised alkaline phosphatase and γ-glutamyl transferase levels should prompt further investigation for primary sclerosing cholangitis, a condition that develops in 5% of patients with ulcerative colitis (see page 276). Concentrations of perinuclear antineutrophil cytoplasmic antibodies (p-ANCA) are commonly elevated in primary sclerosing cholangitis.

Stool tests

Stool glutamate dehydrogenase and microscopy, culture and sensitivity (M,C&S) tests are performed to exclude coexisting infection. The level of faecal calprotectin is useful for distinguishing inflammatory bowel disease from functional bowel disorders (e.g. IBS) and assessing disease activity. An elevated level indicates active gut inflammation.

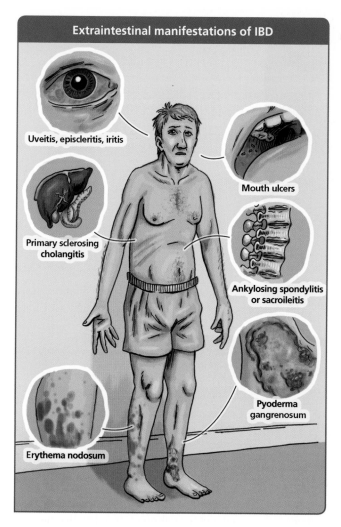

Figure 6.6 Extraintestinal manifestations of IBD.

Imaging

An abdominal radiograph occasionally shows mucosal oedema and 'thumb-printing'. Faecal loading is often seen proximal to an area of active bowel inflammation. This occurs due to more rapid stool transit in areas of colitis due to a failure of water absorption. The radiograph is also used to exclude toxic megacolon in patients with features of severe colitis (**Figure 6.7**). Toxic megacolon is diagnosed if the colon is over 6 cm in diameter.

> **Thumb-printing is the appearance of a thumb outline in the bowel wall, on an abdominal radiograph.** It is caused by oedema in the wall of the large bowel.

Endoscopy

Flexible sigmoidoscopy is the preferred initial investigation when patients present acutely (**Figure 6.8**).

Colonoscopy allows an assessment of disease extent and is used in the surveillance of ulcerative colitis to exclude pre-malignant (dysplasia) and malignant changes. Long-standing inflammation within the large intestine often results in benign inflammatory pseudopolyps. A 'backwash ileitis' is inflammation and ulceration of the terminal ileum, which is occasionally seen in patients with a pancolitis.

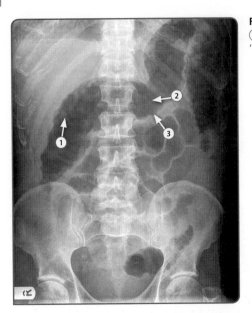

Figure 6.7 Radiographic findings in toxic megacolon. ① Mucosal islands. ② Dilated transverse colon. ③ 'Thumb print'.

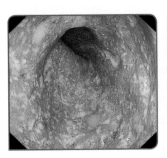
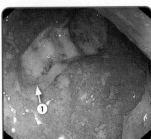

Figure 6.8 Endoscopic appearances of severe colitis. ① Deep ulcers.

In patients with acute severe ulcerative colitis, sigmoidoscopy without enema preparation is undertaken rather than colonoscopy: full bowel preparation, prolonged inflation of air and mechanical pressure from a colonoscope increase the risk of perforation when the large intestine is fragile due to inflammation and ulceration.

Histology

Biopsies of the large intestine show acute and chronic inflammatory cells within the lamina propria and crypts, causing cryptitis. Crypt abscesses are typically seen.

Management

Treatment aims to induce and maintain remission. This allows the mucosa to heal, prevents complications developing and reduces the risk of colorectal malignancy.

Medication

The treatment of ulcerative colitis and Crohn's disease is similar and varies with the site and extent of the disease (see Table 2.31):

■ **Corticosteroids** –these are used to induce remission but are not used as maintenance therapy owing to their long term side-effects (see page 140). They are prescribed with calcium supplements to protect the bones. Intravenous steroids (e.g. hydrocortisone) are used to treat acute severe colitis. Steroid suppositories and enemas are topical medications used in the treatment of left sided (distal) ulcerative colitis and Crohn's disease.

- **Aminosalicylates** (see Figure 2.32) – oral 5-ASA preparations act topically on the mucosa of the large intestine to reduce inflammation. This group of drugs is more effective for ulcerative colitis than Crohn's disease. Rectally administered 5-ASA suppositories and enemas are used as a topical treatment in left sided disease.
- **Immunomodulators:**
  - Thiopurines (azathioprine, 6-mercaptopurine) – used in patients who require frequent courses of steroids and patients with active ulcerative colitis despite treatment with 5-aminosalicylic acid. The level of the enzyme thiopurine methyl transferase (TPMT), which is involved in the metabolism of azathioprine, is checked before starting treatment. This is because deficiency of this enzyme causes metabolism to follow alternative routes that produce toxic metabolites (product of metabolism). These increase the risk of side-effects such as bone marrow suppression. Regular full blood count and liver function tests are required during treatment to monitor for the side effects of marrow suppression and leucopenia.
  - Ciclosporin – used as a treatment in patients with acute severe ulcerative colitis that is not improving with intravenous corticosteroids.
- **Biological agents** – used for moderate and severely active ulcerative colitis. If they prove beneficial, they are continued as maintenance treatment (see Table 2.33).

> Patients considering treatment options for inflammatory bowel disease need detailed counselling on side-effects. Some side-effects are particularly significant in certain patient groups, for example the teratogenic effects of methotrexate in women of child-bearing age and the risk of reactivating tuberculosis and hepatitis B when using biological agents.

Surgery

Around 20–30% of individuals with ulcerative colitis require surgery at some stage. Subtotal colectomy is indicated when medical treatment has failed or local complications affecting the intestine require treatment (**Table 6.8**). Surgery is curative if the entire large intestine is removed, such as in cases of malignancy occurring as a complication of longstanding disease.

Complications

Complications are caused by the underlying disease:

- Thromboembolism – there is an increased risk of deep venous thrombosis and pulmonary embolism. This occurs due to the affect of inflammatory cytokines on coagulation processes, immobility during hospitalisation and dehydration resulting from severe diarrhoea. Thromboprophylaxis with subcutaneous heparin is advised in severe colitis
- Toxic megacolon – this leads to significant morbidity and mortality. Prompt referral to a colorectal surgeon is required, because there is a risk of perforation
- Colonic perforation – the risk is increased with toxic megacolon and bowel preparation used for endoscopy
- Massive rectal bleeding – occurring as a result of severe inflammation and ulceration
- Colorectal carcinoma – patients with ulcerative and Crohn's colitis have a slightly increased risk of dysplasia in the large intestine (pre-malignant change) and carcinoma. This is related to the extent (at least left-sided disease or >50% of the large intestine involved) and duration of the disease (> 10 years), and to the presence of active mucosal inflammation seen at endoscopy or on histology. The risk is higher in those with a family history of colorectal malignancy and primary sclerosing cholangitis. Surveillance colonoscopy is offered at 1–5 yearly intervals depending upon the presence of

Indications for surgery in inflammatory bowel disease		
	Indication	Procedure
Ulcerative colitis	Acute flare not responding to medical therapy	Subtotal colectomy and end-ileostomy (in which end of small bowel is brought to skin)
	Toxic megacolon or imminent perforation	
	Chronic persistent disease not responding to medication	Ileoanal pouch
		Panproctocolectomy and end-ileostomy
	Dysplasia/cancer on surveillance colonoscopy	
Crohn's disease	Failure of medical therapy	Limited intestinal resection
		Ileorectal anastomosis
	Complications, e.g. stricture, obstruction, fistulae, dysplasia/cancer	Limited intestinal resection
		Stricturoplasty (widening of strictures)
	Perianal sepsis	Examination under anaesthesia and drainage of sepsis
		Insertion of a seton if a fistula has formed (see page 247)

Table 6.8 Indications for surgery in patients with inflammatory bowel disease

risk factors and the degree of inflammation seen at endoscopy, and on biopsy of the large bowel. Pancolonic chromoendoscopy (spraying the whole large intestine with dye) is used to highlight abnormal areas of mucosa suggestive of dysplasia, which is confirmed on biopsy. Dysplasia is either treated endoscopically or surgically with colectomy, following a decision by the cancer multidisciplinary team.

Prognosis

The clinical course typically involves periods of relapse and remission. Acute severe colitis remains a potentially life-threatening illness due to the risk of complications such as intestinal perforation.

Crohn's disease

The hallmark of Crohn's disease is patchy transmural inflammation, which affects any part of the GI tract from the mouth to the anus. The features distinguishing it from ulcerative colitis are listed in **Table 6.6**. Around one third of Crohn's patients have inflammation confined to the small intestine (see page 210).

Epidemiology

Crohn's disease is twice as common in smokers as non-smokers. Smoking cessation is probably the most effective factor in maintaining remission and reducing the risk of relapse and is strongly advised.

Smoking increases the risk of Crohn's disease and worsens its course but has a protective effect with respect to the development and severity of ulcerative colitis. Symptoms of the latter frequently develop soon after smoking cessation (nevertheless smoking is remains inadvisable due to its long-term health risks). The mechanism for these associations has been well studied but remains unknown.

Clinical features

Approximately 20% of patients have disease affecting the large intestine alone, 50% have involvement of the small and large intestine, and the remaining patients have involvement of the small intestine, perineum or upper GI tract.

The symptoms depend upon the site affected:

- Upper GI tract (oesophagus and stomach) – vomiting, weight loss and abdominal pain
- Small intestine – abdominal pain, diarrhoea and weight loss
- Large intestine – clinical features similar to those of ulcerative colitis. The inflammation and ulceration sometimes extends beyond the intestinal wall, producing fistulae or abscesses (see page 211)
- Perianal – perianal pain, discharge and bleeding

Examination sometimes reveals abdominal tenderness and associated extraintestinal signs (**Figure 6.6**). Perianal examination occasionally reveals skin tags, ulceration, fistulae and abscesses (see page 245).

Diagnostic approach

As with ulcerative colitis, the diagnosis is based on a combination of blood tests, radiology and endoscopic findings with a corroborative history. It is then confirmed by histology.

Investigations

Initial investigation follows a similar approach to ulcerative colitis (see page 232).

Imaging

Pelvic MRI is useful in assessing perianal complications such as fistulae and abscesses.

Endoscopy

Colonoscopy and ileoscopy are used to help diagnose large intestinal and terminal ileal disease. The thickened oedematous bowel wall with deep ulcers often gives a 'cobblestone' appearance.

Histology typically shows patchy transmural inflammation with a chronic inflammatory cell infiltrate and granulomas (see Figure 5.7).

Management

As with ulcerative colitis, treatment aims to induce and maintain remission.

Medication

Corticosteroids remain the mainstay of treatment for acute disease flares and for induction of remission. Unlike ulcerative colitis, aminosalicylates have a limited role. Immunomodulators such as azathioprine and 6-mercaptopurine are used to maintain remission in patients requiring repeated courses of corticosteroids. Methotrexate is used as second-line therapy in patients who are intolerant of or do not respond to azathioprine. It is used in caution, with counselling required for women of child-bearing age due to teratogenic side effects.

Biologic agents (see page 140) are used in moderate to severely active Crohn's disease not responding to conventional therapy. They are also effective for refractory disease or when other immunosuppressants have failed. In addition, they are useful for fistulating and perianal disease once any sepsis has been treated. Antibiotics, for example ciprofloxacin and metronidazole, are used to treat complications such as perianal abscesses and fistulae.

For patients who smoke, smoking cessation is as effective as any medical therapy for preventing relapses.

Surgery

Up to 80% of patients require surgery at some stage, usually when medical treatment has failed or local complications need to be treated. Indications for surgery in Crohn's disease are given in **Table 6.8**. Operations used to treat inflammatory bowel disease, as well as other common colorectal disorders, are outlined in **Table 6.9**.

Complications

These are the same as for ulcerative colitis:

- Thromboembolism
- Toxic megacolon
- Colonic perforation
- Massive rectal bleeding
- Colorectal carcinoma

See page 235 for further detail.

Prognosis

The mortality rate is the same as for the general population. However, Crohn's disease sometimes considerably affects patients' quality of life and daily activities, particularly after major surgery.

Surgical procedures for colorectal pathology		
Procedure	Description	Common indications
Abdominoperineal resection	Removal of anus, rectum and part of sigmoid colon, with formation of a permanent colostomy	Low rectal cancer
Anterior resection	Removal of rectum and part of sigmoid colon, leaving anal sphincters intact	Mid to upper rectal cancer
Sigmoid colectomy	Removal of sigmoid colon	Sigmoid cancer Diverticular disease
Left hemi-colectomy	Removal of distal transverse, descending and sigmoid colon	Left colon cancer
Right hemi-colectomy	Removal of part of terminal ileum and right colon: ileum is then connected to transverse colon	Right colon cancer
Ileocaecectomy	Removal of terminal ileum and caecum	Terminal ileal Crohn's disease
Subtotal colectomy	Removal of part or all of colon except rectum	Synchronous colonic cancers Polyposis syndromes, e.g. familial adenomatous polyposis Refractory or acute severe colitis (ulcerative colitis or infective) Colitis with dysplasia
Panproctocolectomy	Removal of rectum and colon, with formation of an end-ileostomy	Synchronous colonic cancers Polyposis syndromes Colitis with dysplasia
Ileorectal anastomosis	Removal of colon with connection of ileum to rectum	Colitis (refractory or dyplasia) Polyposis syndromes
Ileoanal pouch	Removal of colon and rectum. A pouch is then made out of distal small bowel	Polyposis syndromes Colitis (refractory, acute severe or dysplasia)

Table 6.9 Commonly-performed surgical procedures used in the treatment of conditions of the large intestine. The commonest indications for each procedure are also outlined.

Microscopic colitis

Microscopic colitis is divided into two types, lymphocytic and collagenous colitis. The aetiology is unknown. However, up to half of all cases are associated with autoimmune conditions (e.g. rheumatoid arthritis, coeliac disease, thyroid disease) or medications such as NSAIDs, proton pump inhibitors and statins. Both types of microscopic colitis have a female predominance with a peak incidence in the sixth decade.

Clinical features

Presentation is with continuous watery, non-bloody diarrhoea lasting several months or a more chronic relapsing course. Despite this, electrolyte disturbance is uncommon. There are usually no abnormal findings from a clinical examination and blood, stool and radiological investigations.

Colonoscopy is the investigation of choice as it allows biopsies of the macroscopically normal large intestine to be taken. Diagnosis is made histologically by an increased number of intraepithelial lymphocytes in lymphocytic colitis or a thickened subepithelial collagenous plate in collagenous colitis.

Biopsies are taken during lower GI endoscopies for symptoms of chronic watery diarrhoea, even if the mucosa has a normal appearance. If this is not done, microscopic colitis will be missed.

Management

Initial management involves excluding precipitating factors such as proton pump inhibitor and NSAID medications and treating associated autoimmune conditions such as coeliac and thyroid disease.

Medication

The anti-diarrhoeal agent loperamide is used to treat diarrhoeal symptoms. Budesonide corticosteroid is the treatment of choice, used in combination with calcium supplements to protect the bones. Up to 60% of patients have coexisting bile salt malabsorption and usually benefit from treatment for this (see page 133). Other medications occasionally used to treat the microscopic inflammation are 5-aminosalicylic acids and immunomodulators.

Surgery

Rarely, surgery is required for severe cases unresponsive to medical therapy. The operations performed are similar to those performed for ulcerative colitis (see page 238).

Prognosis

Microscopic colitis does not increase the mortality rate.

Diverticular disease

Diverticulae are pouches protruding from the intestinal wall that are formed when the mucosa and submucosa herniate through the muscle layer at weak points, usually where blood vessels enter. Diverticulae occur anywhere in the GI tract but are usually found in the descending and sigmoid colon where the muscles contract with greater force to propel the more solid stool. They are usually multiple.

Diverticulosis is more common in individuals over the age of 60 and in developed countries, which is thought to occur secondary to a lower fibre intake.

> **Diverticular disease is rarer in Asian populations.** When it does occur, the presentation is different from that seen in Western countries as it is often found in younger age groups and is more common in the right colon than the left. It has been proposed that it has a genetic basis in this population.

Clinical features

Most people with diverticulosis are asymptomatic. A quarter have symptoms very similar to those of irritable bowel syndrome, i.e. colicky left iliac fossa pain, bloating, flatulence, constipation and/or diarrhoea.

Complicated diverticular disease sometimes causes significant problems (**Figure 6.9**) such as:

- Painless, fresh rectal bleeding
- Diverticulitis causing significant pain and fever
- Diverticular colitis
- Abscesses
- Fistulae – most commonly with the bladder (colovesicular) or vagina (colovaginal)
- Perforation
- Strictures leading to obstructive symptoms

> **Diverticulosis** = asymptomatic diverticula (common)
>
> **Diverticular disease** = diverticula with symptoms such as colicky abdominal pain, bloating, change in bowel habit and occasionally fresh rectal bleeding (less common)
>
> **Diverticulitis** = inflammation of areas of diverticulosis, which sometimes results in severe pain and fever, requiring acute admission to hospital. It may lead to complications such as abscesses, fistulae and strictures (rare)

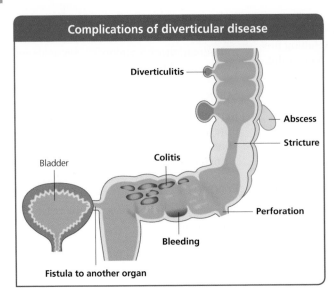

Complications of diverticular disease

Diverticulitis
Abscess
Stricture
Colitis
Bladder
Perforation
Bleeding
Fistula to another organ

Figure 6.9 Complications of diverticular disease.

Investigation

Diverticulae are diagnosed, often incidentally, on colonoscopy or during CT imaging.

Blood tests

Inflammatory markers including white cell count, ESR and CRP are elevated in diverticulitis and if an abscess is present.

Management

In asymptomatic patients, no treatment is required. It is probably good general health advice to suggest an increase in fibre intake for patients with diets low in fibre. If there are symptoms, a high-fibre diet is advised long term, with the addition of fibre supplements such as ispaghula.

Medication

Broad-spectrum antibiotics are prescribed for diverticulitis. Hospital admission is sometimes required for supportive treatment such as intravenous fluids and painkillers. Diverticulitis often settles but often recurs, requiring further antibiotic courses.

Surgery

A few patients require immediate surgery due to emergencies such as perforation or bowel obstruction. Elective surgery is sometimes required for symptomatic patients with complications such as strictures (**Table 6.9**).

Prognosis

Diverticular disease does not affect life expectancy.

Colorectal neoplasia

Colorectal cancer is the third most common cancer worldwide, accounting for 10% of all cancer diagnoses. It occurs sporadically or arises secondary to recognised genetic mutations in high-risk conditions such as familial adenomatous polyposis. Bowel cancer screening programmes have been introduced internationally to reduce the incidence of colorectal cancer, through the detection and removal of benign polyps before they become malignant.

Epidemiology

Over one million new cases of colorectal cancer are diagnosed annually worldwide, with a higher incidence in developed countries.

The incidence is slightly higher in men than women (1.4:1.0). The prevalence of colorectal adenomas increases with age, peaking in patients aged 60–80 years.

Aetiology

Colorectal cancer arises when certain types of benign colorectal polyp, for example adenomas or serrated polyps, progress to adenocarcinoma. Mutations of a variety of tumour suppressor genes (e.g. adenomatous polyposis coli gene), oncogenes (e.g. *KRAS*) and genes responsible for mismatch repair enzymes cause the progression (**Figure 6.10**).

Several characteristics of polyps are related to an increased risk of malignancy:

- Histological type – a villous polyp has the highest risk, a tubulovillous polyp intermediate risk and a tubular polyp lowest risk
- Histological grade of the dysplasia – high-grade dysplasia carries a higher risk of malignant transformation than low-grade dysplasia
- Size – the risk of malignancy increases for polyps measuring 1 cm or more in diameter
- Number of polyps – the risk increases as the number of polyps increases

A diet high in red meat, smoking and alcohol each increases the risk of colorectal cancer. Risk also increases with the number of family members diagnosed with colorectal cancer and a younger age at diagnosis.

> Surveillance colonoscopy is recommended for patients with colorectal adenomas, previous colorectal cancer, polyposis syndromes or a family history of colorectal cancer. Polyp surveillance guidelines in the UK are based upon the number and size of polyps detected. Surveillance guidance based upon family history varies internationally but broadly divides patients into moderate-risk and high-risk groups; the latter are listed in Table 6.10.

Prevention

Colorectal cancer screening strategies vary internationally. Most countries use a guaiac faecal occult test (FOB) that detects blood in the stool or the more specific faecal immuno-chemical test (FIT). If either test is positive, colonoscopy is undertaken as the gold standard investigation allowing biopsy or removal of any polyps. CT pneumocolon is used as an alternative if the patient has significant comorbidity.

Preventive surgery

Due to the inevitability of cancer, individuals with familial adenomatous polyposis are advised to undergo prophylactic surgery in

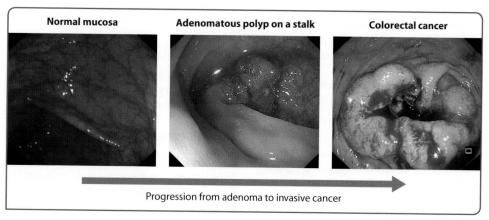

| Normal mucosa | Adenomatous polyp on a stalk | Colorectal cancer |

Progression from adenoma to invasive cancer

Figure 6.10 Adenoma–carcinoma sequence. A series of genetic mutations and chromosomal instability causes normal intestinal epithelial cells to progress initially to adenomas and then on to carcinoma (cancer).

Genetic disorders raising the risk of colorectal cancer		
Genetic disorder	Genetic mutations	Characteristic features
Hereditary non-polyposis colorectal cancer (HNPCC)	Mismatch repair genes including *MLH1, MSH2, MSH3, MSH6, PMS1* and *PMS2*	Predominantly right colon cancers
Familial adenomatous polyposis (FAP)	Adenomatous polyposis coli (APC) gene	Multiple (100s–1000s) polyps in the large intestine. Increased risk of small bowel malignancy
MUTYH-associated polyposis (MAP)	Human *mutY* homologue gene	–
Serrated polyposis syndrome (SPS)	*BRAF* and *KRAS* oncogene mutations	–
Juvenile polyposis	*SMAD4 (DPC4)* and *BMPR1A (ALK3)* genes	Multiple (50+) hamartomatous polyps affecting small and large intestine
Peutz–Jeghers polyposis	*STK11 (LKB1)*	Perioral pigmentation. Hamartomatous polyps usually affecting small intestine

Table 6.10 Hereditary disorders associated with a high risk of developing intestinal cancer

early adulthood. Surgical options are colectomy with ileorectal anastomosis or a proctocolectomy with formation of an ileoanal pouch (**Table 6.9**). The pouch is a reservoir formed from loops of ileum to replace the rectum.

Clinical features

Colorectal polyps are usually asymptomatic and identified incidentally during the investigation of bowel symptoms, during a surveillance procedure if there is a family history of bowel cancer or as part of a bowel screening programme. Larger polyps in the left side of the large intestine occasionally present with rectal bleeding or mucus.

Sporadic colorectal cancer most commonly arises in the left colon. It sometimes presents acutely with features of bowel obstruction including abdominal distension, colicky pain and vomiting. Bowel obstruction is sometimes complicated by a perforation. However, most patients present more generally unwell with the following:

- Symptoms of iron deficiency anaemia, such as tiredness and shortness of breath
- Change in bowel habit
- Weight loss – usually gradually over several months
- Bleeding – fresh blood if the malignancy is in the distal colon, darker red if from the

proximal colon or occasionally melaena in cancers of the caecum or ascending colon
- Tenesmus - a recurrent sensation of needing to evacuate the bowels, occurring with large rectal polyps and cancer
- Abdominal pain – occurs directly at the site of the cancer if it is locally advanced or colicky if the malignancy is causing bowel obstruction

Clinical examination is often normal or shows features of iron deficiency anaemia such as koilonychia and pale conjunctivae. Sometimes an abdominal or rectal mass is noted during abdominal palpation or rectal examination. In cases of bowel obstruction, the abdomen is distended, resonant on percussion and the bowel sounds are prominent or tinkling.

Diagnostic approach

Suspicion of malignancy is raised by the clinical history, examination findings or the presence of iron deficiency anaemia.

Investigations

Diagnosis is made using a combination of blood tests, endoscopic and radiological investigations. Patients presenting acutely with bowel obstruction who require emergency surgery are investigated with blood tests and CT alone.

Blood tests

Low haemoglobin and ferritin levels, mean corpuscular volume and mean corpuscular haemoglobin indicate iron deficiency anaemia. Elevated liver enzymes or calcium levels raise the possibility of liver or bone metastases.

> The tumour maker carcinoembryonic antigen is not a reliable screening or diagnostic test for colorectal cancer, but it is used to monitor disease status during treatment or signs of recurrence after surgery. It is sometimes slightly elevated in smokers, although the reason for this is unknown.

Lower GI endoscopy

Colonoscopy is the gold standard investigation as it allows the resection of benign polyps, biopsy of suspected cancers and the injection of black ink tattoo markings into the lining of the bowel wall (**Figure 6.11**). Seen from the serosal surface of the large intestine during surgery, these tattoos identify the site of the cancer, ensuring the correct segment of intestine is removed.

Sigmoidoscopy only detects abnormalities up to the splenic flexure. Therefore it should only be used instead of colonoscopy if there is concomitant radiological investigation (e.g. CT pneumocolon) to visualise the proximal colon.

Radiological investigations

The rate of identifying pathology is the same for CT pneumocolon and colonoscopy but CT pneumocolon does not allow biopsy. A minimal preparation CT of the abdomen and pelvis is used to exclude large colorectal polyps or cancer in patients with significant co-morbidity or frailty (Table 2.22).

Barium enema is an alternative investigation but is inferior to colonoscopy or CT in diagnosing pathology, as it is reliant on the adequate coating of the colon with barium liquid and operator skill. It is therefore no longer performed in most centres.

A CT scan of the thorax, abdomen and pelvis is performed to look for metastases in patients with colorectal cancer. Positron-emission tomography scans are also used to evaluate for metastatic disease. An MRI of the pelvis is used in the local staging of rectal tumours. Staging is summarised in **Table 6.11** and is based upon:

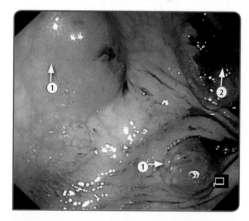

Figure 6.11 Endoscopic image of colonic cancer with tattoos ①. Margin of colorectal cancer ②.

Colorectal cancer staging

Dukes stage	Equivalent TNM stage	Tumour extent	5-Year survival
A	T1, N0, M0 or T2, N0, M0	Invasion into the bowel wall but not through it	93%
B	T3, N0, M0 or T4, N0, M0	Invasion through the bowel wall but not involving the lymph nodes	77%
C	Any T, N1, M0 or Any T, N2, M0	Involvement of lymph nodes	48%
D	Any T, any N, M1	Widespread metastases	6%

TNM, tumour, node, metastases.

Table 6.11 Staging of colorectal cancer

- The degree of invasion of the bowel wall
- The involvement of local lymph nodes
- The presence of metastases

Management

The management depends on the pathology and most commonly involves endoscopic or surgical treatments.

Medication

Medical treatments for ulcerative colitis and colonic Crohn's disease reduce the incidence of colorectal cancer. Long-term aspirin also reduces the risk of colorectal cancer, but it has to be taken regularly for over 20 years to gain this benefit. The NSAID sulindac significantly reduces the number of polyps in familial adenomatous polyposis but does not replace the need for surgery.

Endoscopy

Benign polyps are removed by endoscopic mucosal or submucosal resection. Removal of polyps reduces the incidence of colorectal cancer, by preventing their progression to carcinoma (**Figure 6.10**). Early cancers are resected if there is no evidence of local or distant spread on staging scans.

In bowel obstruction secondary to colonic cancers, self-expanding metal stents are inserted to open up the bowel lumen.

Surveillance colonoscopy is performed after colorectal surgery for cancer to monitor for new colorectal polyps and disease recurrence.

Surgery

Surgery with the aim of cure is performed either laparoscopically or as an open operation. The type of surgery depends upon the tumour location (**Table 6.9**). Isolated liver metastases are also resected.

Patients presenting with bowel obstruction and widespread metastases can be treated with a palliative defunctioning ileostomy or colostomy.

Chemoradiotherapy

Preoperative short-course and long-course radiotherapy reduce the risk of local tumour recurrence. It is often given in combination with chemotherapy to reduce the size of the cancer and the risk of cancer recurrence following surgery.

Palliative chemotherapy reduces the disease burden in metastatic disease. Palliative radiotherapy is used in advanced malignancy to treat bleeding or pain.

Prognosis

The prognosis varies with the tumour stage (**Table 6.11**). The overall 5-year survival for colorectal cancer is approximately 59%.

Anorectal disorders

Anorectal disorders are conditions that occur at the junction of the anal canal and rectum. The majority are benign and have a similar presentation of bleeding and pain. However, careful evaluation is required to exclude malignancy.

The most common anorectal disorders are:

- Haemorrhoids – prominent vascular 'cushions' in the anal canal (**Figure 6.12**). They sometimes prolapse through the canal on defaecation
- Abscess – a collection of pus located in or around the internal and external anal sphincter and perianal muscles

- Fistula – a communication between the perianal skin and anal canal or low rectum, passing through or around the internal and external anal sphincter muscles
- Fissure – a tear in the anal mucosa; 90% occur posteriorly and 10% anteriorly
- Anal cancer – 80% are squamous cell cancers, 16% adenocarcinomas and 4% other types including melanomas and basal cell carcinomas
- Rectal prolapse – prolapse of the rectal mucosa through the anal canal
- Pruritus ani – itching of the anus and perianal region as a result of local causes

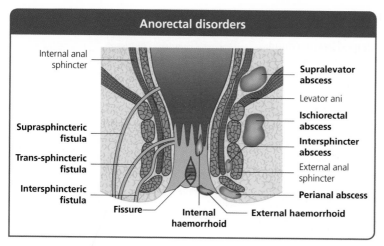

Figure 6.12
Anorectal disorders.

(e.g. poor hygiene, worms), dermatological conditions (e.g. candidiasis) or systemic diseases (e.g. diabetes, jaundice). It is also sometimes idiopathic
- Proctalgia fugax – a sharp anorectal pain lasting from seconds to minutes that occurs secondary to smooth muscle dysfunction

Epidemiology

Haemorrhoids are present in up to 25% of the population and are among the most common cause of rectal bleeding. Among the other anorectal disorders, anal fissures and pruritis ani are the most common. The incidence rate of anal cancer is 1–2 per 100,000, with a female predominance.

Aetiology

Underlying causes of the different types of anorectal disorder are listed in **Table 6.12**.

Clinical features

The features of the disorder depend on the underlying aetiology:

- Rectal bleeding – fresh blood is often noted on the clothing, on wiping or in the toilet pan
- Discharge – pus discharges from fistulae and abscesses

Anorectal disorders	
Disorder	Underlying cause
Abscess	Inflammatory bowel disease
	Infections – HIV, tuberculosis
	Malignancy
Anal cancer	Squamous cell carcinoma – human papillomavirus, HIV
	All types of cancer – immunosuppressant medication
Fissure	Inflammatory bowel disease
	Infections – syphilis, tuberculosis, AIDS
	Malignancy – carcinoma, leukaemia
Fistula	Inflammatory bowel disease
	Diabetes
	Tuberculosis
Haemorrhoids	Constipation
Pruritis ani	Infections – threadworms, pinworms, fungal infection
	Dermatological conditions – eczema, lichen sclerosis
Ulcer	Inflammatory bowel disease
	Behçet's syndrome

Table 6.12 Aetiology of common anorectal disorders

- Pain – suggestive of a fissure if experienced during defaecation. It also occurs with anal cancer and haemorrhoids. Haemorrhoid thrombosis presents with significant rapid-onset pain

■ Anal mass – from prolapsed haemorrhoids, rectal prolapse or anal cancer. This is sometimes noticed on wiping. A visible swelling can indicate an abscess.

Anal cancer may present with any of these features.

Diagnostic approach

A clinical history and examination, including a rectal examination, provide information to guide the diagnosis. A combination of blood tests, endoscopy and radiological investigations are required.

> **Because it is often hard to differentiate between benign and malignant anal disorders,** all patients presenting with anorectal symptoms require especially careful examination.

Investigations

Blood tests

Iron deficiency anaemia sometimes occurs with chronic or significant rectal bleeding. Raised inflammatory markers and a raised platelet count suggest an abscess or an underlying inflammatory condition such as Crohn's disease.

Stool tests

Microscopy of the stool excludes parasitic infection, which sometimes causes symptoms of pruritus ani.

Endoscopy

Proctoscopy and rigid sigmoidoscopy allow direct visualisation of the rectum and anal canal. Flexible sigmoidoscopy is performed if a more proximal source of bleeding is suspected.

Imaging

CT staging is required for anal cancers to assess for local and distant metastases, using the

Anorectal conditions and treatment	
Anorectal disorder	**Treatment**
Abscess	Surgery – incision and drainage of larger abscesses, seton insertion
	Antibiotics – used alongside surgery but ineffective as a single treatment
Anal cancer	Chemoradiotherapy (radiotherapy alone may cure early squamous cell carcinoma)
	Surgery – local excision, abdominoperineal resection
Fissure	Laxatives to avoid straining
	Topical glyceryl trinitrate or diltiazem cream (see page 141)
	Botulinum toxin injected to relax internal anal sphincter to stop spasm
	Surgery – sphincterotomy, excision of fissure
Fistula	Treatment of underlying condition, e.g. Crohn's disease
	Fibrin glue
	Surgery – fistulotomy, seton insertion
Haemorrhoids	Topical corticosteroid, local anaesthetic cream
	High-fibre diet
	Banding
	Injection of sclerosant
	Infrared photocoagulation
	Surgery – excision or stapling haemorrhoidectomy
Proctalgia fugax	Salbutamol inhaler (mechanism unknown)
	Analgesics, e.g. amitriptyline
Pruritis ani	Good perianal hygiene
	Treatment of underlying cause
	Topical steroids
Rectal prolapse	Laxatives to avoid straining
	Surgery, e.g. Delorme's procedure
Ulcer	Treatment of underlying cause

Table 6.13 Treatment of anorectal disorders

TNM system (see Figure 2.28). MRI and ano-rectal ultrasonography provide local cancer staging and also help to define the anatomy of complex abscesses and fistulae.

Surgery

Examination under anaesthetic enables detailed examination of the anus and perineum and biopsy of any lesions to exclude malignancy.

Management

Management is tailored to the condition (**Table 6.13**).

In cases where a fistula forms, a non-absorbable thread called a seton is passed through the fistula tract and left in place to prevent the accumulation of pus by keeping the tract of the fistula open.

Prognosis

Anal cancer has an overall 5-year survival of 60–75%; survival depends on disease stage and ranges from 80% for T1N0M0 disease to 10% for M1 (metastatic disease). All other anorectal conditions are benign and do not affect life expectancy.

Answers to starter questions

1. The cause of polyps in the large intestine remains uncertain, although it is likely due to genetic and lifestyle factors. Mutations in certain genes, such as tumour suppressor genes and oncogenes, cause disruption in cell proliferation, migration and differentiation resulting in polyp formation. These factors, in addition to DNA mutation during replication, cause the progression of benign adenomas to adenocarcinoma.

2. Colorectal cancer cannot be prevented unless the large intestine is completely removed, for example in management of ulcerative colitis. However, not smoking, not drinking alcohol to excess and avoiding a diet high in red meat all reduce the risk. In the UK, the NHS Bowel Cancer Screening programme offers biennial screening to everyone aged 60–74 years using either guaiac faecal occult tests (FOB) that detect blood in the stool or the more specific faecal immunochemical test (FIT). If either is positive colonoscopy is performed to remove adenomatous and serrated polyps, preventing their progression to adenocarcinoma.

3. Irritable bowel syndrome (IBS) is a multifactorial condition and the exact cause remains unknown. The role of food is unclear, although patients often report symptoms are exacerbated by certain dietary triggers. Food intolerances, particularly gluten sensitivity and carbohydrate malabsorption, are thought to play a part. For example, FODMAPs are carbohydrates which are poorly absorbed in the small intestine and so pass through to the large intestine where they are fermented by bacteria, resulting in bloating and other symptoms. Restricting these from the diet can be an effective way of treating IBS.

4. Diverticulae are sac like protrusions in the lining of the GI tract, most commonly the left colon. A low fibre diet plays a pivotal role in their development, explaining the wide variation in prevalence worldwide. Slower colonic transit time and reduced stool bulk results in a narrowed colonic lumen and the need for higher intraluminal pressures to propel the stool. This can result in herniation of the mucosa through weak points in the bowel wall causing diverticulae to form. These weak points occur naturally where the vasa recta arteries pass through the circular muscle layer, particularly in the sigmoid colon where there is a lack of complete longitudinal muscle layer. Loss of collagen through aging may also play a role.

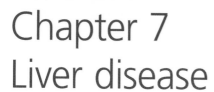

Chapter 7
Liver disease

Starter questions

Reading this chapter will enable you to answer the following questions. Answers are on page 284.

1. Why do only some people who are obese develop chronic liver disease, and is it possible to predict?
2. Is liver damage reversible?
3. Why doesn't an elevated cholesterol level in primary biliary cholangitis increase cardiovascular risk?

Introduction

The liver plays a major role in the breakdown of toxins (including drugs), in digestion and in lipid, carbohydrate and protein metabolism. Consequently it is essential for maintaining health. Significant damage has a range of potentially life-threatening consequences. However, symptoms of liver damage often take a long time to appear. Most people with abnormal liver function tests have non-specific symptoms or are completely well.

Liver injury is either acute (e.g. due to viruses and medications) or the result of chronic damage over a period of time, leading to cirrhosis – fibrosis and scarring of liver tissue – and its potential complications, such as ascites, varices and hepatocellular carcinoma. Many patients with chronic liver damage display the classic stigmata of liver disease (**Figure 7.1**).

Chronic liver diseases are becoming more common, mainly due to increasing rates of alcohol intake and non-alcoholic fatty liver disease (NAFLD). As a result, the death rate from liver disease has risen significantly over the last few decades despite the improvements in care and treatment that have led to falling mortality rates from other conditions such as cancer and ischaemic heart disease.

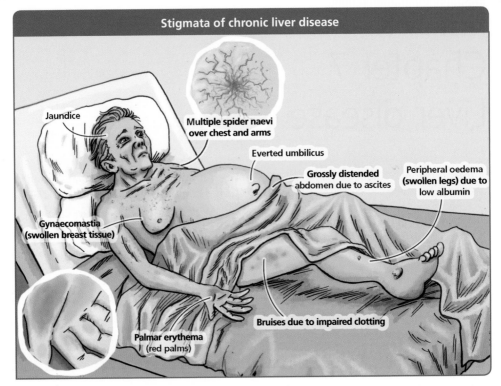

Stigmata of chronic liver disease

Jaundice

Multiple spider naevi
over chest and arms

Everted umbilicus

Grossly distended
abdomen due to ascites

Peripheral oedema
(swollen legs) due to
low albumin

Gynaecomastia
(swollen breast tissue)

Bruises due to impaired clotting

Palmar erythema
(red palms)

Figure 7.1 Stigmata of chronic liver disease.

Case 8 Jaundice

Presentation

Luke Jennings, a 20-year-old man, makes an emergency appointment to see his general practitioner (GP). Luke has been feeling unwell for several days but over the last 24 hours he has developed jaundice.

Initial interpretation

Luke is young and has a relatively short history of being unwell prior to developing jaundice, which suggests an acute liver injury. To help determine the cause of the jaundice, more details about his illness are required, including any history of abdominal pain, medication use and other symptoms.

History

Over the previous week, Luke has had 'flu-like' symptoms with a fever, lethargy and generalised aches and pains. His urine and stool are a normal colour. There has been some upper abdominal discomfort. He has been taking regular paracetamol for the symptoms. He originally became unwell towards the end of a month's holiday travelling around India.

Interpretation of history

The history is highly suggestive of an infection and the travel history is relevant. There is a high rate of both hepatitis A and E on the Indian subcontinent, as well as some other parts of the world. There are no symptoms of cholestasis, such as dark urine or pale stool, so biliary tree disease is less likely (see Chapter 2, page 88). In patients with jaundice, it is essential to ask about other risk factors of liver disease, such as intravenous drug use and unprotected sex.

Further history

Luke has taken no more than six paracetamol tablets a day since becoming unwell and has not used any other medications (prescribed, over-the-counter, herbal or illicit). He did not receive any vaccinations before going abroad as the trip was arranged at very short notice. He has never had any previous episodes of jaundice. He is usually fit and well, and has no significant past medical or psychiatric history. There is no family history of liver or autoimmune disease.

Luke is currently at university. He has not had a sexual relationship for over 6 months and is a non-smoker. His alcohol intake is variable but he binge drinks fairly regularly, consuming over 8 units of alcohol in one go.

Examination

Luke is jaundiced (**Figure 7.2**). There are no stigmata of chronic liver disease (see **Figure 7.1**) and no tattoos. The liver is moderately enlarged and tender to deep palpation. There are no abnormal findings on cardiovascular and respiratory examination.

Interpretation of findings

The history and examination are in keeping with an acute illness involving the liver. Infection is the likely cause, but further investigations are required to confirm this and exclude other aetiologies.

Investigations

The GP requests liver function tests to assess the type of jaundice. He receives the results the next day after which he phones the infectious diseases team for advice (**Table 7.1**). After discussing Luke's presenting symptoms and reviewing these results they recommend performing a liver screen, including viral hepatitis serology (**Table 7.2**) and monitoring his liver function carefully.

> An international normalised ratio (INR) and prothrombin time is always checked in patients with an acute liver injury. A prolonged time or increased ratio is a sign of acute liver failure and specialist help is advised.

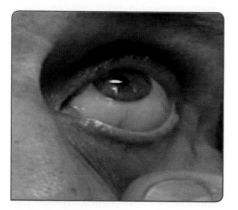

Figure 7.2 Yellow sclera due to jaundice.

Results of liver function tests

Test	Result (normal range)
Bilirubin	220 µmol/L (1–22 µmol/L)
Alkaline phosphatase	145 U/L (45–105 U/L)
Alanine transaminase	954 U/L (5–35 U/L)
γ-Glutamyl transferase	214 IU/L (<50 U/L)
Albumin	36 g/L (37–49 g/L)
International normalised ratio	1.5 (1.0–1.3)

Table 7.1 Luke's liver function and INR test results

Case 8 *continued*

Liver screen	
Blood tests	Viral serology: ■ Hepatitis A IgM and IgG ■ Hepatitis B Surface antigen (HBsAg) ■ Hepatitis C antibody ■ Hepatitis E IgM and IgG If clinical history and symptoms are suggestive, consider : ■ Monospot for Epstein–Barr virus ■ 'Atypical' serology including *Legionella, Mycoplasma*, herpes simplex and cytomegalovirus ■ Leptospirosis – if renal failure is present
	Liver autoantibodies: ■ Anti-smooth muscle antibody (ASMA) ■ Antinuclear antibody (ANA) ■ Antimitochondrial antibody (AMA) ■ Anti neutrophil cytoplasmic antibody (ANCA)
	Ferritin or transferrin saturation (if chronic disease is suspected)
	Copper or caeruloplasmin level (only if <40 years old)
	α_1-Antitrypsin level (if chronic disease suspected)
	Glucose (HbA1c) and lipid concentrations
	Immunoglobulins
	Prothrombin time or INR
	Paracetamol level (if acute toxicity is a possibility)
Radiology	Ultrasonography of the liver, including portal vein Doppler scanning

INR, international normalised ratio.

Table 7.2 Liver screen: this is tailored according to the presentation and the pattern of liver enzymes, as demonstrated by liver function tests

Ultrasonography of the liver shows mild hepatomegaly but no focal abnormality. The bile ducts and other abdominal structures appear normal.

The differential diagnoses include:

■ Hepatitis A or E is the most likely diagnosis, due to Luke's recent travel to Indian subcontinent
■ Blood-borne viral infections such as hepatitis B, C and D, although there are no obvious risk factors for these from Luke's clinical history
■ Epstein–Barr virus, which causes glandular fever, especially in younger patients
■ An overdose of paracetamol or secondary to medications (e.g. NSAIDs and nitrofurantoin), which causes a similar biochemical profile
■ Autoimmune hepatitis, although this is more common in women
■ Alcohol excess is a possible cause of the abnormal liver function tests, although this very rarely causes such a significantly elevated transaminase level
■ Underperfusion of the liver, e.g. after a cardiac arrest or pronounced hypotensive episode, which would also produce such a significant hepatitis.

Luke's hepatitis A IgM antibody result is positive, indicating acute infection. Negative results are reported for hepatitis B, C and E, the Monospot test (for Epstein–Barr virus) and liver autoantibodies.

> **Alcohol excess sometimes causes a hepatitis, but rarely causes the transaminase level to increase to more than 10 times the upper value, i.e. aspartate transaminase (AST) and alanine transaminase (ALT) concentrations remain below 500 U/L.**

Diagnosis

After receiving the viral hepatitis serology results from the virology lab, the infectious diseases team contact the GP and explain that Luke has acute hepatitis A.

Case 8 *continued*

The prodromal illness before the onset of jaundice is characteristic of viral hepatitis.

Luke's GP tells him that hepatitis A is a self-limiting infection that does not cause chronic disease. He is advised to have a few weeks away from his studies until he feels well enough and the liver function tests are improving on follow up blood tests. He is told that he will make a full recovery.

Treatment is supportive with low dose paracetamol for the fever and pain. Hospital admission is rarely required unless there are signs of acute liver failure, such as hepatic encephalopathy. As the hepa-

titis virus appears in the faeces for 1 week before and 2 weeks after the onset of jaundice, Luke is told to adopt strict personal hygiene to reduce the risk of transmitting the infection to others.

A few days later, the local public health authority contacts Luke. They ask detailed questions about the history of his illness to ensure there is no clustering of cases. They also reiterate advice to him about how to minimise the risk of transmission to friends and relatives.

Luke has weekly liver function tests performed at his GP surgery over the next few weeks until the tests have returned to normal.

Case 9 Swollen abdomen

Presentation

Andrew O'Grady is a 53-year-old man who presents to his GP with a 4-week history of abdominal distension and ankle swelling. He has no past medical history and has never experienced similar symptoms previously. He last visited his doctor over 2 years ago.

Initial interpretation

Abdominal distension is a common presenting symptom that usually occurs secondary to one of the '5 Fs' (see page 90). Distension that fluctuates over a period of time suggests a bowel-related cause such as flatus or constipation. Fluid results in progressive abdominal distension and can accumulate secondary to abdominal diseases and right-sided heart failure.

Further history

Andrew has no change in his bowel habit. However, his appetite is poor as the abdominal distension causes him to feel

full quickly. He eats a reasonable diet and was exercising regularly until his symptoms began. He has recently started to feel breathless during simple activities like climbing the stairs. There is no family history of GI disease.

On further discussion, he admits to feeling low in mood and drinking 2 litres of cider most evenings since he was made redundant 2 years ago.

> **Prior and current alcohol excess sometimes cause liver disease.** Remember that patients are not always truthful about their alcohol intake. An elevated mean corpuscular volume or γ-glutamyl transferase level, and a low urea concentration suggest ongoing alcohol consumption.

Examination

Andrew has a grossly distended abdomen (see **Figure 7.1**) and requires braces to hold his trousers up. He has palmar erythema and eight spider naevi over

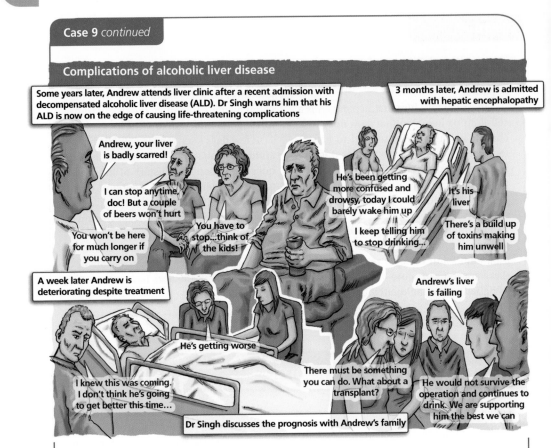

Case 9 *continued*

Complications of alcoholic liver disease

Some years later, Andrew attends liver clinic after a recent admission with decompensated alcoholic liver disease (ALD). Dr Singh warns him that his ALD is now on the edge of causing life-threatening complications

3 months later, Andrew is admitted with hepatic encephalopathy

Andrew, your liver is badly scarred!

I can stop anytime, doc! But a couple of beers won't hurt

You won't be here for much longer if you carry on

You have to stop...think of the kids!

He's been getting more confused and drowsy, today I could barely wake him up

I keep telling him to stop drinking...

It's his liver

There's a build up of toxins making him unwell

A week later Andrew is deteriorating despite treatment

He's getting worse

I knew this was coming. I don't think he's going to get better this time...

Andrew's liver is failing

There must be something you can do. What about a transplant?

He would not survive the operation and continues to drink. We are supporting him the best we can

Dr Singh discusses the prognosis with Andrew's family

his upper arms and chest wall. There is shifting dullness on abdominal percussion. Pitting leg oedema is present up to the thighs. He is not jaundiced and has no signs of encephalopathy. There are no abnormal findings on respiratory and cardiovascular examination.

Interpretation of findings

The progressive nature of the symptoms and examination findings is suggestive of chronic liver disease with ascites. The absence of cardiorespiratory symptoms and examination findings make diseases of these systems unlikely.

Investigations

Andrew's GP arranges blood tests to assess his liver function and severity of liver disease, the results of which are shown in **Table 7.3**.

Abdominal ultrasound shows a small nodular liver and gross ascites. No focal liver lesions are identified, and the portal and hepatic veins have a normal Doppler blood flow.

Abdominal ultrasonography with portal and hepatic vein Doppler studies is performed in all patients with new or rapidly accumulating ascites, to exclude underlying thrombosis as a potential cause.

Andrew is urgently referred to the hepatology clinic for further assessment.

Here, further blood tests are taken for a full liver screen to exclude viral and metabolic causes of liver disease (**Table 7.2**). A diagnostic ascitic tap shows a high

Case 9 continued

Blood test results	
Test	Result (normal range)
Haemoglobin	131 g/dL (130–180 g/L)
Platelets	83 x 10⁹/L (150–400 x 10⁹/L)
Mean corpuscular volume	101 fL (80–96 fL)
Sodium	134 mmol/L (137–144 mmol/L)
Urea	1.2 mmol/L (2.5–7.0 mmol/L)
Creatinine	64 µmol/L (79–118 µmol/L)
Albumin	24 g/L (37–49 g/L)
Alanine transaminase	60 U/L (5–35 U/L)
γ-Glutamyl transferase	210 U/L (<50 U/L)
International normalised ratio	1.4 (1.0–1.3)

Table 7.3 Andrew's blood test results

serum–ascites albumin gradient (SAAG), which is consistent with portal hypertension. There is no evidence of infection, or malignant cells on cytology.

> **A diagnostic ascitic tap** is an essential investigation in any patient with signs of chronic liver disease who presents with ascites.

Diagnosis

The clinical history and investigations suggest a diagnosis of decompensated alcoholic liver disease (i.e. liver disease with additional complications). The consultant hepatologist advises complete abstinence from alcohol and commences the diuretic spironolactone to treat the ascites and peripheral oedema. Andrew's GP is asked to monitor his renal function while taking this medication, for electrolyte imbalance and acute kidney injury.

Andrew is reviewed by a substance misuse specialist and referred to community alcohol support services for counselling. A dietitian provides advice on a high-protein and no-added-salt diet, which prevents protein calorie malnutrition and reduces the rate of accumulation of ascites.

At a follow-up 3 weeks later, Andrew has lost 8 kg in weight due to a reduction in the amount of ascitic fluid and leg oedema, resulting in an improvement in his abdominal distension.

Acute liver failure

Acute liver failure refers to the rapid failure of the liver's synthetic and metabolic function in the absence of known pre-existing liver disease. It is an uncommon but serious condition, requiring specialist and critical care input, and has a high mortality rate if left untreated.

Classification of acute liver failure is based on the interval between the initial onset of jaundice and the development of encephalopathy:

- **hyperacute** – within 7 days
- **acute** – between 8 and 28 days
- **subacute** – between 29 days and 12 weeks

In the UK, the most common cause is paracetamol overdose; worldwide it is acute viral hepatitis.

The investigation and management of acute liver failure are discussed further in Chapter 10 (see page 322).

Portal hypertension

Portal hypertension is increased blood pressure in the hepatic portal circulation above its normal level of 7 mmHg (see Figure 1.36), independent of systemic blood pressure.

Aetiology

Portal hypertension is caused by any pathology that prevents blood flowing through the portal vein into and through the liver into the hepatic vein:

- **Hepatic causes**: cirrhosis is the commonest overall cause of portal hypertension; other causes include schistosomiasis, hereditary haemorrhagic telangiectasia (HHT) and conditions causing liver infiltration (e.g. malignancy and sarcoidosis)
- **Prehepatic causes**: portal or splenic vein blockage, e.g. by thrombosis or infiltration of these vessels by surrounding tumour (e.g. pancreatic cancer)

- **Posthepatic causes**: thrombosis of the hepatic vein (see page 277) or inferior vena cava, or cardiac disease

Clinical features and investigation

Portal hypertension is often asymptomatic. Otherwise it manifests with varices or ascites. There may also be visible collateral vessels on the abdominal wall (**Figure 7.3**) and splenomegaly.

In patients with ascites, portal hypertension is diagnosed if the SAAG value is ≥11 g/L (see page 128).

Management

Management is directed at the cause of the portal hypertension, e.g. cirrhosis , and relieving the consequences, e.g. by draining ascites or insertion of a transjugular intrahepatic portosystemic shunt to reduce the pressure (TIPS – see page 262).

Cirrhosis

Cirrhosis is caused by chronic inflammation or insults to the liver, for example due to alcohol leading to fibrosis and scarring (see **Figure 7.9**). The consequent reduction in normal liver function and altered blood flow leads to complications such as ascites.

Epidemiology

The prevalence of cirrhosis is estimated to be 76 per 100,000 population in the UK and accounts for approximately 2% of all deaths in Europe.

Aetiology

The most common cause in the UK is alcohol. Other causes of cirrhosis include:

- Viral hepatitis: hepatitis B and C – see pages 265–268

- Metabolic disorders: non-alcoholic fatty liver disease (page 270), haemochromatosis (page 272), Wilson's disease (page 273), α_1-antitrypsin deficiency (page 274)
- Autoimmune disorders, e.g. autoimmune hepatitis and primary biliary cholangitis (page 274–275)
- Primary sclerosing cholangitis (PSC; page 276)
- Drugs such as methotrexate

Sometimes the cause is unknown, in which case the disorder is termed cryptogenic cirrhosis.

Clinical features

Cirrhosis is sometimes asymptomatic and therefore only detected during radiological investigation. Alternatively, it presents with a variety of features:

- Disorientation, confusion or drowsiness – due to hepatic encephalopathy (see Complications below), in which there is often a liver flap, or hyponatraemia
- Bruising – secondary to a coagulopathy and low platelet level (thrombocytopenia). Cirrhosis causes portal hypertension, which results in splenomegaly (see **Figure 7.3**) and consequently leads to increased consumption of platelets by the spleen, lowering the platelet level. The coagulopathy is due to a reduced production of clotting factors by the liver
- Abdominal distension – due to ascites (see Complications below)
- Unsteady gait and muscle weakness – from poor nutrition or as a result of cerebellar atrophy secondary to alcohol misuse

Clinical examination shows features of chronic liver disease (see **Figure 7.1**), for example palmar erythema and Dupuytren's contracture (see Figure 2.8). The liver often becomes shrunken and nodular in patients with cirrhosis, and is therefore not palpable. Occasionally chronic liver disease raises the oestrogen level and resulting in gynaecomastia (spironolactone diuretic therapy sometimes has the same effect).

Complications in decompensated liver disease

Compensated cirrhosis is the presence of scarring of the liver without loss of normal functions such as metabolism and the removal of toxins. Patients with cirrhosis are described as becoming decompensated when the liver is not capable of performing all its normal functions, leading to a number of complications:

- Hepatic encephalopathy
- Varices
- Ascites
- Other less common complications, as outlined in **Table 7.4**

Hepatic encephalopathy This is a diffuse disturbance of brain function related to liver disease. Its presentation varies considerably:

- Grade 1 – short attention span and some cognitive impairment
- Grade 2 – lethargy, disorientation and personality change
- Grade 3 – confusion and somnolence
- Grade 4 – comatose.

Increased intestinal absorption of ammonia and its reduced metabolism in the cirrhotic liver, leads to an increased level of ammonia in the blood. The ammonia crosses the blood–brain barrier where it is detoxified to form glutamine. This results in swelling of the astrocyte brain cells and mild cerebral oedema, leading to the symptoms and signs of hepatic encephalopathy. Hepatic encephalopathy is usually precipitated by an underlying cause such as electrolyte disturbance (e.g. due to diuretics), infection (e.g. spontaneous

Less common complications of cirrhosis		
Condition	Description	Cause
Spontaneous bacterial peritonitis	Bacterial infection of ascitic fluid: neutrophil count >250/mm³ or positive culture results	Translocation of bacteria from colonised blood and gut into ascitic fluid
Hepatocellular carcinoma	Liver tumour ± raised α-fetoprotein level	See page 278
Hepatorenal syndrome	Renal impairment in patient with advanced liver disease in absence of identifiable cause	Changes in renal blood flow and cardiac function
Hepatic hydrothorax	Pleural effusion in patient with portal hypertension Usually right-sided	Translocation of ascitic fluid from peritoneal to pleural cavity through defects in diaphragm
TIPS, Transjugular intrahepatic portosystemic shunt.		

Table 7.4 Less common complications of cirrhosis (see text for the more common complications, e.g. encephalopathy, varices and ascites)

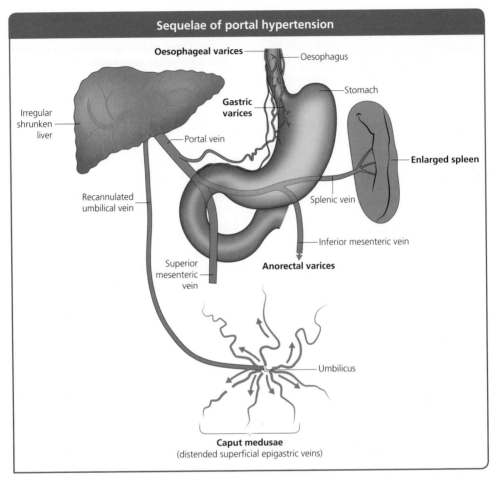

Sequelae of portal hypertension

Oesophageal varices — Oesophagus

Stomach

Gastric varices

Irregular shrunken liver — Portal vein

Enlarged spleen

Recannulated umbilical vein

Splenic vein

Inferior mesenteric vein

Superior mesenteric vein

Anorectal varices

Umbilicus

Caput medusae
(distended superficial epigastric veins)

Figure 7.3 Sequelae of portal hypertension (sequelae are in bold). The liver often becomes shrunken in patients with cirrhosis. Caput medusae radiate out from the umbilicus across the abdominal wall.

bacterial peritonitis), GI bleeding, constipation or drugs (e.g. benzodiazepines or opiates).

Varices These are dilated submucosal veins in the oesophagus, stomach, rectum and abdominal wall (caput medusae), which occur secondary to portal hypertension (see **Figure 7.3**). The most common site is the oesophagus. Patients with bleeding from oesophageal and gastric varices present with large-volume fresh haematemesis and melaena and have a 20% mortality rate. Rectal varices occasionally bleed resulting in large-volume rectal bleeding

Ascites Dilatation of systemic blood vessels occurs in patients with cirrhosis, which

causes a reduced effective blood volume and stimulation of the renin–angiotensin–aldosterone system. This results in fluid retention and the formation of ascites, categorised as:

- Grade 1 – mild ascites only detected by ultrasonography
- Grade 2 – moderate abdominal distension
- Grade 3 – gross ascites with marked abdominal distension

Peripheral (leg) oedema occurs due to low albumin levels, which reduce the oncotic pressure in the blood vessels and results in leakage of fluid into surrounding body tissues.

> **Spontaneous bacterial peritonitis (SBP) is infection of the ascitic fluid.** The risk of renal impairment, encephalopathy and variceal bleeding is increased in patients with SBP.

Diagnostic approach

A diagnosis of cirrhosis is usually made using a combination of blood tests and radiology. Occasionally a liver biopsy is required to obtain histology to determine the underlying cause.

Investigations

Blood tests and radiological investigations are required to determine the aetiology of cirrhosis and screen for complications.

> **Slightly abnormal liver function tests are very common and have many causes,** for example obesity, poorly controlled diabetes, alcohol excess or drugs. They are often found in asymptomatic individuals undergoing blood tests to monitor conditions such as diabetes or to investigate non-specific symptoms such as lethargy.

Blood tests

In cirrhosis, liver function tests are almost always abnormal. Low serum albumin and a deranged coagulation profile (a prolonged prothrombin time and high INR) demonstrate impaired synthetic hepatic function. The pattern of abnormality in the liver enzymes, e.g. a hepatocellular or cholestatic pattern, varies with the underlying aetiology. A liver screen is performed to identify the potential cause of the cirrhosis (**Table 7.2**). Alanine transaminase (ALT) and alkaline phosphatase (ALP) levels are often normal or only mildly elevated in advanced cirrhosis, due to damage to the hepatocytes. Hyponatraemia occurs in a quarter of patients with cirrhosis and ascites.

The level of α-fetoprotein (AFP) is assessed to screen for hepatocellular carcinoma, a complication of cirrhosis. An elevated AFP of > 400 kU/L in the presence of a liver nodule is diagnostic of hepatocellular carcinoma. Testicular and ovarian germ cell tumours also sometimes cause a raised AFP.

> **Patients with cirrhosis sometimes develop hyponatraemia due to fluid overload (dilutional) or diuretic treatment.** Dilutional hyponatraemia is treated by fluid restriction.

Imaging

Abdominal ultrasonography usually shows a nodular liver outline consistent with cirrhosis and signs of portal hypertension such as splenomegaly. This test is also used to screen the liver for masses due to hepatocellular carcinoma. Portal and hepatic vein Doppler ultrasonography is important to exclude thrombosis as a precipitant of ascites or variceal bleeding in patients with cirrhosis.

MRI or CT imaging of the liver is considered if a liver lesion is suspected or the level of alpha-fetoprotein is elevated, as these tests help to identify malignancy. Hepatocellular carcinoma appears as a hypodense mass on CT, with central areas of necrosis. On MRI scan they are identified as high signal lesions, surrounded by a thin fibrous capsule.

Ascitic fluid

Fluid is sent for a neutrophil count and culture to exclude spontaneous bacterial peritonitis (SBP). This is diagnosed if the neutrophil count is >250/mm³ or if the cultures grow a specific bacterial organism. A SAAG value (SAAG = serum albumin concentration - ascitic fluid albumin concentration) is calculated to assess for portal hypertension, which is diagnosed if the value is ≥11 g/L (see page 128). Cytology is requested if there is a clinical suspicion of malignancy.

Histology

Liver biopsy is undertaken via a percutaneous or transjugular vein approach (see page 127). Histology shows fibrosis (see **Figure 7.9**) and regenerative nodules. Specific blood test results and histological features and special stains confirm autoimmune or hereditary metabolic aetiologies.

Endoscopy

Surveillance upper GI endoscopy is performed in patients with cirrhosis to look for oesophageal and gastric varices.

Other changes visible at endoscopy due to portal hypertension include portal hypertensive gastropathy and gastric antral vascular ectasias (GAVE), which are dilated blood vessels arising in the gastric antrum. GAVE is an uncommon cause of iron deficiency anaemia and chronic GI bleeding.

Management

Management is directed towards the treatment of each complication and prevention of any continuing liver damage, for example by recommending alcohol cessation. It is summarised in **Table 7.5** and the individual elements of treatment are described in more detail below.

Nasogastric tube feeding is considered if patients are unable to meet their dietary calorie requirements, as assessed by a dietician (see Chapter 2, page 146). It is also used to provide nutrition and medications such as lactulose (see below) to patients with hepatic encephalopathy who are too drowsy to eat and drink.

> **Spironolactone is the diuretic of choice when treating fluid overload in liver disease.** This is because it is an aldosterone antagonist and there is an inappropriate over-activation of the renin–angiotensin–aldosterone pathway in patients with cirrhosis.

Medication

Medication is tailored to the complication.

- **Lactulose** is used in the treatment of hepatic encephalopathy. It is a non-absorbable disaccharide laxative that is not metabolised until it reaches the colon, where it is broken down into components which reduce the production and absorption of ammonia. The dose is increased until 2–3 bowel actions are achieved each day
- **Sodium phosphate enema** (see Table 2.29) is used to treat patients with hepatic

Treatment of cirrhosis complications

Condition	Treatment
Hepatic encephalopathy	Treat precipitating cause (e.g. electrolyte disturbance)
	Lactulose (aim for 2–3 bowel actions/day)
	Sodium phosphate enema
	Rifaximin (see page 142)
Varices	Beta-blocker (e.g. propranolol, carvedilol)
	Oesophageal banding
	TIPS
Ascites	Diuretics
	Fluid restriction if hyponatraemic
	No-added-salt diet
	Therapeutic paracentesis
	TIPS
Spontaneous bacterial peritonitis	Antibiotics
	Human albumin solution
Hepatocellular carcinoma	See page 278
Hepatorenal syndrome	Stop diuretics
	Human albumin solution
	Terlipressin (see page 132)
Hepatic hydrothorax	As with ascites

TIPS, transjugular intrahepatic portosystemic shunt.

Table 7.5 Treatment of the complications of cirrhosis

encephalopathy who are too drowsy to take lactulose, as constipation is one of the commonest precipitants of this condition
- **Antibiotics** are used to treat spontaneous bacterial peritonitis and, by reducing infection, to improve the survival of patients presenting with suspected or confirmed variceal bleeding. Treatment begins with intravenous third-generation cephalosporins (e.g. cefotaxime and ceftriaxone) then the antibiotic choice is changed according to sensitivities of bacteria cultured from ascitic fluid. Rifaximin is used in the treatment of hepatic encephalopathy: because it is non-absorbable it reduces the number of ammonia-forming bacteria in the colon. Prophylactic antibiotics (e.g. ciprofloxacin)

are given to patients following treatment for SBP or a low ascitic protein level, because of the risk of infection of the ascitic fluid

- **Non-cardioselective beta-blockers** (e.g. propranolol or carvedilol) are used to reduce portal pressure in patients with large asymptomatic varices and following endoscopic treatment for bleeding varices. The dose is increased to the highest tolerated dose or until a heart rate of 50 bpm is achieved

- **Oral diuretics** are used in the treatment of ascites and leg oedema occurring as a complication of cirrhosis. Spironolactone is the first-line treatment, due to its action as an aldosterone antagonist. It is often given in combination with furosemide, a loop diuretic. Diuretic dosage is gradually increased until the patient starts to lose weight, which indicates fluid loss. Frequent urea and electrolyte testing of blood is required to avoid diuretic-induced electrolyte disturbance and acute kidney injury: treatment is usually discontinued if the Na$^+$ falls to < 125 mmol/L

- **Ascitic paracentesis** is used in patients with large volume ascites and those with recurrent ascites who are intolerant to or don't respond to diuretic medication (see Chapter 2, page 155). Intravenous human albumin solution is given as the ascites is drained to avoid an acute kidney injury

- **Terlipressin** (see page 132) is used to reduce portal pressure and increase the mean arterial pressure in variceal bleeding and hepatorenal syndrome

- **Human albumin solution**, as an intravenous infusion of salt-poor albumin, is used as an intravascular volume expander in patients with spontaneous bacterial peritonitis, hepatorenal syndrome and during ascitic paracentesis. Albumin reduces the risk of renal impairment and the mortality rate in patients with SBP

Endoscopy

Upper GI endoscopy is used to provide endoscopic treatment to bleeding varices:

- **Oesophageal varices** are almost always treated with endoscopic banding. Each varix is sucked up into a plastic cap placed on the tip of the gastroscope in turn, after which a rubber band is deployed around its base (**Figure 7.4**). The bands fall off within a few weeks, causing local ulceration and scarring which reduces the size of the varix. After the initial treatment, banding is performed as an outpatient every few weeks until the varices disappear

- **Gastric varices** are treated using an injection of cyanoacrylate (tissue adhesive) or thrombin (enhances clotting) into the varix using an injection needle inserted through the gastroscope

A Sengstaken tube is inserted if variceal bleeding cannot be controlled during endoscopy (see page 321). This only acts as a short-term measure to stabilise the patient whilst definitive treatment, e.g. a transjugular intrahepatic portosystemic shunt (TIPS), is undertaken.

Bleeding from GAVE is treated by cauterisation of the blood vessels in the gastric antrum usually by argon plasma coagulation therapy (see Chapter 2, page 152–153).

Radiological

A transjugular intrahepatic portosystemic shunt (TIPS) is used in the treatment of

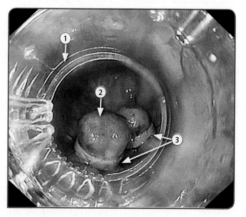

Figure 7.4 Endoscopic image of banded oesophageal varices. (1) Banding device attached to the end of the endoscope. (2) Banded varix. (3) Rubber bands placed on the bases of the varices.

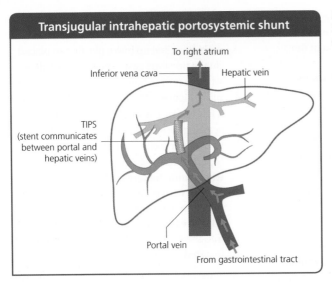

Figure 7.5 Transjugular intrahepatic portosystemic shunt (TIPS).

variceal bleeding that cannot be controlled endoscopically, ascites not responding to medical treatments (e.g. diuretics) and hepatic hydrothorax (**Figure 7.5**). A metal shunt is inserted under X-ray guidance to connect the hepatic and portal veins, thereby lowering the pressure within the portal system.

Surgery

Cadaveric or living donor liver transplantation is considered in individuals with liver tumours or chronic liver disease when there are significant complications (e.g. recurrent ascites or encephalopathy) and limited life expectancy. Long-term immunosuppressant medication is required after transplantation to prevent liver rejection.

Prognosis

In Europe, cirrhosis and its complications cause around 170,000 deaths per year. The prognosis depends on a modification of lifestyle and risk factors, for example alcohol abstinence if there is alcoholic liver disease. The development of ascites in patients with cirrhosis indicates a poor prognosis, with a mortality rate of 50% at 2 years.

Alcoholic liver disease

Alcohol is a group of organic compounds containing common structural components. Ethanol is the main type present in alcoholic beverages. Alcohols are also used in other areas of medicine as an antiseptic (e.g. alcohol-based hand gel) or preservative. Use of the term alcohol throughout this chapter will make reference to alcohol ethanol. Excess alcohol consumption is more common in men and young people, and sometimes results in dependence. Misuse results in a broad spectrum of liver conditions ranging from acute alcoholic hepatitis to chronic liver disease and cirrhosis.

Epidemiology

The harmful use of alcohol accounts for around 6% of all deaths worldwide. A quarter of all deaths in 20- to 39-year-olds in the UK are related to alcohol, including liver disease.

Aetiology

Following ingestion, alcohol is absorbed in the proximal small intestine (duodenum and proximal jejunum) by simple diffusion. It is distributed throughout the body in the blood, with more vascular organs such as the brain reaching higher concentrations more quickly. Alcohol (ethanol) cannot be stored by the body and is predominantly broken down within the liver, where it undergoes several oxidative processes to form water and carbon dioxide or through alternative pathways to form fatty acids. The toxic effects of alcohol occur secondary to its effect on fat metabolism resulting in a fatty liver and the depletion of antioxidants. Fatty liver results in inflammation of the liver tissue, progressing to fibrosis and ultimately cirrhosis.

Binge drinking is the episodic consumption of excessive amounts of alcohol. The risk of cirrhosis is higher in individuals drinking more than 12 g of alcohol per day, particularly amongst women. One unit equates to approximately 8 g of alcohol (see Figure 2.5).

Clinical features

Alcoholic liver disease is sometimes asymptomatic. Alternatively, it presents with a variety of features depending on the severity of disease:

- Reduced appetite – alcohol consumption suppresses appetite
- Diarrhoea – due to accelerated gut transit or complications such as pancreatic insufficiency (see Table 8.5)
- Nutrient deficiencies (see Table 5.6) – lead to consequences such as peripheral neuropathy
- Sweats, tremor, nausea and hallucinations due to alcohol withdrawal
- Features of chronic liver disease

Physical examination can be normal or show signs of liver disease, for example palmar erythema. Alcoholic hepatitis and fatty liver sometimes result in hepatomegaly. Findings in cirrhosis are described on pages 250 and 256.

Complications

These occur either acutely due to alcohol withdrawal or chronically secondary to sustained alcohol misuse:

- Delirium tremens ('DTs') – confusion, agitation, disorientation, sweats, fever, hallucinations, tachycardia
- Seizures – secondary to alcohol withdrawal

- Alcoholic hepatitis – jaundice, ascites with or without hepatic encephalopathy
- Cognitive impairment – Wernicke's encephalopathy, Korsakoff's psychosis, alcoholic dementia
- Peripheral neuropathy – impaired sensation of the limbs due to nerve damage
- Cirrhosis and its complications (**Table 7.4**). Hepatocellular carcinoma resulting from alcoholic cirrhosis has an incidence of up to 16% after 5 years

Alcohol withdrawal syndrome This is a severe medical condition occurring in alcohol-dependent patients, who suddenly stop or decrease their alcohol intake. It sometimes results in seizures, coma, cardiac arrest and death.

Two disorders seen almost exclusively in alcoholics who are also malnourished are:

Wernicke's encephalopathy is a triad of neurological symptoms secondary to vitamin B deficiency: confusion, ataxia (unsteady body movements) and ophthalmoplegia (weakness of the eye muscles).

Korsakoff's psychosis is a lack of vitamin B in the brain, resulting in amnesia, confabulation and apathy. Usually it occurs as a progression of untreated Wernicke's encephalopathy, when it is called Wernicke–Korsakoff syndrome.

Diagnostic approach

The diagnosis is usually made from the clinical history in combination with blood tests and radiology.

Investigations

Further tests are required if there is evidence of cirrhosis.

Blood tests

ALT and γ-glutamyl transferase concentrations are often elevated in patients with alcohol misuse and alcoholic steato-hepatitis (fatty infiltration and inflammation of the liver). Alcoholic hepatitis causes a raised ALT and often a raised bilirubin level, with associated coagulopathy (elevated prothrombin time and INR). A full liver screen is required if the aetiology of abnormal liver function is unclear (**Table 7.2**). AFP is monitored in patients with alcohol-related cirrhosis to screen for hepatocellular carcinoma, which occurs as a complication of cirrhosis.

Imaging

Abdominal ultrasonography is sometimes normal or shows a 'bright' liver with increased echogenicity consistent with fatty liver. In patients with cirrhosis, the surface of the liver is usually irregular. CT or MR imaging is performed to assess liver lesions when abnormalities are identified on ultrasound. Transient elastography imaging measures liver stiffness to identify fibrosis.

Histology

Liver biopsy and histology in patients with alcoholic hepatitis show Mallory bodies (damaged protein filaments found within the liver cells), ballooning degeneration of the hepatocytes and inflammatory changes. Features of alcoholic liver disease include steatosis (fatty infiltration), fibrosis and ultimately cirrhosis (**Figure 7.6**).

Management

The principal treatment is either reduction of or abstinence from alcohol depending on the degree of liver disease (see page 149). Community-based alcohol support services provide medical detoxification, individual or group counselling sessions and medications to support abstinence from alcohol. Patients at high risk of alcohol withdrawal syndrome are sometimes electively admitted to specialist centres to provide this treatment. Substance misuse specialists also provide information and support to patients admitted acutely to hospital with alcohol related conditions.

Medication

Alcohol withdrawal syndrome is managed using long-acting benzodiazepines, such as diazepam or chlordiazepoxide, to protect against seizures or delirium. High-dose vitamin B replacement in the form of Pabrinex, a proprietary intravenous combination of vitamin B (thiamine, riboflavin, nicotinamide and pyridoxine) with ascorbic acid, or oral thiamine is given to prevent and treat Wernicke's encephalopathy.

The principal treatment for alcoholic hepatitis is with the corticosteroid prednisolone. Pentoxifylline is also occasionally used off license, to suppress the raised anti-tumour necrosis factor levels present in alcoholic liver disease. The decision to commence and continue treatment is based upon prognostic scoring systems using blood tests such as bilirubin, prothrombin time, urea and white cell count.

Several drugs are used to support abstinence from alcohol. Disulfiram causes a physical reaction if alcohol is consumed. Acamprosate and naltrexone are used to prevent relapse in individuals who have achieved abstinence (see page 149). The use of both drugs is off-label in the UK.

Complications of alcohol-related liver disease are managed as outlined on page 260.

Surgery

Liver transplantation is considered for patients with complications of cirrhosis, such as recurrent ascites or encephalopathy. A 6-month period of abstinence from alcohol is generally recommended, due to the potential for patients to relapse and to allow time for reversible elements of the liver disease to recover, so that patients are in optimal fitness if transplantation is required.

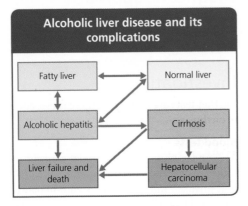

Figure 7.6 Alcoholic liver disease and its complications.

Prognosis

This depends on the stage of the liver disease. Reducing or abstaining from alcohol is one of the principal factors influencing prognosis. The prognosis is worse for individuals with cirrhosis combined with alcoholic hepatitis than for those with either condition alone.

Viral hepatitis

Several different viruses have been identified as causing hepatitis. These include hepatitis A–E (**Table 7.6**) and Epstein–Barr virus (**Table 7.2**). Hepatitis B, C and D can cause chronic disease that leads to cirrhosis and its consequences.

Epidemiology

Hepatitis A and E can be acquired anywhere in the world but are more common in travellers to the Middle and Far East, Africa, South America and Eastern Europe, where epidemics occur.

Characteristics of viral hepatitis					
	A	**B**	**C**	**D**	**E**
Genome	RNA	DNA	RNA	RNA	RNA
Transmission	Faecal–oral	Blood or infected body fluids	Blood	Blood	Faecal-oral
Incubation period (weeks)	2–6	6–25	2–20	4–8	2–8
Serology test	Hep A IgM antibody shows acute infection IgG antibody indicates immunity	HBsAg See Table 7.7 for further testing	Hep C antibody shows infection at some point PCR to determine viral load	Hep D IgM antibody shows acute infection IgG antibody indicates immunity	Hep G IgM antibody shows acute infection IgG antibody indicates immunity
Chronic infection (frequency after acute infection)	No	Yes (<20%)	Yes (75%)	Yes (<50%)	No
Vaccination and target groups	Available: travellers to high-prevalence areas	Available: Childhood vaccination in some countries and selective vaccination in others, e.g. health care workers including students and other high-risk individuals	No vaccine	No vaccine	No vaccine
Reducing risk	Good hygiene and sanitation Safe drinking water, well-cooked food	Not sharing needles, razors or toothbrushes Condom use Avoiding unlicensed premises for tattoos or piercings			Good hygiene and sanitation Safe drinking water, well-cooked food

HBsAg , hepatitis B surface antigen; Hep, hepatitis; PCR, polymerase chain reaction.

Table 7.6 Characteristics of viral hepatitis types A–E

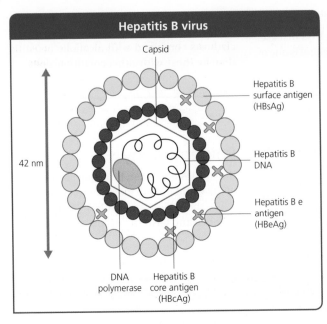

Hepatitis B virus

Capsid

Hepatitis B surface antigen (HBsAg)

42 nm

Hepatitis B DNA

Hepatitis B e antigen (HBeAg)

DNA polymerase

Hepatitis B core antigen (HBcAg)

Figure 7.7 Hepatitis B virus structure. Serological testing for hepatitis B determines levels of the antigens (or antibodies to them), in a way that helps determine the stage of infection (see **Figure 7.8** and **Table 7.7**).

In developed countries, hepatitis B (**Figure 7.7**) and C are mainly seen in higher risk groups, for example intravenous drug users. However, they are far more common in other parts of the world, such as East Asia and sub-Saharan Africa. Over 240 million people worldwide have chronic hepatitis B and 150 million have chronic hepatitis C. Each year, over 1 million people die from complications of hepatitis B.

Aetiology

Hepatitis A and E are acquired from contaminated food (especially seafood in the case of hepatitis A) and water.

Hepatitis B, C and D are contracted via infected blood or blood products (**Table 7.6**). They are more common in intravenous drug users who share needles, people who have had tattoos and those who received blood transfusions before routine screening began in 1990. Hepatitis B (in particular) and C is transmissible through unprotected sex via semen and vaginal fluids. Hepatitis B can also spread vertically from an infected mother to her baby during childbirth and through breast milk. Hepatitis D only survives in the presence of hepatitis B, where it increases the risk of cirrhosis.

Viral hepatitis (types B and C) is the most common cause of cirrhosis worldwide, while alcohol is currently the most common cause in developed countries.

Clinical features

The presentation varies widely between the five types of hepatitis virus (**Table 7.6**):

Acute infection

- Initially, non-specific viral symptoms occur and last for up to a fortnight, e.g. fatigue, loss of appetite, fevers, nausea and muscle pains
- Diarrhoea and vomiting – hepatitis A and E often present with a self-limiting gastroenteritis-type illness and resolve without permanent damage
- Jaundice occurs in most but not all individuals – as a result, some patients with positive serology are not aware that they have had hepatitis. The jaundice starts just as the prodromal symptoms are resolving. It sometimes lasts for several weeks, during which time lethargy and general malaise is often present

- Other than jaundice, physical examination is usually normal but sometimes shows a tender hepatomegaly caused by acute hepatitis
- Acute liver failure is rare. If present, patients are closely monitored in a critical care setting where there is a higher ratio of nursing staff available to monitor their fluid balance, blood glucose and conscious level. Acute liver failure is an indication for possible liver transplantation

Chronic infection

- Chronic infection occurs in a minority of individuals who acquire hepatitis B, but most of those who get hepatitis C. Patients either have no noticeable symptoms or experience non-specific complaints such as tiredness or depression. Of those with chronic hepatitis infection, the risk of liver cirrhosis is up to 30% within 20 years after the infection is acquired
- Hepatitis B and C can result in chronic liver disease and features of cirrhosis

Diagnostic approach

Diagnosis is made through blood testing. A viral cause is considered in any patient with acute hepatitis, particularly if the characteristic prodromal symptoms are present. Tests for hepatitis B (**Figure 7.8**) and C are conducted if there is chronic hepatitis or cirrhosis. These tests are also now carried out in people who are at higher risk of infection, for example intravenous drug users and patients with haemophilia who have received blood products.

Investigations

Blood tests

Liver function tests predominantly show a hepatitis picture and raised bilirubin during the acute illness. Ballooning of the hepatocytes due to inflammation sometimes compresses the small bile ducts. This causes a self-limiting, secondary cholestatic picture to the liver function tests.

Serological testing is summarised in **Table 7.6**. To determine the status of hepatitis B infection, several antigens and antibodies are tested (**Table 7.7**). In patients with hepatitis C antibodies, the polymerase chain reaction shows current infection and determines the viral load. This, together with identification of the hepatitis C genotype (1 to 6), determines the treatment regimen and duration.

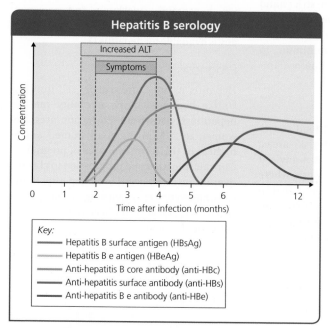

Figure 7.8 Hepatitis B serology. ALT, alanine transaminase.

Interpreting hepatitis B serology					
	HBsAg	HBeAg	Anti-HBs	Anti-HBe	Anti-HBc
Incubation	+	+	–	–	–
Acute hepatitis	+	+	–	+/–	+ (IgM)
Carrier or chronic infection	+	+/-	–	+/–	+ (IgG)
Recovery	–	–	+	+	+ (IgG)
Vaccination	–	–	+	–	–

Table 7.7 Interpreting hepatitis B serology (for abbreviations, see **Figures 7.7** and **7.8**)

Other investigations

In chronic hepatitis B and C, a liver biopsy determines the degree of fibrosis or cirrhosis of the liver (histological staging), used to determine a patient's suitability for antiviral treatment. Liver biopsy is increasingly being replaced by transient elastography as a non-invasive test to assess liver fibrosis (see Chapter 2, page 119). Surveillance for hepatocellular cancer by regular liver ultrasonography and alpha-fetoprotein level is advised.

Management

In acute infections, the treatment is symptomatic. All known cases are reported to local public health authorities. In forms of hepatitis with faecal-oral spread, strict hand washing and personal hygiene reduce the risk to others. It is sensible to recommend that alcohol intake is kept to a minimum, to avoid any additional inflammation or damage to the liver.

Prevention

Careful attention to water and food sources is recommended in high-risk areas. Immunisation against hepatitis A is advised before travelling to parts of the world where it commonly occurs, such as sub-Saharan Africa and the Middle East. It is also recommended for family members and close contacts of those with an acute infection.

A vaccine has been developed for hepatitis E but is not widely available. About 75% of countries have a childhood vaccination programme for hepatitis B. The remaining countries, such as the UK, have a selective immunisation programme for health-care professionals and at-risk individuals (e.g. people who inject drugs, sex workers and patients who receive regular blood products).

Medication

Antiviral agents, as monotherapy or in combination, are effective in providing sustained treatment responses for individuals with chronic infection. Drugs include lamivudine, adefovir, tenofovir, entecavir and pegylated interferon-α for hepatitis B; and telaprevir, boceprevir, sofosbuvir and pegylated interferon-α for hepatitis C. No antiviral therapy is available for hepatitis D.

Prognosis

Hepatitis A and E are usually self-limiting. Unlike hepatitis A, the mortality rate for hepatitis E rises from 1% in non-pregnant women to 20% in pregnant women and is highest in the third trimester of pregnancy. Chronic infection and progression to chronic liver disease can occur with hepatitis B and C, although newer antiviral agents mean that hepatitis C could be eradicated in developed countries by 2030.

Drug-induced liver injury

One of the vital functions of the liver is the metabolism of drugs. Most medications have the potential to cause abnormal liver function tests, and any pattern of acute and chronic liver injury (**Table 7.8**).

Epidemiology

Paracetamol overdose and adverse drug reactions (e.g. NSAIDs, flucloxacillin) account for around 50% of cases of acute liver failure in developed countries. Hepatotoxicity is the most common reason for approved medications to be removed from the market or for warnings about their usage to be issued.

Aetiology

Some drug-induced injuries are dose related, for example with paracetamol overdose. Others (e.g. co-amoxiclav) are more unpredictable (idiosyncratic). These unpredictable reactions often occur in individuals with a genetic susceptibility. They directly affect the cell biochemistry or cause an immune-mediated response.

> **Always think of drugs as a potential cause of abnormal liver function tests.** Ask specifically about over-the-counter medications, illicit drugs and herbal remedies as well as prescribed treatments that have been completed within the past few weeks.

Clinical features

Most individuals are asymptomatic, with abnormalities of the liver function tests seen either incidentally or as part of recommended monitoring, for example of patients taking statins. Features include:

- Jaundice or features of cholestasis such as itching
- Occasionally, a hypersensitivity reaction with a fever and rash

Physical examination is usually normal, but there are sometimes signs of jaundice.

Drug-induced liver injury	
Type	Cause
Hepatitis	Paracetamol overdose
	Statins
	Antiepileptics, e.g. phenytoin, sodium valproate
	Antituberculosis drugs, e.g. isoniazid, rifampicin
	Amiodarone
	Methotrexate
	Halothane (anaesthetic agent)
	NSAIDs
	Herbal preparations
Cholestasis	Antibiotics, e.g. co-amoxiclav (amoxicillin plus clavulanic acid), erythromycin, flucloxacillin
	Hormones: oral contraceptive pill, anabolic steroids
	Angiotensin-converting enzyme inhibitors
	Tricyclic antidepressants
	Chlorpromazine
	NSAIDs
	Herbal preparations
Isolated elevation in γ-glutamyl transferase	Hepatic enzyme inducers, e.g. phenytoin
Fibrosis or cirrhosis	Methotrexate
	Vinyl chloride
Focal nodular hyperplasia or adenomas	Oral contraceptive pill, anabolic steroids
Veno-occlusive disease	Oral contraceptive pill, anabolic steroids

NSAID, non-steroidal anti-inflammatory drug.

Table 7.8 Drug-induced liver injury

Diagnostic approach

A complete and detailed drug history is taken. Questioning is extended beyond currently prescribed treatments as a drug-related injury can occur on the first day of use or several months later. Drugs taken in recent weeks are identified; cholestatic jaundice, for example, sometimes occurs several weeks after completing a course of antibiotics such as flucloxacillin.

Investigations

Liver function tests indicate a hepatitis or cholestatic picture. Additional tests are performed including abdominal ultrasonography to exclude biliary tract dilatation and screening blood tests, for example viral serology, ferritin level and liver autoantibodies (see **Table 7.2**).

Management

This includes identifying potentially involved drugs. A risk/benefit decision has to be taken, involving the indication for the medication and whether any alternatives are available.

In some cases the medication, for example an antibiotic, has already been stopped.

A paracetamol overdose sometimes causes liver damage. Treatment with an N-acetylcysteine infusion is commenced depending upon the paracetamol level and the timing of the overdose (see page 323). However, up to 6% of individuals develop an anaphylactoid reaction to this treatment, with nausea and vomiting, rash and difficulty breathing. In these cases, the treatment is usually successfully restarted at a slower infusion rate without further symptoms.

Prognosis

With most drugs, the liver impairment is self-limiting. Medications such as methotrexate sometimes cause liver fibrosis. Paracetamol occasionally results in fulminant liver failure potentially requiring transplantation.

Non-alcoholic fatty liver disease

Non-alcoholic fatty liver disease (NAFLD) is a spectrum of liver disease which sometimes progresses from benign liver steatosis to non-alcoholic steato-hepatitis (NASH), and ultimately liver fibrosis and cirrhosis (see **Figure 7.9**). Histologically, it is indistinguishable from alcoholic liver disease. Its prevalence, along with that of other obesity-related illness, is increasing, and is a cause of significant patient morbidity and mortality.

Epidemiology

One billion people worldwide, and up to one third of the population in developed countries, have evidence of NAFLD; the vast majority have simple steatosis. However, around 10–30% progress to NASH, where inflammation as well as fatty infiltration occurs. This can progress to liver fibrosis, cirrhosis and its complications.

Aetiology

The exact aetiology remains poorly understood but there is a strong association with underlying insulin resistance and metabolic

syndrome (type 2 diabetes mellitus, hypertension, hyperlipidaemia, central obesity).

A 'two-hit' hypothesis has been proposed in which an initial insult causes steatosis as a result of excess triacylglyceride (triglyceride) accumulation within the liver. These changes then make the liver susceptible to a second insult, which is driven by increased oxidative stress (imbalance between the production of free radicals and the ability of the body to counteract their effects) and leads to inflammation and fibrosis.

> **The incidence of fatty liver disease is rising rapidly worldwide because of a 'westernisation' of lifestyle.** It has been predicted that it will become a more frequent cause of chronic liver disease than alcohol.

Clinical features

The majority of patients are asymptomatic and are identified incidentally by elevated liver function tests. A detailed alcohol history is taken and other forms of liver disease excluded. Some patients have non-specific upper abdominal discomfort.

Examination findings include:

- Hepatomegaly
- Features of metabolic syndrome, e.g. truncal obesity
- Acanthosis nigricans – dark pigmentation occurring in the folds of the skin (e.g. armpits, groins and neck) due to insulin resistance
- Stigmata of chronic liver disease (in cases of progression to cirrhosis)

Diagnostic approach

There is no single diagnostic test for NAFLD or for the progression of simple steatosis to NASH. Diagnosis is made from the clinical history, including an alcohol intake of less than 5 units (40 g) per week, together with an elevated transaminase level and radiological investigations demonstrating a fatty liver.

Investigations

Blood tests

Transaminases are mildly to moderately elevated, ALT usually proportionally more than AST (in contrast to alcoholic liver disease). Fasting lipid and glucose levels are usually elevated in patients with an underlying metabolic syndrome.

A liver screen is performed to look for other aetiologies of liver disease (**Table 7.2**). Scoring systems (e.g. fatty liver index and the NAFLD fibrosis score) help to determine individuals who are more likely to progress to NASH. Risk factors for progression include increasing age, body mass index over than 35 kg/m², diabetes mellitus, a low platelet count and a low albumin concentration.

Imaging

Abdominal ultrasound typically shows a hyperechoic 'bright' liver due to fatty infiltration. Features of cirrhosis or portal hypertension are sometimes evident. Transient elastography is used to assess liver fibrosis.

Liver biopsy

Liver biopsy is often unnecessary. If it is performed, patients with NAFLD typically have macrovesicular steatosis. The histology of NASH is indistinguishable from that of alcoholic steato-hepatitis, with steatosis, hepatocyte injury and lobular inflammation (**Figure 7.9**).

Management

The mainstay of treatment is lifestyle modification, such as increased physical activity and dieting in overweight or obese patient's and control of risk factors, e.g. raised cholesterol. Exercise reduces the liver fat content.

Medication

The following are used alongside lifestyle modification:

- Medication to aid weight loss, e.g. orlistat, an enteric lipase inhibitor that acts by causing malabsorption of dietary fat
- Medication to control underlying hypertension, hyperlipidaemia and diabetes mellitus
- Thiazolidinediones (used in the treatment of type 2 diabetes), which help to improve steatosis, inflammation and even fibrosis
- Vitamin E, an antioxidant, protects the liver against damaging free radicals

Surgery

Bariatric surgery, such as a gastric bypass or gastric balloon insertion (see Figure 2.38), has a role in patients who have not achieved sufficient weight loss using non-surgical measures with the support of specialised hospital services; and who have a BMI of greater than 35 kg/m² with or without significant disease (e.g. type 2 diabetes or hypertension) that would improve with weight reduction. Assessment for liver transplant is appropriate if there are signs of progression to cirrhosis and related complications, e.g. ascites.

Prognosis

Around 8–15% of patients with NASH will progress to cirrhosis within 10 years.

Histology of fatty liver

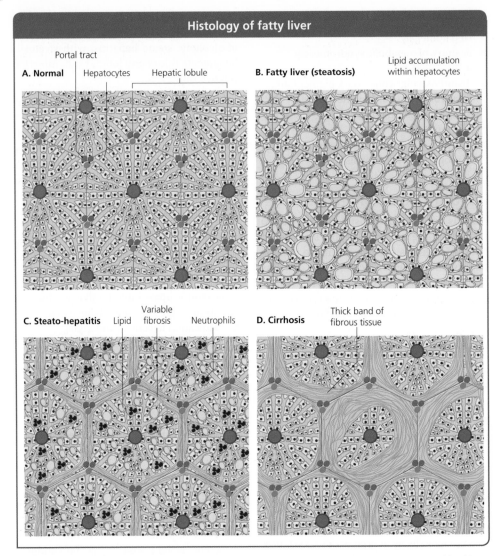

A. Normal — Portal tract, Hepatocytes, Hepatic lobule

B. Fatty liver (steatosis) — Lipid accumulation within hepatocytes

C. Steato-hepatitis — Lipid, Variable fibrosis, Neutrophils

D. Cirrhosis — Thick band of fibrous tissue

Figure 7.9 Histology of fatty liver. In fatty liver there is lipid accumulation within the hepatocytes (B). This also occurs in steato-hepatitis (C), in which it is accompanied by infiltration by neutrophils and a variable amount of fibrosis. In cirrhosis there are much thicker bands of fibrous tissue (D).

Metabolic disorders

There are several types of rare metabolic liver disorder, which are usually hereditary. The most common are haemochromatosis, α_1-antitrypsin deficiency and Wilson's disease.

Haemochromatosis

Haemochromatosis, or iron overload, is either:

■ Primary, due to hereditary haemochromatosis

- Secondary, due to repeated blood transfusions, excess dietary iron or iron supplements, chronic liver disease, congenital haemolytic anaemia, thalassaemia or sideroblastic anaemia

Hereditary haemochromatosis is an autosomal recessive disorder characterised by excess iron accumulation. It has a prevalence of approximately 1 in 400 in white individuals and a heterozygote carrier frequency of 1 in 10 in this patient group. The most common form is caused by a C282Y or H63D mutation of the HFE gene, present on chromosome 6. This leads to excess iron absorption from the small intestine. The iron then accumulates in the liver, pancreas, heart, pituitary and joints.

Clinical features

These include hepatomegaly and cirrhosis with its potential complications such as hepatocellular carcinoma. Systemic features are also sometimes identified:

- Fatigue and malaise
- Bronze discolouration of the skin
- Diabetes mellitus
- Cardiomyopathy and features of heart failure
- Symmetrical polyarthropathy
- Hypogonadism and loss of libido

Women tend to present a decade later than men due to the protective effect of menstrual blood loss. Blood tests show raised levels of ferritin, iron and raised transferrin saturation. Genotypic testing is performed to identify the presence of common gene mutations (C282Y and H63D). Liver biopsy is occasionally performed and identifies iron overload using a Prussian blue stain.

> **A high serum ferritin level is not always a sign of iron overload.** Ferritin is an acute-phase protein that is often elevated in inflammatory conditions. Other causes of a raised ferritin include alcoholic liver disease, diabetes and metabolic syndrome.

Management

Treatment is with regular venesection to reduce iron stores and limit organ damage. Venesection is usually weekly for the first 6–12 months and then three or four times per year. Chelation therapy with desferrioxamine is used for patients who are unable to tolerate repeated venesection (e.g. those with anaemia or cardiac failure). Fasting blood tests for transferrin saturation, ferritin and HFE genotyping are recommended to screen first-degree relatives, so that treatment is available for affected individuals, to reduce the risk of complications.

Prognosis

Cirrhosis commonly develops in untreated disease. There is also an increased risk of hepatocellular carcinoma, particularly if the iron overload is not treated. Life expectancy is normal if treatment is started before the onset of end-organ damage. Once the complications of cirrhosis and arthritis have developed, they are irreversible despite venesection. However, diabetes, hypogonadism, arthralgia, fatigue and raised transaminase liver enzymes sometimes improve or resolve with this treatment.

Wilson's disease

This is a rare autosomal recessive inborn error of copper metabolism that results in copper accumulation in organs including the liver, cornea, basal ganglia and kidneys due to mutation of the *ATP7B* gene present on chromosome 13. Presentation is usually between the ages of 5 and 15 years.

Clinical features

Kayser–Fleischer rings, caused by copper accumulation in Descemet's membrane in the eyes, are often observed, although slit-lamp examination is usually required. Other features include:

- Hepatic – cirrhosis or fulminant hepatic failure

- Neurological – tremor, dysarthria, involuntary movements, dementia
- Renal tubular damage

Blood tests show low serum copper and caeruloplasmin (a plasma protein that carries copper) levels. A 24-hour urine copper level is elevated.

Management

Lifelong penicillamine and trientine are used as copper-chelating agents. Alternatively, these agents are used until the copper level returns to normal, following which oral zinc is started as a long-term treatment, to reduce copper absorption.

> Testing for Wilson's disease is not advised in patients who present with liver disease over the age of 40 years. This is because it is unlikely, owing to the early age of onset of Wilson's disease.

α_1-Antitrypsin deficiency

α_1-Antitrypsin is an inhibitor of trypsin and other protease enzymes, which is synthesised in the liver. α_1-Antitrypsin deficiency is an autosomal recessive condition occurring due to a mutation of the *SERPINA1* gene on chromosome 14. It results in lack of inhibition of these enzymes, causing liver damage.

In adults, α_1-antitrypsin deficiency is usually detected when a liver screen is performed because a patient's liver function tests have demonstrated a mixed hepatocellular and cholestatic picture. Diagnosis is usually made through blood testing, which shows a low serum α_1-antitrypsin level. Additional testing is then required to determine the phenotype of which PiZZ most commonly causes liver disease. Liver biopsy is often not required, but when performed shows a hepatitis with positive periodic acid–Schiff staining.

Treatment is symptomatic, with transplantation considered in patients who develop decompensated liver disease. Hepatocellular carcinoma surveillance is advised due to an increased risk. Due to the hereditary nature of α_1-antitrypsin deficiency, screening of family members is recommended by measuring their α_1-antitrypsin levels.

Autoimmune liver disease

In autoimmune liver disease, an immune response against the liver produces a hepatitis or cholestatic picture on liver function blood tests.

Primary biliary cholangitis (PBC)

This is a chronic condition characterised by progressive destruction of the bile ducts that eventually leads to cirrhosis. It predominantly affects women (10:1) and usually presents in the fourth to sixth decades. The prevalence in the UK is around 24 per 100,000. The exact aetiology is unknown, but immunological mechanisms play a role. Almost all patients have antimitochondrial antibodies, particularly to the M_2 antigen.

> Primary biliary cholangitis was formerly called primary biliary cirrhosis. The name was changed because many patients are not cirrhotic.

Clinical features

Primary biliary cholangitis is often asymptomatic and found incidentally on investigation of abnormal liver enzymes. Features include:

- Pruritus (itching) – the cause is uncertain but potentially related to increased concentrations of bile acids
- Fatigue
- Xanthelasma (yellow coloured fatty deposits) on the eyelids and xanthoma (fatty deposits occurring anywhere in the body)

- Hepatomegaly
- Jaundice – which is a sign of advanced disease
- Osteopenia
- Cirrhosis and its complications, including hepatocellular carcinoma

Clinical examination occasionally reveals multiple excoriation marks, together with the stigmata of chronic liver disease (**Figure 7.1**).

Diagnostic approach

Diagnosis is frequently made with blood tests alone:

- Cholestatic liver function tests (raised alkaline phosphatase and γ-glutamyl transferase)
- Positive antimitochondrial antibodies
- An elevated level of serum IgM, a marker of disease activity

The serum cholesterol level is also often high, but the risk of cardiovascular disease is not increased. Low levels of fat-soluble vitamins (A, D, E and K) sometimes occur as a result of decreased bile acid secretion. Liver biopsy is performed if the diagnosis is uncertain and demonstrates interlobular bile duct destruction.

Management

Treatment is usually symptomatic.

Medication

Ursodeoxycholic acid is the only medication that leads to some improvement in liver function and possibly survival. Obeticholic acid, a semi-synthetic bile acid analogue, has also shown promise. Additional treatments include the replacement of fat-soluble vitamins and calcium supplements, and bisphosphonates for osteopenia and osteoporosis.

Symptoms of pruritus are difficult to treat. The mainstay of treatment is colestyramine, which acts by reducing bile acid absorption in the enterohepatic circulation. Rifampicin and naltrexone are alternatives.

Surgery

Liver transplant is considered with advanced cirrhosis or intractable symptoms.

Prognosis

Median survival from the onset of symptoms is 12 years.

Autoimmune hepatitis

This is a progressive inflammatory condition of the liver with a female preponderance. It is characterised by a chronic active hepatitis that is frequently associated with other autoimmune conditions (**Table 7.9**). Although rare, it is an important differential diagnosis when abnormal liver function tests are present, as there is significant mortality if it is left untreated.

Clinical features

Autoimmune hepatitis is sometimes asymptomatic and detected during the investigation of abnormal liver function tests. Other presenting features include:

- Non-specific symptoms including lethargy, fatigue, arthritis, rash, nausea and abdominal pain

Autoimmune conditions associated with autoimmune hepatitis	
Location	Associated autoimmune conditions
Thyroid gland	Grave's disease
	Autoimmune thyroiditis
Connective tissue	Systemic lupus erythematosus
	Sjögren's syndrome
	Rheumatoid arthritis
	CREST (calcinosis, Raynaud's syndrome, oesophageal dysmotility, sclerodactyly, telangiectasia) syndrome
Stomach	Pernicious anaemia
Liver	Autoimmune hepatitis
	Primary biliary cholangitis
Pancreas	Autoimmune pancreatitis
	Diabetes mellitus
Adrenal gland	Addison's disease
Small intestine	Coeliac disease

Table 7.9 Autoimmune conditions associated with autoimmune hepatitis: occurrence of these conditions is more frequent than in the general population

- Acute or subacute liver failure
- Features of decompensated liver disease, e.g. jaundice and ascites

Diagnostic approach

Autoimmune hepatitis is considered as part of the differential diagnosis in individuals presenting with abnormal liver function tests.

Blood tests

- Elevated ALT, AST and bilirubin
- Positive autoantibodies:
  - Type I autoimmune hepatitis – presence of positive antinuclear or smooth muscle antibodies
  - Type II autoimmune hepatitis – presence of anti-liver-kidney microsomal type 1 or anti-liver cytosolic-1 antibodies
- Elevated serum IgG, which is a marker of disease activity

Liver biopsy

This guides both the diagnosis and assessment of severity. Interface hepatitis (inflammation of hepatocytes at the junction of the portal tract and liver parenchyma) is a typical feature of autoimmune hepatitis seen on histology.

Management

Treatment aims to reduce inflammation and prevent progressive liver fibrosis.

Medication

Corticosteroids (e.g. high-dose prednisolone) are the main agent used to induce remission, after which the dose is gradually reduced. Immunomodulators (such as azathioprine, mycophenolate and tacrolimus) are used alongside long-term, low-dose steroids as steroid-sparing agents to maintain remission and minimise steroid-induced side-effects, such as osteoporosis.

Surgery

A liver transplant is undertaken in patients with acute liver failure or decompensated chronic liver disease due to autoimmune hepatitis. It re-occurs in a fifth of patients with transplanted liver tissue.

Prognosis

If left untreated, autoimmune hepatitis progresses to cirrhosis within 3–5 years.

Primary sclerosing cholangitis (PSC)

This is a chronic cholestatic liver disease characterised by inflammation and fibrosis of both the intrahepatic and extrahepatic bile ducts, which sometimes result in strictures (**Figure 7.10**).

It is more common in men (2:1) and usually presents between the ages of 25 and 40 years. There is a strong association with inflammatory bowel disease (typically ulcerative colitis), which affects up to 80% of patients with PSC.

Clinical features

It is often detected at an asymptomatic stage. Other presenting features include:

- Abdominal pain
- Jaundice
- Signs and symptoms in keeping with underlying inflammatory bowel disease e.g. bloody diarrhoea and pain
- Cirrhosis and its complications

Diagnostic approach

Diagnosis is usually made from a combination of blood tests and radiology.

Blood tests

- Cholestatic liver function tests (raised alkaline phosphatase and γ-glutamyl transferase)
- Positive perinuclear anti-neutrophil cytoplasmic antibody (pANCA) – it is specific but not sensitive for ulcerative colitis

Radiology

Magnetic resonance cholangiopancreatography imaging shows multiple irregular strictures of the intrahepatic and extrahepatic bile ducts.

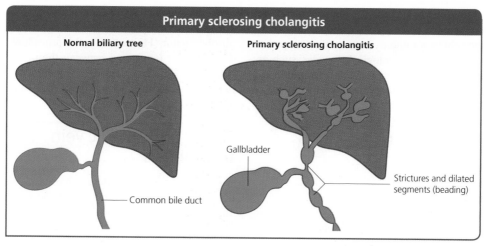

Figure 7.10 Primary sclerosing cholangitis. This affects both the intra- and extrahepatic biliary tree, with dilated segments as well as strictures.

Management

Treatment is mainly symptom based. Ursodeoxycholic acid is prescribed to improve liver function test results in patients with PSC and potentially reduces the risk of colorectal dysplasia in those with ulcerative colitis. Isolated or dominant strictures are dilated or stented at endoscopic retrograde cholangiopancreatography (ERCP), although these treatments confer a high risk of pancreatitis and cholangitis. A liver transplant is indicated in advanced disease, although disease commonly occurs in the transplanted tissue. Complications include:

- Cholangiocarcinoma (10–30%)
- Colorectal cancer – the cumulative colorectal cancer risk in patients with PSC is 33% at 20 years after a diagnosis of ulcerative colitis. Due to this risk, annual surveillance colonoscopy is recommended in those with associated inflammatory bowel disease
- Cirrhosis and liver failure

Prognosis

The 10-year survival following liver transplantation is over 80%. The prognosis of colorectal cancer and cholangiocarcinoma relates to the stage of disease at diagnosis.

> **Primary sclerosing cholangitis is strongly associated with ulcerative colitis.** A colonoscopy should be performed in all patients with PSC to look for signs of underlying inflammatory bowel disease, even in the absence of symptoms.

Vascular liver disorders

Complete disruption of the blood supply to the liver with hepatic infarction is rare because of the liver's dual blood supply (see Figure 1.35). Obstruction of the portal vein or hepatic venous outflow are causes of portal hypertension and often present with abdominal pain.

Budd–Chiari syndrome

This uncommon condition is caused by thrombosis of the hepatic veins. It affects 1 in 100,000 individuals worldwide. It is more common in women, typically presenting in the third or fourth decade.

Risk factors include pregnancy, use of the oral contraceptive pill and obstruction of the vein by a tumour. Some patients have an underlying haematological disorder, such as protein C or S deficiency, anti-thrombin III deficiency or primary proliferative polycythaemia.

Clinical features

These include:

- Abdominal pain
- Gross ascites
- Hepatomegaly
- Sometimes features of acute liver failure

Diagnostic approach

Diagnosis is based on abdominal ultrasonography with Doppler scanning of the hepatic vein, which shows obstruction or reversed flow.

Management

The aim is to identify the underlying cause, alleviating the obstruction and preventing further deterioration in liver function. Anticoagulation is generally advocated. Thrombolysis ('clot-busting') or percutaneous hepatic angioplasty (widening of the narrowed blood vessel) is occasionally used.

A transjugular intrahepatic portosystemic shunt is an alternative method of bypassing the obstruction (**Figure 7.5**). In this procedure, a metal stent is inserted between the portal vein and the hepatic vein. This is sometimes used as an interim measure whilst assessing patient's for liver transplantation.

Portal and splenic vein thrombosis

These are rare disorders characterised by occlusion of the portal or splenic vein. The many causes include decompensated chronic liver disease, intra-abdominal sepsis, malignancies and haematological disorders such as myeloproliferative and clotting disorders.

Clinical features of an acute presentation often include abdominal pain, ascites, hepatic encephalopathy or variceal bleeding. Non-cirrhotic portal hypertension with splenomegaly and oesophageal varices often develops gradually. Doppler ultrasonography is a non-invasive method of confirming the clinically suspected diagnosis. Anticoagulation is the mainstay of treatment for an acute portal vein thrombus. A chronic thrombus does not usually require treatment, because new blood vessels form as collaterals to bypass the occlusion.

Liver neoplasia

Primary tumours of the liver are either benign or malignant. The most common malignant tumours are secondary tumours (metastases), which account for over 90% of liver cancers. The most frequent primary malignant tumour is hepatocellular carcinoma. Haemangiomas (collections of blood vessels) are the commonest type of benign liver tumour.

Epidemiology

Benign liver tumours are usually of limited clinical significance; their epidemiology is summarised in **Table 7.10**. They are often

incidental findings on radiological imaging of the abdomen due to symptoms or abnormal blood tests.

Hepatocellular carcinoma, although relatively rare in developed countries, is the fifth most common neoplasm worldwide. It is particularly prevalent in South-East Asia and sub-Saharan Africa owing to the widespread prevalence of hepatitis B and C.

Aetiology

Hepatocellular adenomas predominantly occur with the long-term use of oral contraceptives, but also occur with anabolic

Benign liver tumours		
Tumour	Incidence	Female:male distribution
Haemangioma (can be multiple)	Up to 10% of population: the most common benign liver lesion	3:1
Focal nodular hyperplasia	Second commonest benign liver lesion	10:1
Hepatocellular adenoma	Uncommon	Females > males (90% of cases associated with long-term oral contraceptives)

Table 7.10 Epidemiology of benign liver tumours

steroids, danazol use, and are associated with glycogen storage diseases. Discontinuation of these medications often causes the adenoma to shrink. Focal nodular hyperplasia is usually cryptogenic (unknown cause) or secondary to trauma, portal vein thrombosis or hereditary haemorrhagic telangiectasia. The aetiology of haemangiomas is unknown.

Hepatocellular carcinoma usually arises in a cirrhotic liver, with hepatitis B infection accounting for 75% of cases worldwide. Other risk factors include hepatitis C, haemochromatosis, alcohol and dietary exposure to aflatoxin.

Secondary liver tumours arise from a primary tumour that is usually in the GI tract, lung or breast.

Clinical features

Many benign and malignant liver tumours are asymptomatic and found incidentally on imaging performed for other indications or during surveillance of patients in at-risk groups (e.g. cirrhosis). Clinical features vary with the type of tumour and include one or more of the following:

- Jaundice
- Right upper quadrant pain
- Hepatomegaly
- Weight loss and/or anorexia, which are usually due to malignant tumours
- Ascites, which is usually due to a malignant tumour if the cause is neoplasia

Focal nodular hyperplasia is sometimes mistaken for cirrhosis due to the nodular appearance of the liver.

Hepatocellular carcinoma usually arises in patients with cirrhosis. As well as the symptoms listed above, these patients have stigmata of chronic liver disease. In secondary liver tumours, firm nodular hepatomegaly is often felt and there is usually jaundice. An arterial bruit or hepatic friction rub is occasionally heard over the liver in patients with primary liver cancer or metastatic disease to the liver.

Diagnostic approach

In symptomatic patients, blood tests are often performed initially. However, the diagnosis is usually made subsequently, based upon characteristic radiological imaging. Ultrasound is almost always performed for hepatocellular surveillance, as it doesn't involve radiation.

> **Surveillance for hepatocellular carcinoma is recommended in patients with cirrhosis**, through 6 monthly abdominal ultrasonography and alpha-fetoprotein measurement.

Investigations

Blood tests

The liver function tests are either normal or the alkaline phosphatase or transaminases are sometimes elevated. The alkaline phosphatase level is often raised if there are liver metastases.

Serum alpha-fetoprotein is a tumour marker used in surveillance for and diagnosis of hepatocellular carcinoma, although the level is sometimes normal. A value that is rising or >400 kU/L is highly suggestive of hepatocellular carcinoma (normal is <10 kU/L). Alpha-fetoprotein is also elevated in other liver conditions such as hepatitis and biliary tract obstruction.

Radiology

Most liver tumours are identified on ultrasonography. CT and MRI (**Figure 7.11**) are useful for assessing the tumour's characteristics and for staging disease. The size and number

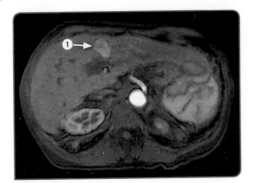

Figure 7.11 MRI image of a focal liver lesion (hepatocellular carcinoma) in a cirrhotic liver ①.

of tumour nodules, along with signs of portal vein invasion, are recorded. CT typically shows an enhancing lesion within the arterial phase, with washout in the portal phase.

Histology

Unlike other cancers, a histological diagnosis is often not required. A percutaneous biopsy also carries the risk of tumour seeding along the needle insertion tract, changing the tumour status from resectable to unresectable. Characteristic imaging and alpha-fetoprotein level are usually sufficient to make a diagnosis.

Management

Benign tumours

Benign liver tumours do not usually require treatment, as most are asymptomatic and have no malignant potential. Potential risk factors need review, such as oral contraceptives in patients with hepatocellular adenomas. Surgical excision is required if:

- An adenoma becomes sufficiently large to rupture (> 5 cm in size) and in men where there is a high risk of malignant transformation
- Focal neoplasia becomes symptomatic

Malignant tumours

Management options for hepatocellular carcinoma are outlined in **Table 7.11**. Options are chosen on the basis of co-morbidities and presence of metastases.

Solitary liver metastasis (e.g. from colorectal or lung cancer) are sometimes amenable to surgical resection. All cases require discussion at a cancer multidisciplinary team meeting to ensure that optimal treatment is offered to the patient following review by different specialists (e.g. hepatobiliary surgeons and oncologists).

Prognosis

Overall, the prognosis for malignant liver tumours is poor unless they are resectable, with a median survival of less than 6 months.

Management of hepatocellular carcinoma		
Treatment option	Suitability	Survival
Surgical resection	Single tumour <2 cm	5-year survival 40–70%
Liver transplant	Single tumour, or 3 nodules each <3 cm	Sometimes treatment is curative
Radiofrequency ablation	Single tumour, or 3 nodules each <3 cm	
Transarterial chemoembolisation*	Multinodular	Median: 20 months
Systemic chemotherapy	Signs of portal vein invasion on imaging	Median: 11 months
Supportive care	Advanced disease	Median: <3 months
	Underlying co-morbidities	

*Injection of cytotoxic drugs into tumour-feeding vessels under fluoroscopic guidance.

Table 7.11 Management options for hepatocellular carcinoma

Infections of the liver

The most common infections of the liver are viral (see page 265–268). However, several bacterial and parasitic infections also occur (**Table 7.12**), which sometimes cause liver abscesses (accumulation of pus) and cysts (fluid filled sac).

Amoebic liver abscess

This is caused by *Entamoeba histolytica*. Although this is uncommon in the UK and Europe except in travellers returning from the tropics (e.g. Mexico, India), worldwide it is the most common cause of liver abscess.

Amoebiasis is common in areas of poor sanitation and is spread by ingestion of water contaminated with *Entamoeba* cysts. These develop into trophozoites (which is the growth stage in the life cycle of a parasite) in the terminal ileum, causing dysentery. They then spread to the liver via the portal circulation, resulting in abscess formation (**Figure 7.12**).

Non-viral liver infections		
Type of infection	Disease	Pathogen
Bacterial	Pyogenic abscess	*Escherichia coli*
		Streptococcus milleri
		Proteus
		Streptococcus faecalis
		Anaerobes
Parasitic	Amoebic abscess	*Entamoeba histolytica*
	Hydatid cyst	*Echinococcus granulosus*
	Liver fluke	*Fasciola hepatica* and *gigantica*
		Clonorchis sinensis
		Opisthorchis viverrini and *felineus*
	Schistosomiasis	*Schistosoma mansoni*
		Schistosoma japonicum

Table 7.12 Causes of non-viral liver infections

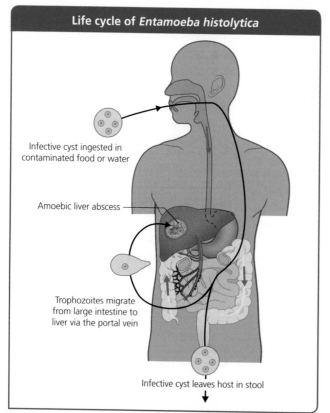

Figure 7.12 Life cycle of *Entamoeba histolytica*.

Life cycle of *Entamoeba histolytica*

Infective cyst ingested in contaminated food or water

Amoebic liver abscess

Trophozoites migrate from large intestine to liver via the portal vein

Infective cyst leaves host in stool

Clinical features

Patients present acutely with:

- Fever
- Weight loss
- Right upper quadrant pain
- Tender hepatomegaly
- Diarrhoea
- Sometimes a reactive right pleural effusion

Diagnostic approach

Blood and stool tests are usually undertaken initially. Radiological investigations are used in both the investigation and treatment of liver abscesses and cysts.

Blood tests

Inflammatory markers such as the CRP, ESR and white cell count are often elevated. Liver function is sometimes normal or shows a cholestatic picture (i.e. raised alkaline phosphatase and γ-glutamyl transferase). The results of serology testing using enzyme immunoassay or antigen detection are usually positive.

Stool test

Trophozoites are sometimes seen in stool.

Radiology

Ultrasonography typically shows a large cystic lesion, more commonly in the right lobe of the liver. Diagnostic aspiration reveals the characteristic 'anchovy sauce' appearance.

Management

Treatment is with metronidazole or tinidazole to kill the active trophozoites, followed by diloxanide to kill remaining intraluminal parasites and reduce the risk of infection recurrence. Cysts that are large or at risk of rupture are treated by radiologically guided drainage.

Pyogenic liver abscess

Although uncommon, this can occur from spread of an intra-abdominal infection via the portal circulation, for example with biliary sepsis, diverticulitis and appendicitis. *Escherichia coli* is the most commonly isolated pathogen.

Clinical features

Symptoms are often non-specific and include a swinging fever, anorexia, malaise and abdominal pain. Tender hepatomegaly, jaundice and features of septicaemia are sometimes seen.

Diagnostic approach

Blood tests

Inflammatory markers are usually elevated, often with a normocytic anaemia (normal mean corpuscular volume). Cholestatic liver function tests are seen if the abscess causes bile duct obstruction. Blood samples are taken for culture.

Radiology

Ultrasonography shows single or multiple cystic lesions within the liver. Microscopy and culture of pus aspirated from these lesions under ultrasound guidance sometimes identifies the causative organism. Further imaging with CT often helps to identify the primary source of infection, e.g. inflammatory change around the appendix or diverticulae.

Management

Treatment is with a combination of:

- Broad-spectrum antibiotics
- Radiologically guided percutaneous drainage

Surgical intervention is rarely required. Complications occur due to the underlying sepsis or rupture of the cyst causing peritonitis. The mortality rate is up to 10% and is worse in patients with multiple liver abscesses.

Hydatid disease

Hydatid disease is caused by the sheep–dog tapeworm *Echinococcus granulosus*. There are estimated to be 2–3 million cases worldwide. It is endemic in some parts of the Middle East and Africa, and is also seen in parts of Europe where sheep farming is common, such as Wales.

Disease is caused by ingestion of the tapeworm and its eggs in contaminated food or water. The embryos hatch in the duodenum and enter the portal circulation, producing hydatid cysts in the liver. Systemic spread sometimes occurs to the lung, kidney and brain.

Clinical features

Hydatid cysts are often asymptomatic. The average time from infection to diagnosis is 5-10 years. Patients sometimes present with hepatomegaly or right upper quadrant abdominal pain from a pressure effect or rupture of the cysts. Rupture often leads to anaphylaxis.

Diagnostic approach

A full blood count sometimes reveals an eosinophilia. Liver function tests are either normal or show a cholestatic picture. Hydatid serology is positive in 85% of cases. Abdominal ultrasonography characteristically shows multilocular cysts and daughter cysts with clearly defined walls.

All focal lesions of the liver are evaluated by a combination of history, blood tests and radiology to determine whether they are benign, malignant or due to abscesses. If there is still doubt about malignancy after appropriate scans, interval imaging is undertaken to look for any change in appearance of the lesions.

Management

If asymptomatic, hydatid cysts are often left untreated and don't require follow up. In symptomatic patients or those with large cysts at risk of rupture, surgery is performed to remove the cyst completely. An alternative to surgery is radiologically guided injection of ethanol, which helps to sterilise the cyst and is used in combination with Albendazole to reduce the risk of seeding of fluid from the cyst within the peritoneal cavity. Albendazole is also used in those patients not fit enough for surgery, a ruptured cyst or disseminated disease.

Liver fluke

This is a worldwide zoonosis due to the ingestion of parasites (*Clonorchis sinensis*, *Opisthorchis* and *Fasciola species*) present in raw or uncooked fish or fresh-water plants (e.g. watercress). The parasites migrate to the biliary tree, where they enlarge in size. Infection is usually asymptomatic, but sometimes patients present with fever, malaise, weight loss, abdominal pain, jaundice, hepatomegaly and rarely pancreatitis.

Eggs from the parasites are identified in the stool or in fluid aspirated from the duodenum or bile. ELISA blood testing is performed to look for antibodies against the *Fasciola* parasite. Defects in the bile ducts are sometimes seen on ultrasound, CT or MRCP.

Treatment of *Clonorchis sinensis* and *Opisthorchis* is with praziquantel or albendazole and *Fasciola* with triclabendazole. Chronic infection with *Clonorchis sinensis* and *Opisthorchis* increases the risk of cholangiocarcinoma up to 14-fold.

Schistosomiasis

The *Schistosoma mansoni* and *japonicum* parasite burrows through the skin of people swimming in infected water, before passing to the portal system within the liver, where they grow in size. Initial presentation is with itching ('swimmer's itch'), followed by a fever, malaise and rash. Chronic infection causes liver fibrosis and portal hypertension (non-cirrhotic) resulting in splenomegaly, oesophageal varices and sometimes ascites.

Diagnosis is made through the presence of ova in the stool, urine or rectal biopsy, or blood tests to detect *Schistosoma* antibodies. Abdominal ultrasound or CT imaging show thickened portal tracts, and splenomegaly if portal hypertension if present.

Praziquantel treatment is given to paralyse the worm after which it is attacked and cleared by the body's natural defence systems.

Answers to starter questions

1. Not all obese people develop features of associated liver disease, although most will have excess triglyceride accumulation in the liver cells causing steatosis. Progression to liver fibrosis and cirrhosis is due to an interplay between environmental insults and underlying genetic susceptibilities. The non-alcoholic fatty liver disease (NAFLD) score can help predict those at greater risk of progression.

2. Many of the early stages of liver disease are reversible. Providing any ongoing liver injury or insult is removed, the liver cells are able to regenerate.

3. Hypercholesterolaemia caused by primary biliary cholangitis doesn't appear to be associated with an increased risk of atherosclerosis or cardiovascular mortality. This is because it is typically high-density lipoprotein HDL (or 'good') cholesterol that is elevated, with a normal level of low-density lipoprotein (LDL). The exact mechanism is not fully understood. However, treatment with statins should still be considered if there are other risk factors for cardiovascular disease present.

Chapter 8
Pancreatic disease

Starter questions

Reading this chapter will enable you to answer the following questions. Answers are on page 302.

1. How does alcohol cause pancreatitis?
2. Do young people get pancreatitis?
3. Why does pancreatic cancer present late?

Introduction

The pancreas has two distinct roles:

- Endocrine cells produce the hormones insulin, glucagon and somatostatin, which play a key role in glucose homeostasis
- Exocrine cells secrete the digestive enzymes amylase, proteolytic enzymes and lipase into the small intestine to aid the breakdown of carbohydrate, protein and lipids respectively

The presentation of pancreatic disease varies depending on whether endocrine or exocrine cells are affected. This chapter discusses the latter; disorders of endocrine function such as diabetes are the subject of endocrinology texts and are not covered here.

In clinical practice, the most common disorders affecting the exocrine pancreas are acute and chronic pancreatitis and pancreatic cancer.

Case 10 Offensive stool and chronic abdominal pain

Presentation

Clive Peters, a 49-year-old man, sees his general practitioner (GP) because of increasing central and upper abdominal pain. He has experienced episodes of this over the last 5 years. Previously, it lasted for several hours each time but over the last few months it has been almost continuous.

Initial interpretation

Chronic upper abdominal (or epigastric) pain is usually due to a disorder of the upper GI tract, biliary tree or pancreas. However, it is sometimes due to a musculoskeletal cause or secondary to small or large intestinal disease (see page 87). Further questioning on the site and nature of the pain, and its exacerbating and relieving factors, will help narrow down the likely causes. It is important to ask about other GI symptoms, such as weight loss, which occur with malignancy and pancreatic exocrine insufficiency (i.e. the production of fewer digestive enzymes). The past medical, drug, family and social histories will need to be obtained.

History

Clive describes the pain as a 'severe ache' that radiates straight through to his back. It often gets worse after meals. He has been admitted to hospital on several occasions with particularly severe attacks. These have always settled after a few days of supportive treatment with intravenous fluids and opioid analgesics. This time, however, there has been no relief from a

Management of chronic pancreatitis

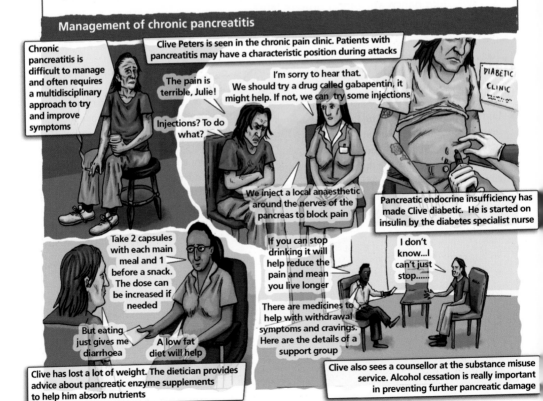

Chronic pancreatitis is difficult to manage and often requires a multidisciplinary approach to try and improve symptoms

Clive Peters is seen in the chronic pain clinic. Patients with pancreatitis may have a characteristic position during attacks

The pain is terrible, Julie!

I'm sorry to hear that. We should try a drug called gabapentin, it might help. If not, we can try some injections

Injections? To do what?

DIABETIC CLINIC

We inject a local anaesthetic around the nerves of the pancreas to block pain

Pancreatic endocrine insufficiency has made Clive diabetic. He is started on insulin by the diabetes specialist nurse

Take 2 capsules with each main meal and 1 before a snack. The dose can be increased if needed

But eating just gives me diarrhoea

A low fat diet will help

If you can stop drinking it will help reduce the pain and mean you live longer

I don't know...I can't just stop......

There are medicines to help with withdrawal symptoms and cravings. Here are the details of a support group

Clive has lost a lot of weight. The dietician provides advice about pancreatic enzyme supplements to help him absorb nutrients

Clive also sees a counsellor at the substance misuse service. Alcohol cessation is really important in preventing further pancreatic damage

proton pump inhibitor and only a little help from the opioid medication.

Interpretation of history

Clive's pain is characteristic of pain originating from the pancreas. It does not respond to acid-suppressant medication, such as a proton pump inhibitor, and frequently requires strong analgesia to control it. Patients often avoid food or restrict the amount of food they eat to reduce the pain.

It is important to ask about symptoms that occur due to chronic pancreatic damage and potential underlying causes such as alcohol misuse.

Further history

Clive says he has loose stool, opening his bowels between six and eight times a day. The stool has a pale appearance and is difficult to flush away. Clive often feels embarrassed because it also smells very offensive. He has lost 8 kg in weight over the last year and feels tired all the time. He has felt very thirsty and has been passing large volumes of urine. He has also had a 'tingling' sensation in his hands and feet for several months.

Clive has no family history of pancreatitis or pancreatic cancer. He is an unemployed factory worker and lives alone, having divorced his wife 7 years ago. He drinks up to a bottle of whisky a day and has done so for many years – up to 40 units of alcohol a day, 280 units a week. He has a 30 pack–year history of smoking.

> It is recommended that men and women drink no more than 14 units of alcohol per week.

Examination

Clive is underweight and looks unwell. His upper abdomen is tender on deep palpation. There are no masses or enlargement of the organs (organomegaly) and his abdomen is not distended. There is reduced sensation to soft touch over the hands and feet in a 'glove-and-stocking' distribution.

Interpretation of findings

The pale, offensive stool (steatorrhoea) must be investigated further. However, it is consistent with malabsorption secondary to exocrine pancreatic insufficiency, which often leads to weight loss. Clive's reduced appetite due to pain may also be contributing. He also has symptoms of hyperglycaemia, i.e. polydipsia (excessive thirst) and polyuria (passage of excess urine).

Clive drinks an excessive amount of alcohol and is at risk of damaging other organs including the liver and brain. Given his employment status and the fact he lives alone, he is likely to be socially isolated. This could lead to concurrent anxiety or depression and make it much harder for Clive to stop drinking, leading to alcoholism. Smoking is known to exacerbate chronic pancreatitis.

Clive is undernourished due to his poor appetite and malabsorption. He has neurological findings typical of a peripheral neuropathy, which sometimes results from diabetes, alcohol excess or haematinic (vitamin B_{12} and folate) deficiencies secondary to malabsorption.

Investigations

Clive's GP arranges some blood tests (**Table 8.1**). Three serial stool tests are performed, which show no evidence of infection (e.g. *Giardia*). This should always be excluded in patients with offensive loose stool.

The coexisting raised γ-glutamyl transferase and mean corpuscular volume are highly suggestive of alcohol excess.

Case 10 *continued*

Initial investigation results	
Test	Result (normal range)
γ-Glutamyl transferase	854 U/L (<50 U/L)
Mean corpuscular volume	110 fL (80–96 fL)
Random plasma glucose	25.2 mmol/L (4–7 mmol/L)
Faecal elastase	15 µg/g stool (>200 µg/g stool)

Table 8.1 Case 10: Clive's investigation results

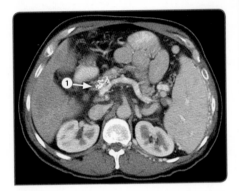

Figure 8.1 Abdominal CT showing calcification in the pancreas gland ① in chronic pancreatitis.

A random glucose level of > 11.1 mmol/L with typical symptoms of hyperglycaemia is diagnostic of diabetes.

The GP refers Clive to the gastroenterology clinic and diabetic specialist nurse for further investigation and management. Abdominal CT shows pancreatic calcification and atrophy (**Figure 8.1**). A faecal elastase test is performed to investigate the diarrhoea and confirms pancreatic insufficiency (**Table 8.1**).

Diagnosis

The gastroenterologist tells Clive that the clinical history and investigation results suggest chronic pancreatitis due to his long-standing alcohol excess. He advises Clive that alcohol and smoking cessation are crucial to his prognosis.

Repeated damage to the pancreas has resulted in diabetes and pancreatic exocrine insufficiency. His GP and the diabetes specialist nurse manage the diabetes and peripheral neuropathy. A gastroenterology specialist (or pancreatic surgeon) is also involved in Clive's care and oversees his investigations and treatment of the pancreatic exocrine insufficiency. A dietician provides advice about how to take the enzyme supplements and maintain his weight.

Clive will require much support to address his alcoholism and depression. A psychologist, counsellor and patient group programmes help individuals deal with these issues and with living with an incurable disorder. An antidepressant (e.g. selective serotonin reuptake inhibitor) will help, as Clive's mood disorder also needs to be addressed.

Case 11 Painless jaundice

Presentation

Raymond Humphries is a 78-year-old man who presents to his GP with jaundice, anorexia and a 5 kg weight loss. He has also noticed that his urine is darker than usual.

Initial interpretation

Jaundice has pre-hepatic, hepatic or post-hepatic causes (see page 89). The presence of obstructive symptoms, such as pale stool and dark urine, helps to narrow the differential diagnosis to a cholestatic cause.

Mr Humphries' symptoms are considered further in terms of time of onset, the presence of abdominal pain and any other factors related to his symptoms. Unintentional weight loss of 5 kg is concerning, raising the possibility of malignancy.

Further history

Mr Humphries reports a 2-week history of progressive jaundice. He also describes itching that keeps him awake at night. He has no abdominal pain but he feels nauseous and his appetite has disappeared. In addition to his urinary symptoms, he has also noticed pale stools.

There has been no recent change in medication, antibiotic prescriptions or foreign travel as potential causes of the jaundice. Mr Humphries was diagnosed with diet-controlled type 2 diabetes mellitus 3 months ago. There is no history of change in bowel habit or inflammatory bowel disease.

Examination

Mr Humphries appears thin with muscle wasting (cachectic). He has yellow sclerae and discoloration of his skin due to jaundice. There are no features of chronic liver disease or palpable lymph nodes.

No organomegaly or masses are felt on abdominal examination. There are several scratch marks on his arms because of itching.

Interpretation of findings

The combination of progressive painless jaundice and weight loss suggests a possible underlying malignancy.

Investigations

The GP arranges some blood tests, the results of which are outlined in **Table 8.2**. The liver function tests show a cholestatic picture (i.e. raised alkaline phosphatase and γ-glutamyl transferase) and the INR is raised due to biliary obstruction. The pancreatic tumour marker CA19-9 is also elevated.

Mr Humphries is referred for an abdominal ultrasound, which shows a dilated common bile duct (13 mm in diameter compared with a normal diameter of less than 6 mm). There is intrahepatic and extrahepatic duct dilatation, and a hypoechoic irregular mass within the head of the pancreas.

Initial investigation results	
Parameter	Result (normal range)
Haemoglobin	103 g/L (130–180 g/L)
Albumin	28 g/L (37–49 g/L)
Bilirubin	258 μmol/L (1–22 μmol/L)
Alanine transaminase	45 U/L (5–35 U/L)
Alkaline phosphatase	673 U/L (45–105 U/L)
γ-Glutamyl transferase	525 U/L (<50 U/L)
CA19-9	891 kU/L (<33 kU/L)
International normalised ratio	1.8 (1.0–1.3)
CA19-9, cancer antigen 19-9.	

Table 8.2 Mr Humphries' investigation results

Case 11 *continued*

Mr Humphries is referred to the pancreatic surgical team and a CT scan is arranged. This confirms a 6 cm mass in the head of the pancreas, compressing the common bile duct (**Figure 8.2**) and several enlarged lymph nodes at the porta hepatis (see Chapter 1, page 44).

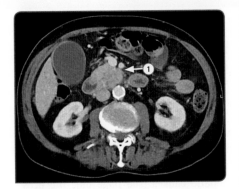

Figure 8.2 Abdominal CT showing a cancer mass in the head of the pancreas ①.

Diagnosis

The results are discussed at a weekly pancreatic multidisciplinary meeting and a diagnosis of locally advanced pancreatic cancer is made. An endoscopic retrograde cholangiopancreatography (ERCP) is recommended to relieve the jaundice, at which a stent is inserted into the common bile duct. After this, the oncologist arranges to see Mr Humphries and his wife to discuss the option of palliative chemotherapy.

> **Courvoisier's law states that, in the presence of painless jaundice, a palpable gallbladder is unlikely to be due to gallstones.** The most likely cause is malignancy of the gallbladder, bile duct or pancreas.

Acute pancreatitis

In acute pancreatitis, there is excessive conversion of trypsinogen to the digestive enzyme trypsin within the acinar cells. This increased level of trypsin overwhelms the pancreas glands' normal mechanisms to inactivate this enzyme, resulting in the further conversion of pro-enzymes such as trypsinogen and elastase precursors to cause local inflammation, swelling and damage to blood vessel linings, resulting in the death of some acinar cells.

Acute pancreatitis is a common reason for admission to hospital with acute abdominal pain. It ranges in severity from severe to mild. Severe disease is associated with a significantly increased mortality rate of approximately 20% and with a higher risk of complications.

Epidemiology

The incidence of acute pancreatitis varies between 13 and 45 cases per 100,000 population across the world. In the UK and Europe it is about 25 per 100,000.

Aetiology

The two most common causes of acute pancreatitis are gallstones, which account for approximately half and alcohol around a fifth of all presentations. Gallstones sometimes obstruct the bile ducts, preventing the release of pancreatic enzymes into the duodenum.

Alcohol misuse is a well-recognised cause of pancreatitis; however, the mechanism is uncertain. It is potentially due to alcohol promoting the synthesis of digestive enzymes and autodigestion of the pancreas.

Less common causes of acute pancreatitis are:

- Vascular - e.g. systemic arteritis
- Infection - e.g. mumps, cytomegalovirus
- Trauma – due to blunt or penetrating abdominal injury, arising post-ERCP (see below) or following abdominal surgery
- Metabolic - e.g. hypercalcaemia or hypertriglyceridaemia due to a serum triglyceride level over 10 mmol/L (normal level < 1.94 mmol/L)
- Hereditary
- Neoplastic - benign or malignant pancreatic mass
- Medications - e.g. azathioprine, 6-mercaptopurine, antiepileptics, corticosteroids
- Other – idiopathic or very rarely due to scorpion stings

ERCP can cause acute pancreatitis if mechanical injury results from the insertion of instruments in and around the pancreatic duct and from the injection of contrast agents to highlight the biliary tree during the procedure.

Clinical features

Patients with acute pancreatitis present with any of the following:

- Abdominal pain: this is almost always present. It is often severe, located in the epigastric region and sometimes radiates through to the back
- Nausea and vomiting: this often occurs and is sometimes profuse
- Circulatory collapse (tachycardia and poor peripheral perfusion): this occasionally occurs due to the release of inflammatory cells, the loss of fluid into tissues around the pancreas and vomiting

Abdominal examination often reveals epigastric or upper abdominal tenderness with or without guarding. Jaundice is usually present when there is obstruction of the bile ducts. Bruising seen in the abdominal flanks 1–2 days after the initial presentation is termed Grey Turner's sign (**Figure 8.3**). This is seen in severe pancreatitis when pancreatic necrosis and haemorrhage occurs. It is rarely (1% of cases) associated with Cullen's sign, which is bruising around the umbilicus (**Figure 8.3**).

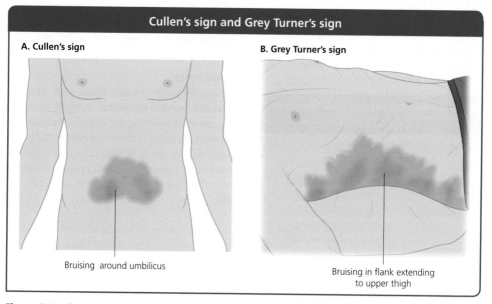

Cullen's sign and Grey Turner's sign

A. Cullen's sign

Bruising around umbilicus

B. Grey Turner's sign

Bruising in flank extending to upper thigh

Figure 8.3 Cullen's sign and Grey Turner's signs of bruising due to severe pancreatitis with pancreatic necrosis and haemorrhage.

The criteria used to define the severity of pancreatitis are given in **Table 8.3**.

> **Guarding and rebound tenderness are often absent in the early stages of acute pancreatitis**. This is because the inflammation is largely retroperitoneal, where part of the pancreas is located.

Complications

The complications of acute pancreatitis result from any of the potential causes. Local complications include:

- Peri-pancreatitic fluid collection
- Pancreatic and peripancreatic necrosis – this is either sterile or infected and may require endoscopic, radiological or surgical drainage
- Pancreatic pseudocyst – a collection of fluid containing pancreatic enzymes, blood and necrotic tissue that is usually located in the lesser sac

Drainage is required for symptomatic pseudocysts that are increasing in size.
Systemic complications of acute pancreatitis include:

- Systemic inflammatory response syndrome
- Multiorgan dysfunction
- Acute respiratory distress syndrome
- Hyperglycaemia or hypoglycaemia

The revised Atlanta criteria for acute pancreatitis	
Severity grade	Indicators
Mild	Absence of organ failure
	Absence of local or systemic complications
Moderately severe	Transient organ failure resolving within 48 hours ± local or systemic complications without persistent organ failure
Severe	Persistent organ failure (>48 hours)

Table 8.3 Assessing the severity of acute pancreatitis: the revised Atlanta criteria

- Acute kidney injury
- Hypocalcaemia
- Disseminated intravascular coagulation
- Portal vein thrombosis

Diagnostic approach

The diagnosis is made from a combination of clinical history and features, blood tests and radiological imaging. Establishing the underlying cause guides future management. The presence of at least two of the following is usually sufficient for diagnosis:

- Abdominal pain
- Serum amylase or lipase levels more than three times the upper limit of normal
- Characteristic radiological findings

Hereditary pancreatitis should be considered in young patients presenting with acute pancreatitis, particularly when there is a family history of pancreatic disease.

Investigations

Investigations help to establish the severity of pancreatitis and the underlying aetiology. The Ranson's and Glasgow criteria are scoring systems used to predict the disease severity and prognosis. These use the patient's age, white cell count, lactate dehydrogenase, glucose, aspartate transaminase, calcium, albumin, plasma urea levels, and partial pressure of oxygen in the blood.

Blood tests

Serum amylase and/or lipase are usually elevated, but are normal in a small number of patients. However, the degree of elevation does not correlate with the severity of the pancreatitis. It needs to be kept in mind that amylase is also elevated in other conditions such as renal failure, severe diabetic ketoacidosis and abdominal conditions such as a perforated peptic ulcer, acute cholecystitis or ruptured ovarian cyst, which also present with abdominal pain. The clinical history (e.g. dyspeptic symptoms or past history of diabetes) and investigations (e.g. urea and electrolytes, blood glucose and abdominal radiological imaging) help exclude these as potential causes.

Inflammatory markers including white cell count and C-reactive protein level are elevated. A raised plasma urea and creatinine indicates an acute kidney injury due to fluid loss resulting from vomiting and sepsis.

> **Amylase is rapidly excreted by the kidneys so the level usually returns towards normal around 48 hours after the onset of symptoms.** A persistently high serum amylase level is sometimes the sign of a complication such as a pancreatic pseudocyst (see page 295).

Imaging

An erect chest radiograph should be performed to exclude other causes of acute abdominal pain, such as a perforated peptic ulcer. An abdominal ultrasound is often performed as an initial investigation to exclude gallstones or a dilated common bile duct. The pancreas sometimes appears swollen on ultrasound imaging, but is often difficult to visualise owing to its retroperitoneal position and overlying bowel gas.

Pancreatic CT is indicated when the diagnosis is uncertain or when there is clinical deterioration or sepsis. CT imaging shows pancreatic oedema and inflammatory changes in the fat surrounding the pancreas with acute pancreatitis. It visualises the pancreas to provide information about complications such as necrosis of the pancreas, which shows as areas of non-opacification following intravenous contrast. It is also used to assess benign and malignant pancreatic masses, with pancreatic carcinoma occurring more commonly in older patients. Magnetic resonance cholangiopancreatography (MRCP) and endoscopic ultrasonography (EUS) are used to assess the bile ducts of patients with recurrent pancreatitis of unknown cause, or when the bile ducts are dilated on ultrasound but in the absence of visible gallstones.

Management

Management of acute pancreatitis focuses on:

- Early resuscitation with intensive intravenous fluid replacement
- Assessment of disease severity (**Table 8.3**) – patients with severe disease often require observation and treatment in critical care due to the potential for acute deterioration. There are increased numbers of nursing staff available to closely monitor patient vital signs and fluid balance
- Identification and treatment of the underlying cause
- Identification of complications

Medication

There is no specific medication to treat acute pancreatitis. Opioid analgesia is often required to ease the pain and antiemetics to treat symptoms of nausea and vomiting. The use of antibiotics is controversial, but they are given if there is cholangitis (see Chapter 9, page 310), bacteraemia or complications such as infected pancreatic necrosis. Medications (e.g. corticosteroids) that are thought to have precipitated an episode of acute pancreatitis are discontinued where possible.

In the absence of contraindications such as peptic ulceration, rectal non-steroidal anti-inflammatory drugs are given prior to ERCP to inhibit the mediators of inflammation, reducing the risk of post-ERCP pancreatitis.

Early enteral nutrition with nasogastric feeding is considered in patients with severe disease because many have a limited oral intake. Prophylactic subcutaneous heparin is given to all patients to reduce the risk of thromboembolism secondary to reduced mobility, dehydration and active inflammation.

Endoscopy

An urgent ERCP (see Chapter 2, page 125) is performed in patients presenting with acute severe pancreatitis secondary to gallstone disease if there is jaundice, cholangitis or a dilated common bile duct. This almost always includes a sphincterotomy procedure to allow the easier passage of gallstones and drainage of the bile ducts. It involves the use of a wire cutting device inserted through the endoscope to cut the sphincter muscle where the common bile duct joins the duodenum. In cases where ERCP does not allow gallstones to be removed, a plastic stent is inserted into the common bile duct to allow drainage of the bile, to relieve the biliary obstruction.

Surgery

Laparoscopic or open cholecystectomy is recommended within 2 weeks of an episode of gallstone pancreatitis, to prevent future recurrence.

Prognosis

In the majority of patients, acute pancreatitis is self-limiting. Overall mortality increases from 1% in mild pancreatitis to 20% in severe cases with the presence of complications.

Chronic pancreatitis

Long-standing repeated inflammation of the pancreas leads to replacement of the acinar cells by fibrotic tissue. Chronic pancreatitis either presents with typical symptoms of pancreatitis or with complications, such as symptoms of pancreatic exocrine insufficiency. It often significantly impairs a patient's quality of life.

Epidemiology

Chronic pancreatitis is most commonly seen in middle-aged men but occasionally occurs in children with cystic fibrosis or other genetic syndromes. The increasing prevalence over recent decades is linked to trends in alcohol consumption.

Aetiology

In developed countries, the cause is long-term alcohol excess in over 75% of patients with chronic pancreatitis. Other causes are listed in **Table 8.4**. In up to 20% of patients, no cause is identified.

Diagnostic clues in chronic pancreatitis	
Cause	Diagnostic clues
Alcohol misuse	Patient (or relative) confirms alcohol excess
	Compatible blood tests (raised γ-GT and MCV), signs of chronic liver disease
Cystic fibrosis	Young age and concurrent lung disease, e.g. bronchiectasis
Hereditary	Starts any time from childhood to early adulthood
	Family history of pancreatitis
Autoimmune	Other autoimmune diseases present, e.g. Sjögren's syndrome, primary sclerosing cholangitis or inflammatory bowel disease – these are not necessarily present in autoimmune chronic pancreatitis but do increase risk
Congenital	May present at a young age
	Congenital anatomical deformities of the pancreas which cause chronic pancreatitis (e.g. annular pancreas or pancreas divisum) are often not identified until radiological imaging is performed
Hyperparathyroidism	Features of hypercalcaemia, e.g. aches and pains, history of renal stones or low mood
	Often apparent only when blood tests show hypercalcaemia and raised parathyroid hormone level
Hypertriglyceridaemia	Often no clues
	Patients or family members occasionally have ischaemic heart disease or cerebrovascular disease at a young age

Table 8.4 Diagnostic clues to the cause of chronic pancreatitis

Clinical features

Symptoms arise from the chronic pancreatitis or from its complications (**Table 8.5**):

- Abdominal pain – central pain radiating through to the back that is generally worse after meals. It often becomes constant and in the late stages disappears
- Diarrhoea
- Steatorrhoea
- Anorexia
- Weight loss – due to reduced oral intake secondary to symptoms or related complications such as pancreatic exocrine insufficiency
- Nausea and vomiting

Diagnostic approach

The history is often highly suggestive of chronic pancreatitis and there are a number of diagnostic clues as to the underlying cause (**Table 8.4**). However, further investigation is always required to confirm the diagnosis, its underlying aetiology and any conditions resulting from it.

Investigations

Diagnosis of chronic pancreatitis is made using a combination of blood tests and imaging. Additional testing is also done to identify complications of the disease.

Blood tests

Amylase is usually normal but is sometimes elevated in acute-on-chronic pancreatitis. The fasting lipid profile and serum calcium concentration are checked to investigate for hypertriglyceridaemia and hypercalcaemia, which are potential causes of chronic pancreatitis. Immunoglobulin G_4 is elevated in autoimmune pancreatitis.

A genetic screen (*CFTR* for cystic fibrosis, PRSS1 and *SPINK1* for hereditary pancreatitis) is considered if there are additional clinical features, for example respiratory disease, or if there is no history of alcohol excess.

Blood tests for complications of chronic pancreatitis: The following are tested:

- Plasma glucose and HbA1c (glycated haemoglobin) if there are symptoms of diabetes
- CA19-9 (a tumour marker for pancreatic cancer): a progressive rise sometimes indicates cancer, but it can also be elevated in pancreatitis alone

If pancreatic exocrine insufficiency arises as result of a complication, there is an increased risk of vitamin A, D, E and K deficiencies because they are malabsorbed. There are blood tests to measure the levels of vitamin A, D and E, and also none to measure the level of vitamin K which is best checked by the prothrombin time, which is prolonged when it is deficient.

Complications of chronic pancreatitis	
Complication	**Clue from presentation**
Diabetes (due to endocrine insufficiency); occurs in 50% of patients	Weight loss, polyuria and polydipsia
	Diabetes is sometimes asymptomatic and only found on blood testing
Pancreatic exocrine insufficiency (reduced enzyme production)	Diarrhoea
	Steatorrhoea (requires loss of 90% of pancreatic exocrine function)
Pancreatic cancer	Weight loss
	Obstructive jaundice (occurs if mass is in pancreatic head)
	Sometimes difficult to distinguish from pancreatitis on basis of symptoms and imaging
Pancreatic pseudocyst	Prolonged pain or bloating
Portal or splenic vein thrombosis	Haematemesis or melaena due to bleeding from oesophageal varices

Table 8.5 Complications of chronic pancreatitis.

Stool tests

Because chronic pancreatitis causes pancreatic exocrine insufficiency in a proportion of patients, the faecal elastase level is checked in those with symptoms of diarrhoea or steatorrhoea. The elastase level is low in patients with this complication (see Chapter 2, page 114).

> A falsely low faecal elastase result occurs if other causes of diarrhoea have produced watery stool, diluting the level of elastase.

Imaging

Pancreatic calcification is sometimes identified on a plain abdominal radiograph. An abdominal CT scan will show pancreatic atrophy, a dilated and irregular pancreatic duct and calcification; the latter is particularly found when alcohol is the cause. Abdominal CT is also used to look for pancreatic cancer and portal or splenic vein thrombosis, which occur as a complication of chronic pancreatitis.

MRCP or EUS are helpful in defining the anatomy of the pancreatic duct and excluding other causes for its dilatation such as malignancy. A fine needle aspiration is performed during EUS if an abnormality (e.g. tumour) is seen or to take samples of a fluid from pancreatic pseudocysts, which sometimes occur as a complication of chronic pancreatitis, to exclude malignant cells.

> A CT scan is often required for optimal visualisation of the pancreas. This is because its deep-seated position means it is frequently covered by overlying bowel containing gas, which prevents it being seen well on an ultrasound scan.

Management

Chronic pancreatitis is incurable. Management focuses on lifestyle modification and the treatment of the underlying cause, symptoms and complications. Abstinence from alcohol is crucial in reducing further pancreatic damage. Smoking cessation is also beneficial.

Corticosteroids such as prednisolone are given as a treatment for autoimmune pancreatitis. Hypertriglyceridaemia is treated with fibrates, e.g. bezafibrate. Hypercalcaemia occurring due to primary hyperparathyroidism is treated by surgical removal of the parathyroid glands. The complications of chronic pancreatitis are treated as outlined in **Table 8.6**.

Treatment of complications of chronic pancreatitis	
Complication	Treatment
Diabetes	Insulin and dietary modification
Pancreatic exocrine insufficiency	Pancreatic enzyme supplements containing protease, lipase and amylase
	Dietary advice to eat low-fat foods
Pancreatic cancer	Often palliative, e.g. analgesia, ERCP to insert a stent if the common bile duct is blocked
	Surgery or chemotherapy in a minority of patients
Pancreatic pseudocyst	May resolve spontaneously
	Can be drained under CT guidance or surgery
Portal or splenic vein thrombosis	In acute setting consider anticoagulation, but usually just the consequences are treated, e.g. varices

ERCP, endoscopic retrograde cholangiopancreatography.

Table 8.6 Treatment of complications of chronic pancreatitis

> Patients with chronic pancreatitis who develop diabetes are prone to recurrent hypoglycaemic episodes. This is because there is a coexisting deficiency of glucagon, the action of which is to increase the plasma glucose level.

Opioids are often required but pain is difficult to control, requiring involvement of chronic pain services. Amitriptyline, gabapentin and selective serotonin reuptake inhibitors often help. If these treatments are unsuccessful other options are a coeliac axis nerve block, in which local anaesthetic is injected around the aorta, or a splanchnicectomy, in which splanchnic nerves are cut in the chest. A partial or total pancreatectomy is considered if the pain is intractable.

Upper GI endoscopy is performed to treat patients with variceal bleeding resulting from splenic or portal vein thrombosis as a complication of chronic pancreatitis.

Prognosis

Around 75% of patients with chronic pancreatitis from alcohol are alive at 10 years if they abstain from drinking. For those who do not, the survival rate falls to around 40%.

Pancreatic neoplasia

Benign and malignant neoplasms sometimes arise within the pancreas. The vast majority of malignant pancreatic tumours are adenocarcinomas arising from the exocrine ductal or acinar cells (see Chapter 1, page 56).

> Pancreatic cancer has a poor prognosis because usually it does not cause symptoms until it is advanced.

Epidemiology

Pancreatic cancer is the 10th most common cancer in the UK, with around 16 new cases per 100,000 population diagnosed each year. Men and women are equally affected.

Aetiology

The cause of malignant pancreatic neoplasms is unknown, although several risk factors have been identified. These include cigarette smoking, chronic pancreatitis and hereditary pancreatitis. The risk is also increased by familial cancer syndromes such as Peutz–Jeghers syndrome, familial adenomatous polyposis, hereditary non-polyposis colorectal cancer, familial breast cancer and familial atypical multiple-mole melanoma syndrome.

The main types of pancreatic neoplasia:

- Ductal adenocarcinoma – this accounts for more than 90% of all exocrine pancreatic tumours. Of these, 60% arise within in the head of the pancreas, 15–20% in the body and 10% in the tail
- Ampullary tumours arise from the ampulla of Vater
- Cystic lesions – benign serous cyst adenoma and mucinous cyst adenoma. There is a small risk of malignant transformation
- Intraductal papillary mucinous neoplasms (IPMN) are premalignant lesions that occur within the main pancreatic duct or a side branch and secrete mucus

Clinical features

Malignant neoplasms are often advanced by the time of presentation. The clinical features (**Figure 8.4**) depend on the tumour site and include:

- Obstructive jaundice (due to obstruction of the common bile duct at the ampulla of Vater) (**Figure 8.5**). This is often painless in the early stages
- Abdominal pain – typically epigastric pain that radiates to the back, which usually indicates posterior capsule invasion and unresectability of the tumour
- Weight loss
- Anorexia and lassitude
- Nausea or vomiting – which is occasionally due to a mass effect causing duodenal obstruction
- Pruritus – secondary to biliary obstruction and increased level of bile acids

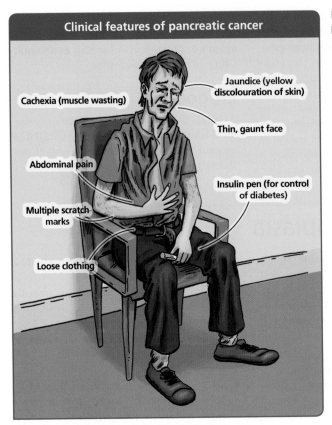

Clinical features of pancreatic cancer

Jaundice (yellow discolouration of skin)

Cachexia (muscle wasting)

Thin, gaunt face

Abdominal pain

Insulin pen (for control of diabetes)

Multiple scratch marks

Loose clothing

Figure 8.4 Clinical features of pancreatic cancer.

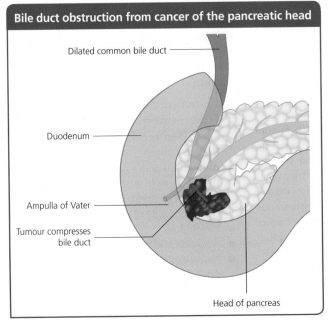

Bile duct obstruction from cancer of the pancreatic head

Dilated common bile duct

Duodenum

Ampulla of Vater

Tumour compresses bile duct

Head of pancreas

Figure 8.5 Bile duct obstruction secondary to cancer of the pancreatic head.

- Diabetes mellitus – around 5% of patients develop this within the 2 years prior to diagnosis
- Acute pancreatitis
- Trousseau's syndrome – migratory thrombophlebitis or venous thromboembolism
- Splenic vein obstruction – occurring either due to compression or direct tumour invasion of the vein

Patients often appear cachectic. The gallbladder is occasionally dilated and easily palpable due to back pressure caused by the tumour. Supraclavicular lymph nodes and the liver (hepatomegaly) are sometimes palpable due to metastases from the pancreatic cancer. Ascites occurs in one-fifth of patients with pancreatic cancer due to obstruction of the diaphragmatic lymphatic drainage and production of exudate from the tumour.

Benign pancreatic neoplasms are usually asymptomatic and often found incidentally during radiological investigations. However, they occasionally cause symptoms of abdominal pain due to a mass effect.

Diagnostic approach

The diagnosis of suspected pancreatic cancer usually relies on radiological imaging and supporting blood tests.

> When a mass is identified on radiological imaging, it is sometimes difficult to distinguish between cancer and chronic pancreatitis. This usually requires a tissue sample (e.g. at EUS) or follow-up imaging to see if it has resolved.

Investigations

Blood tests

Bilirubin and alkaline phosphatase levels are usually elevated due to biliary obstruction.

CA19-9 is a tumour marker that is often raised in exocrine pancreatic tumours. It is also sometimes elevated in benign conditions such as pancreatitis and hepatic dysfunction.

Radiology

Abdominal CT will diagnose most pancreatic neoplasms (**Figure 8.2**) as well as identifying local nodal spread or metastases in malignant disease. If there is an intraductal papillary mucinous neoplasm (IPMN) on CT imaging, it is seen arising from the main pancreatic duct or a side branch, but is sometimes difficult to distinguish from a pancreatic pseudocyst.

Ultrasonography tends to be less sensitive than CT, particularly for identifying lesions within the body and tail of the pancreas. This is because this area is often partially obscured by gas in overlying bowel. Lesions in the pancreatic head, common bile duct dilatation and liver metastases are more easily identified.

Endoscopy

EUS is helpful in visualising the head of the pancreas to provide local staging of malignant tumours. It enables biopsies and fine-needle aspiration to be taken to confirm a diagnosis. The aspiration and analysis of fluid from pancreatic cysts is also used in the diagnosis of mucinous cyst adenomas.

ERCP allows a stent to be placed into the common bile duct to relieve jaundice. With ampullary tumours, it also often used to obtain brushings for cytology.

Management

The management of malignant pancreatic tumours depends upon co-morbidities and the type of cancer and its stage according to the TNM (tumour, node, metastases) classification (see page 127). A multidisciplinary team jointly determines and provides the most appropriate treatment.

Pancreatic exocrine insufficiency occurring as a result of malignant tumours is treated with enzyme replacement therapy. Benign pancreatic neoplasms (serous cyst adenoma, mucinous cyst adenoma, IPMN) are usually monitored through surveillance radiological imaging to assess for the change in size that would indicate the need for further investigation or treatment.

Curative

Surgery is sometimes performed for malignant tumours to obtain a cure, but few patients are suitable for this because the cancer is often advanced at presentation. The operation of choice is a Whipple's procedure, which consists of a partial gastrectomy, duodenectomy and partial pancreatectomy (**Figure 8.6**) or pylorus-preserving pancreaticoduodenectomy. This is a major operation with significant morbidity and mortality. Adjuvant chemotherapy is often given to treat 'micro-metastases' and reduce the risk of cancer recurrence following surgery.

Patients with malignant ampullary tumours usually present earlier because of painless obstructive jaundice. These tumours are usually treated with a Whipple's procedure, if the patient is fit enough for major surgery.

Surgery for benign pancreatic neoplasms is occasionally required if the patient is symptomatic or the lesion is increasing in size.

Palliative

As pancreatic cancer is often advanced at presentation, the treatment is mostly palliative. The palliative care team should be involved early on to help ensure adequate symptom control.

Palliative chemotherapy alone or in combination with radiotherapy is offered to patients unsuitable for surgery to treat locally advanced and metastatic disease. Radiotherapy shrinks the tumour to relieve pressure on the nerves and improve intractable pain.

Other palliative approaches include:

- ERCP with insertion of a stent to relieve jaundice
- Opiate analgesics or a coeliac axis block for pain relief
- Duodenal bypass or an endoscopically placed stent to relieve duodenal obstruction

Prognosis

The overall prognosis of pancreatic adenocarcinoma is poor, with a 5-year survival of less than 5%. The median survival of patients with locally advanced disease is 6–10 months. Benign pancreatic neoplasms do not alter a patient's life expectancy unless they become malignant.

Neuroendocrine tumours (NETs)

Neuroendocrine tumours (NETs) stem from the endocrine cells of the pancreas. They are sometimes seen as part of multiple endocrine

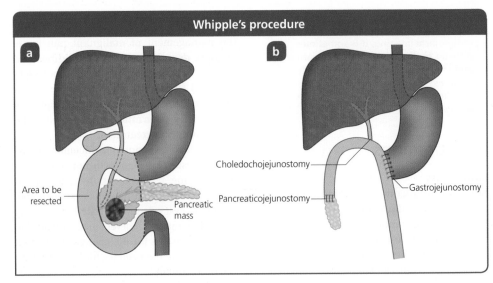

Whipple's procedure

Area to be resected

Pancreatic mass

Choledochojejunostomy

Pancreaticojejunostomy

Gastrojejunostomy

Figure 8.6 (a) Before a Whipple's procedure. (b) Postoperative anatomy after a Whipple's procedure.

neoplasia (MEN) alongside tumours of the pituitary and parathyroid glands.

Epidemiology

The incidence of pancreatic NETs in the UK is 0.3 cases per 100,000 population annually. They can occur at any age, but have the highest incidence in patients aged over the age of 50 years old.

Aetiology

The aetiology of NETs is poorly understood. Most occur sporadically, but they occasionally form part of a familial syndrome, e.g. MEN. Types of pancreatic neuroendocrine tumour:

- Gastrinoma – G-cells
- Insulinoma – β cells
- VIPoma (vasoactive intestinal peptide) – Non-β islet cells
- Glucagonoma – α cells
- Somatostatinoma – δ cells

Clinical features

The clinical features of NETs of the pancreas vary, depending on whether the cells are functional (hormone secreting) or non-functional. The clinical features of functioning tumours reflect the hormone they produce (**Table 8.7**). Sixty per cent of NETs are non-functioning and usually present with pain and weight loss, or with biliary obstruction caused by a local mass effect.

> **Zollinger–Ellison syndrome occurs as a result of ectopic gastrin secretion by pancreatic neuroendocrine tumours. Presentation is with abdominal pain, diarrhoea and severe peptic ulceration.**

Diagnostic approach

The diagnosis is made using a combination of blood tests and specialised radiological and nuclear imaging.

Blood tests

Functioning neuroendocrine tumours are usually detected by measuring the fasting plasma levels of gut hormones:

Pancreatic neuroendocrine tumours	
Type	Clinical features
Gastrinoma (Zollinger–Ellison syndrome)	Gastrointestinal bleeding
	Recurrent severe peptic ulceration
	Diarrhoea
Insulinoma	Fasting hypoglycaemia
VIPoma	Profuse watery diarrhoea
	Hypokalaemia
	Hypercalcaemia
	Metabolic acidosis
	Flushing, hypotension
	Dehydration
Glucagonoma	Necrolytic migratory erythema
	Venous thrombosis
	Neuropsychiatric manifestations
Somatostatinoma	Diabetes mellitus
	Steatorrhoea
	Hypochlorhydria
	Weight loss

Table 8.7 Clinical features of pancreatic neuroendocrine tumours

- In gastrinoma: gastrin is elevated
- In insulinoma: c-peptide is elevated and blood glucose is < 2.2 mmol/L following a 72-hour fast
- In VIPoma: vasoactive intestinal peptide is elevated
- In glucagonoma: glucagon is elevated
- In somatostatinoma: somatostatin is elevated

Radiology

CT imaging with intravenous contrast is used in the diagnosis and staging of pancreatic NETs, to assess for the invasion of local structures and metastases. MRI is also used to provide local information about the tumour and has the advantage of involving no radiation.

Nuclear imaging

An octreotide scan (somatostatin receptor scintigraphy) is performed in the nuclear medicine department. Octreotide is a drug similar to somatostatin; it is labelled with a small dose of a radioactive material and injected into the patient's bloodstream. It attaches to cells with somatostatin receptors on their surface, which are then visible on a special scanner. It is used to locate the primary tumour and any metastases.

Endoscopy

Endoscopic ultrasound improves the detection of small pancreatic NETs. Its main role is to obtain tissue samples from a tumour to provide a diagnosis.

Management

Surgical management

Depending upon the fitness of the patient, surgery is performed to obtain a cure if the tumour is localised and if metastases are resectable. Operations include local removal of the tumour or part of the pancreas gland (e.g. distal pancreatic resection) or Whipple's procedure (**Figure 8.6**).

Medical management

Somatostatin analogues, e.g. lanreotide and mTOR (serine/threonine kinase) inhibitors, e.g. everolimus are used to treat symptomatic functioning NETs. Systemic chemotherapy is used in metastatic disease. Zollinger–Ellison syndrome is treated with very high-dose PPI therapy.

Prognosis

The overall 5-year survival for NETS of the pancreas is around 40%.

Answers to starter questions

1. The pathophysiology is poorly understood, but it is thought a predisposing insult, such as long term alcohol excess, causes pancreatitis by inappropriate activation of pancreatic enzymes. Trypsinogen is converted into trypsin, which causes a further cascade of digestive enzymes to be activated resulting in cell damage. These damaged cells release activated enzymes into the surrounding tissues, as well as inflammatory mediators and cytokines into the systemic circulation. This causes local inflammation and swelling of the pancreas gland that results in symptoms of pancreatitis, such as abdominal pain, vomiting and, occasionally, circulatory collapse.

2. Yes, pancreatitis can present at a young age because it isn't always the result of alcohol misuse or gallstones. A hereditary cause should always be considered in a young patient; there may be a family history of pancreatitis or pancreatic cancer. Mutations in three genes account for most cases of hereditary pancreatitis: *PRSS1*, *CFTR* and *SPINK1*. Other causes include trauma, viral infection or medications.

3. Pancreatic cancer typically presents late, usually at an incurable stage. This is because symptoms only tend to develop when tumours have reached a certain size or there is local invasion of surrounding structures resulting in biliary obstruction and jaundice. Back pain can be a sign of invasion of the coeliac plexus and vomiting a sign of duodenal obstruction. There is no screening test currently reliable enough for population-based screening. Doctors therefore need to be vigilant when assessing patients with upper abdominal symptoms.

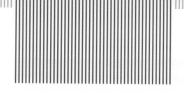
Chapter 9
Biliary tract disease

Starter questions

Reading this chapter will enable you to answer the following questions. Answers are on page 315.

1. How do blocked bile ducts cause itchy skin?
2. Does removal of the gallbladder (cholecystectomy) prevent gallstones forming?
3. Do we need a gallbladder?
4. Why does biliary neoplasia have a late presentation?

Introduction

Problems in the biliary tract are most commonly caused by gallstones. These are usually asymptomatic but can characteristically lead to abdominal pain. Depending on where they are situated in the biliary tree, they also cause bacterial infection, pancreatitis and obstructive jaundice.

Other biliary tract conditions result from strictures, parasitic infections or medical intervention. Biliary tree cancers have a poor prognosis as they often do not present until they are incurable.

A range of diagnostic and therapeutic imaging techniques are used in biliary tract disease, as listed in **Table 9.1**.

Diagnostic and therapeutic imaging of the biliary tree			
Investigation	Diagnostic or therapeutic	Invasive or non-invasive	Features
Ultrasonography (US)	Diagnostic	Non-invasive	Good visualisation of biliary tree
CT	Diagnostic	Non-invasive	Poorer visualisation of biliary tree than US
			Good for assessing pancreatic and hepatic causes of biliary obstruction
MRCP	Diagnostic	Non-invasive	Visualises biliary and pancreatic ducts, using bile as contrast
ERCP	Therapeutic	Invasive	Allows therapeutic interventions to relieve or prevent biliary obstruction, e.g. sphincterotomy, balloon trawl and stent insertion
			Allows collection of samples for cytology
PTC	Therapeutic	Invasive	Stents are inserted percutaneously to treat strictures particularly after failed ERCP
EUS	Diagnostic	Invasive	Further visualisation of biliary tree

ERCP, endoscopic retrograde cholangiopancreatography; EUS, endoscopic ultrasonography; MRCP, magnetic resonance cholangiopancreatography; PTC, percutaneous transhepatic cholangiography.

Table 9.1 Diagnostic and therapeutic imaging of the biliary tree

Case 12 Jaundice and abdominal pain

Presentation

Mary Lewis, aged 68 years, is admitted to hospital with a 5-day history of progressive jaundice. This was initially noticed by her husband, who saw that the whites of her eyes were yellow.

Initial interpretation

Jaundice has many different causes. Further questioning can help to determine the anatomical site (e.g. liver or bile ducts) and the likely cause. It is important to ask specifically about abdominal pain, as its presence or absence helps to narrow down the likely underlying cause.

History

For the last week, Mrs Lewis has experienced bouts of colicky, right upper quadrant pain radiating around to her back.

She has had a similar pain on and off for a number of years. It tends to occur about 30 minutes after meals. She finds that greasy foods often precipitate an attack so tries to avoid them. This time the pain is persistent and feels more intense.

Interpretation of history

'Painful' jaundice (i.e. when abdominal pain and jaundice occurs at the same time) is almost always caused by gallstones which are in the extrahepatic biliary tree. These obscure the flow of bile and produce excessive smooth muscle contractions which try to move the stone forward. Mrs Lewis's preceding history is characteristic of stones in the gallbladder.

Further history

Mrs Lewis has noticed darker urine, pale stools and generalised itching, but no

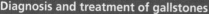

Case 12 *continued*

Diagnosis and treatment of gallstones

Mrs Lewis's GP elicits symptoms of obstructive jaundice and arranges admission to hospital for further investigation

A week later, Dr Sim, the consultant gastroenterologist explains the ultrasound findings and discusses the need for endoscopic retrograde cholangiopancreatography (ERCP)

I've had sharp pains in my stomach the last few weeks and yesterday my husband noticed my skin and eyes have become yellow

Have you noticed any other symptoms?

Well, um...my urine has become dark and my stools are pale

The scan shows you have gallstones in your bile duct, where bile from the liver drains into the gut. Stones are collections of different material that block the duct, causing pain and your yellow skin. We will arrange a special camera test called an ERCP to look more closely and release the blockage if needed

I feel much better, thank you! I'm so relieved it was nothing more serious

Okay, I've removed the blockage

Good! To prevent another blockage, we can arrange an operation to remove your gallbladder...

ERCP is performed and the stones are removed from the common bile duct with a balloon trawl and sphincterotomy

2 weeks later, Mrs Lewis is reviewed in clinic and the role of cholecystectomy is discussed

weight loss. She has not had any previous episodes of jaundice or hospital admissions. She takes no medication and drinks less than 10 units of alcohol per week.

Examination

Mrs Lewis is overweight, with a body mass index of 29 kg/m². She has a temperature of 37.8°C. She is jaundiced with yellow sclerae and discoloration of her skin. There are no stigmata of chronic liver disease. There is tenderness in the right upper quadrant of the abdomen but no palpable masses.

Interpretation of findings

These clinical findings along with the history of abdominal pain suggest jaundice caused by biliary disease. Mrs Lewis is seen on the surgical assessment unit and further investigation is arranged.

Investigations

Mrs Lewis's liver function tests (**Table 9.2**) have a 'cholestatic' pattern indicative of biliary obstruction with raised alkaline

Initial liver function test results	
Test	Results (normal range)
Bilirubin	126 µmol/L (1–22 µmol/L)
Alkaline phosphatase	642 U/L (45–105 U/L)
Alanine transaminase	48 U/L (5–35 U/L)
γ-Glutamyl transferase	487 U/L (<35 U/L)

Table 9.2 Liver function test results for Mrs Lewis

Case 12 *continued*

phosphatase and γ-glutamyl transferase levels. The white cell count and C-reactive protein (CRP) concentration are also high.

She is given analgesia to help her pain and is commenced on intravenous fluids and broad-spectrum antibiotics to treat biliary infection which often occurs in this situation.

An abdominal ultrasound scan is performed. This shows multiple stones in the gallbladder. The common bile duct is 11 mm in diameter, which means it is dilated (normal <6 mm). However, no apparent cause (i.e. a mass in the head of the pancreas or abnormality within the bile duct) is identified.

Because the cause of the biliary dilation is not apparent on ultrasonography, the consultant requests a magnetic resonance cholangiopancreatography (MRCP). This is non-invasive and very effective at outlining the structure of the gallbladder and biliary tree (**Figure 9.1**). It shows an 8 mm stone in the distal common bile duct.

Diagnosis

The consultant explains to Mrs Lewis that she has obstructive jaundice with pain caused by a stone in the common bile

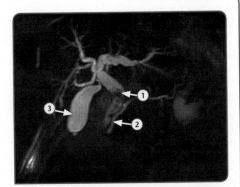

Figure 9.1 Magnetic resonance cholangiopancreatography showing a gallstone in the common bile duct ①. Pancreatic duct ②, and gallbladder ③.

duct. He advises an endoscopic retrograde cholangiopancreatography (ERCP) to remove the stone. A sphincterotomy (incision of the ampulla of Vater) is often performed to allow further stones to pass through it. If the common bile duct cannot be cleared, a plastic stent is inserted. This is placed beyond the stone to allow bile to drain into the duodenum and relieve the jaundice.

After the ERCP, Mrs Lewis is discharged with plans for an urgent outpatient cholecystectomy to reduce the risk of future problems with gallstones.

Gallstones and cholecystitis

Gallstones (or cholelithiasis) are formed usually within the gallbladder from an aggregation of bile components. Symptoms arise when stones become impacted and cause inflammation or when they migrate to a part of the biliary tree where the lumen is narrow and the stone lodges or causes infection.

Around 8% of the UK population over the age of 40 years have gallstones. Risk factors include older age, female sex (2–3:1), obesity and multiparity.

The 'Fs' of gallstones are classically used to describe the people most likely to develop gallstones:

Female

Fair

Fat

Forty (or 'Fertile')

Aetiology of gallstones

Type of gallstone	Cause	Risk factors
Cholesterol	Increased cholesterol ± decreased bile salt excretion	Female, older age, obesity or rapid weight loss, oral contraceptives, low-fibre diet, multiparity, cirrhosis, total parenteral nutrition, terminal ileal resection
Black pigment	Increased bilirubin + calcium excretion into bile	Haemolysis (sickle cell disease, spherocytosis, prosthetic heart valve)
Brown pigment	Bacterial infection with hydrolysis of bilirubin conjugate	Sclerosing cholangitis, biliary parasites

Table 9.3 Aetiology of the different types of gallstone

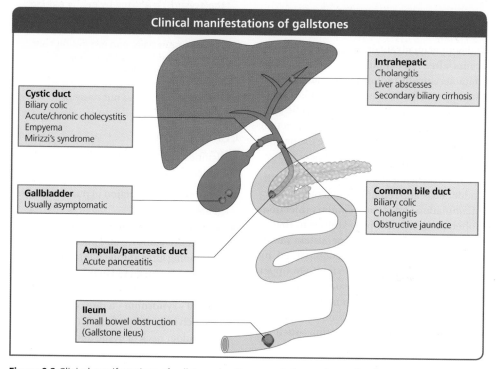

Clinical manifestations of gallstones

Intrahepatic
Cholangitis
Liver abscesses
Secondary biliary cirrhosis

Cystic duct
Biliary colic
Acute/chronic cholecystitis
Empyema
Mirizzi's syndrome

Gallbladder
Usually asymptomatic

Common bile duct
Biliary colic
Cholangitis
Obstructive jaundice

Ampulla/pancreatic duct
Acute pancreatitis

Ileum
Small bowel obstruction
(Gallstone ileus)

Figure 9.2 Clinical manifestations of gallstones by site: presentation and complications.

Aetiology

There are three types of gallstone (**Table 9.3**):

- cholesterol stones
- black pigment stones
- brown pigment stones

In developed countries, the majority (80%) of gallstones are cholesterol stones or mixed stones. Although the exact pathogenesis is unclear, stones are thought to form due to a combination of:

- Bile stasis
- Raised cholesterol level in the bile
- Crystallisation-promoting glycoproteins within the bile

Clinical features (Figure 9.2)

The vast majority of gallstones are asymptomatic and are detected incidentally on abdominal imaging for another reason. The clinical presentation of symptomatic gallstones depends upon their location (**Table 9.4**). The two most common acute presentations are biliary colic and acute cholecystitis. Ascending cholangitis, pancreatitis and small bowel obstruction are also relatively common (**Figure 9.2**). Intrahepatic gallstones are rarely associated with infection by the fluke *Clonorchis sinesis*.

> Asymptomatic gallstones detected incidentally are left alone unless they start to cause symptoms.

Biliary colic

Right upper quadrant or epigastric pain often occurs after fatty foods or a large meal. It characteristically radiates to the back or right shoulder and lasts several hours. It is caused by temporary obstruction of the cystic duct by a stone; the gallbladder contractions that occur normally after eating cause the pain.

Acute cholecystitis

This arises when a stone impacts in the gallbladder neck and remains impacted, causing inflammation and often secondary infection. It often presents with pain similar to that of biliary colic. This is usually persistent rather than intermittent, and is accompanied by nausea, vomiting and anorexia. Right upper quadrant tenderness is usually found on examination, and there is sometimes 'guarding' (i.e. rigidity) of the abdomen on palpation. Systemic signs of infection, such as fever, are often present.

Around 5% of patients have acute acalculous (i.e. without a stone) cholecystitis. The cause is uncertain but it is more common in severely ill patients, such as those on critical care units.

Chronic cholecystitis

Chronic cholangitis presents with similar symptoms to acute cholecystitis. Recurrent episodes of inflammation of the gallbladder cause thickening of its wall.

> Murphy's sign (pain caused by cholecystitis) is elicited by gently placing two fingers on the right hypochondrium and asking the patient to take a breath in. This causes pain, and inspiration halts so the patient 'catches' their breath. The result is regarded as positive if repeating the manoeuvre in the left hypochondrium does not cause pain.

Complications

Gallstones are associated with a number of complications:

- **Empyema** – a collection of pus within the gallbladder
- **Ascending cholangitis** – painful obstructive jaundice and infection developing after a stone has migrated to and become impacted in the common bile duct
- **Mirizzi's syndrome** – a rare complication in which impaction of a gallstone in the gallbladder neck or cystic duct causes

Presentations of gallstones		
Site of gallstone	Presentation	Clinical features
Gallbladder	Incidental	Asymptomatic
Neck of gallbladder or cystic duct	Biliary colic Acute cholecystitis	Right upper quadrant pain, nausea, vomiting
Common bile duct	Ascending cholangitis (see page 310)	Obstructive jaundice, pain, fever
Ampulla of Vater or pancreatic duct	Pancreatitis	Epigastric pain radiating through to the back, nausea, vomiting
Ileum (from a cholecystoduodenal fistula)	Small bowel obstruction	Abdominal pain, distension, vomiting

Table 9.4 Presentations of gallstones

obstructive jaundice as a result of external compression of the common bile duct

- **Gallstone ileus** – a rare complication in which a large gallstone erodes through the gallbladder wall into the duodenum to form a fistula (cholecystoduodenal fistula). This becomes impacted in the small intestine resulting in small bowel obstruction
- **Gallbladder cancer** (see page 312) – cancer risk is increased with chronic cholecystitis
- **Acute pancreatitis** (see page 290)
- **Secondary biliary cirrhosis**
- **Liver abscesses**

> **'Chole' refers to bile or the biliary tree, hence:**
>
> Cholangitis – infection in the biliary tree
>
> Cholecystectomy – surgical removal of the gallbladder
>
> Cholecystitis – inflammation of the gallbladder
>
> Choledocholithiasis – migration of a gallstone into any duct
>
> Cholelithiasis – gallstone formation

Diagnostic approach

Patients with suspected gallstone disease are usually investigated using a combination of blood tests and abdominal ultrasonography.

Investigations

Blood tests

Concentrations of inflammatory markers (white cell count, CRP) are often raised in cholecystitis. Liver function tests are usually abnormal if there are complications, such as common bile duct stones. The amylase level is checked; during acute pancreatitis, greater amounts than normal are released into the blood from the inflamed pancreas although it occasionally is slightly raised in biliary colic or cholecystitis.

Stool tests

Clonorchis sinesis eggs are identified by microscopic examination of the stool (page 283).

Radiology

Abdominal ultrasound (**Table 9.1**) is the initially diagnostic test and detects more than 90% of gallstones. It also helps to identify complications such as inflammation of the gallbladder and bile duct stones.

An abdominal radiograph is not usually helpful as only 10% of gallstones are radiopaque. HIDA (hydroxyl iminodiacetic acid) scans are radioisotope scans that assess gallbladder function and detect blockages in the cystic duct or common bile duct from the delay in bile excretion (**Figure 9.3**).

Abdominal CT, MRCP or endoscopic ultrasound scans sometimes are required to identify extrahepatic biliary stones.

Management

If gallstones are found incidentally without symptoms, then no further treatment is required. The risk of gallstones becoming symptomatic is approximately 2% per year.

Medications

The pain from biliary colic usually subsides spontaneously or with simple analgesia, e.g. an opioid or nonsteroidal anti-inflammatory drug such as ibuprofen. A low fat diet reduces episodes of biliary colic.

Broad-spectrum antibiotics are indicated if there are features of acute cholecystitis. Intravenous fluids, analgesia and antiemetics are also usually required to treat symptoms and support the patient.

The bile acid ursodeoxycholic acid is sometimes used to try to dissolve cholesterol stones in patients who decline or are too high risk for surgery. However, it is rarely effective, a lengthy course of treatment is usually required and the stones frequently recur.

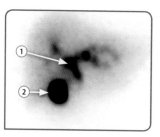

Figure 9.3
HIDA (hydroxyl iminodiacetic acid) scan. ① Tracer being excreted from the liver. Gallbladder ②.

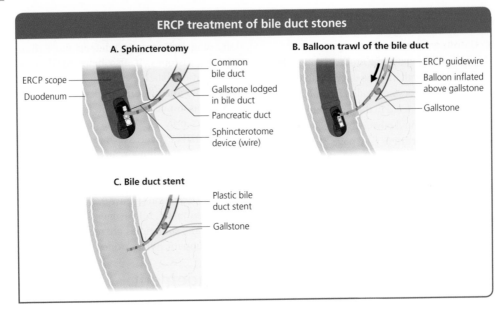

Figure 9.4 Endoscopic retrograde pancreatography (ERCP) treatment of bile duct stones.

Praziquantel is the drug of choice to treat *C. sinesis infection*.

Endoscopy

Stones within the common bile duct are removed by ERCP (**Figure 9.4**), often using a balloon or basket to trawl the duct. A sphincterotomy is usually performed to allow further stones to pass once the bile duct has been freed from obstruction. If the stone cannot be removed, a stent is inserted to relieve the biliary obstruction.

Surgery

'Cholecystectomy' (surgical removal of the gallbladder) is the treatment of choice for symptomatic gallstones. It is usually undertaken laparoscopically. In acute cholecystitis, it is ideally performed within 7 days of presentation; this shortens the hospital stay and without any increased risk of surgical complications.

Prognosis

Patients usually have no symptoms in the years after cholecystectomy but occasionally experience diarrhoea due to bile salt malabsorption. It is important to note, however, that stones are still occasionally produced without a gallbladder – they rarely form in the common bile duct which leads to obstructive jaundice, etc.

Ascending cholangitis

Ascending cholangitis is bacterial infection of the biliary tree, usually secondary to bile duct obstruction. The most frequent cause is obstruction by gallstones: infection complicates around 1% of patients with gallstones. Other causes of ascending cholangitis are listed in **Table 9.5**.

Clinical features

Patients commonly present with a set of features known as Charcot's triad:

- Pain in the right upper quadrant of the abdomen
- Fever
- Jaundice

Causes of ascending cholangitis		
Type of infection	Precipitating factor	Underlying cause or organism
Bacterial	Gallstones	–
	Stricture	Primary sclerosing cholangitis Postoperative Cholangiocarcinoma
	Medical procedures	Post-ERCP Biliary stent
Parasitic	Ingestion of parasite, e.g. eating raw fish in endemic area in the Far East Most common in sub-Sarahan Africa, South America, Far East	*Ascaris lumbricoides* (roundworm) *Clonorchis sinensis* (liver fluke)

Table 9.5 Organisms that cause ascending cholangitis and precipitating factors

Ascending cholangitis also causes rigors and features of systemic sepsis including shock.

> **Rigors (shaking of the whole body) is often due to deep-seated sepsis that produces bacteraemia.** Common causes are cholangitis and pyelonephritis.

Clinical examination shows yellow sclerae due to jaundice and right upper quadrant tenderness.

Complications

These are reduced by prompt treatment and include:

- Consequences of sepsis, e.g. multiorgan failure
- Liver abscesses (see **Figure 9.2**), which require a prolonged course of antibiotics over several weeks to adequately clear the infection

Diagnostic approach

Diagnosis is based upon a combination of clinical features and blood tests.

> **Ascending cholangitis sometimes presents with a pyrexia of unknown origin.** Liver function tests should be performed in all patients with a fever.

Investigations

If ascending cholangitis is suspected, blood tests, blood cultures and imaging is performed in all patients.

Blood tests

A raised CRP concentration and white cell count indicate infection. Liver function tests show raised bilirubin, alkaline phosphatase and γ-glutamyl transferase, to indicate biliary obstruction and inflammation.

Blood cultures are taken to determine appropriate antibiotic therapy. Gram-negative bacterial species that are normally seen in the GI tract (e.g. *Escherichia coli*, *Klebsiella* and *Enterobacter*) are most commonly identified, followed by Gram-positive cocci (e.g. *Enterococcus*). Anaerobic organisms are less frequently found. Stool samples are taken to look for parasites if the patient has travelled to endemic areas (**Table 9.5**).

Imaging

Abdominal ultrasound and MRCP will identify biliary dilatation due to bile duct stones or strictures. Endoscopic ultrasonography (EUS) should be considered if small gallstones are clinically suspected but not seen on other imaging.

Management

Treatment is with intravenous fluid replacement, analgesics and treatment of the infection and the underlying cause (**Table 9.6**).

Antibiotics

Broad-spectrum antibiotics (e.g. cephalosporins) to cover commonly identified organisms are the initial therapy for bacterial infection. The antibiotic choice is then reviewed, and if necessary adjusted, in response to blood culture results.

Parasitic infection is treated by mebendazole (for A. *lumbricoides*) and *praziquantel* (for C. *sinensis*).

Prognosis

Mortality mainly results from the consequences of infection. The risk of death is high if the infection is left untreated but low if prompt antibiotic therapy is given and there is early removal of the obstruction or drainage, via ERCP for example.

Treating underlying causes of bacterial ascending cholangitis	
Underlying cause	Treatment
Gallstones	ERCP to perform sphincterotomy and remove any stones from bile duct; a biliary stent is inserted to relieve bile duct obstruction. Cholecystectomy is considered later
Stricture	Decompression of biliary system by dilatation of the stricture or insertion of a plastic stent at ERCP
Medical procedures and stents	Prophylactic antibiotics pre and post-procedure
	Antibiotics during infection
	Removal or change of biliary stent if infected

ERCP, endoscopic retrograde cholangiopancreatography.

Table 9.6 Treating the underlying cause of bacterial ascending cholangitis

Biliary tract neoplasia

Tumours of the biliary tree are either malignant or benign. Gallbladder cancer is the fifth most common GI tract malignancy worldwide and commonest biliary tree malignancy, followed by cholangiocarcinoma. Gallbladder polyps are the commonest type of benign tumour.

- Chronic cholecystitis
- Obesity and smoking
- Gallbladder polyps (see page 314)
- Chronic typhoid (*Salmonella typhi* and S. *paratyphi*) infection of the gallbladder – the risk of gallbladder cancer is increased up to 200 fold

Gallbladder cancer

The most common gallbladder cancer is adenocarcinoma, which arises from the glandular cells of the gallbladder and accounts for around 80% of cases. Less common forms include squamous and small cell carcinomas. Gallbladder cancer is more common in women (ratio 3:1) and people over 70 years old. It is a common type of malignancy in Japan, northern India, central and Eastern Europe and central and South America. Gallstones are present in 75% of patients with gallbladder cancer. Other risk factors and associations include:

Clinical features

20% of all cases are found coincidentally in patients undergoing cholecystectomy for other reasons e.g. biliary colic. Early gallbladder cancer is often asymptomatic. Patients with symptoms usually present with right upper quadrant pain, vomiting and weight loss. Jaundice is sometimes present if there is obstruction of the bile ducts by the tumour. Examination is usually normal but sometimes reveals a hard mass in the right upper quadrant.

Blood tests are usually normal, but occasionally demonstrate a cholestatic jaundice with raised bilirubin, alkaline phosphatase and γ-glutamyl transferase if there is obstruction of the biliary tree.

Abdominal ultrasound shows a mass in the gallbladder, or a gallbladder replaced by tumour. Obstruction of the bile ducts by tumour causes their dilatation above this level. CT imaging is used for staging of the tumour using the TNM classification (see page 127).

Management

Most tumours present late. Furthermore, the rich lymphatic and venous drainage of the gallbladder leads to early spread and means that tumours are not surgically resectable.

Chemotherapy and radiotherapy

Chemotherapy and radiotherapy are occasionally used either on their own or in combination with surgery.

Endoscopy

ERCP and biliary stent insertion is undertaken in patients with jaundice, to relieve obstruction of the bile duct. Percutaneous transhepatic cholangiogram (PTC) is used when ERCP is not possible e.g. if there is a very tight stricture that cannot be crossed. Contrast medium is injected into the bile duct through a needle inserted through the abdominal wall. Under x-ray visualisation a stent is then inserted into the bile duct to relieve the biliary obstruction.

Surgery

Curative surgery is only an option for patients presenting early. The gallbladder is removed along with a partial hepatectomy (liver resection) and removal of local lymph nodes. If gallbladder cancer is identified co-incidentally during cholecystectomy, further surgery is often required.

Prognosis

The overall 5-year survival is less than 5%. This rises to 80% in patients with localised disease.

Cholangiocarcinoma

Cholangiocarcinoma develops from bile duct epithelium within the intrahepatic or extrahepatic biliary tree. Intrahepatic cholangiocarcinoma is the second most common primary liver cancer worldwide and has a rising incidence. The prevalence of cholangiocarcinoma is higher in Africa and East Asia where it is associated with liver fluke infection by a mechanism that is not understood. Other risk factors include:

- primary sclerosing cholangitis
- congenital cystic liver disease
- choledochal cysts
- bile duct adenomas
- viral infection (hepatitis B virus, hepatitis C virus, HIV)

Clinical features

Presentation is usually with jaundice and pruritus secondary to biliary obstruction. Pale stool and dark urine are often reported. Non-specific symptoms include weight loss and upper abdominal pain.

Apart from jaundice, the physical examination is normal or there is hepatomegaly or a mass in the right upper quadrant.

Blood tests demonstrate cholestatic jaundice with raised bilirubin, alkaline phosphatase and γ-glutamyl transferase. There is a coagulopathy, shown by a raised prothrombin time and international normalised ratio. The level of tumour marker CA19-9 is usually elevated.

Dilated bile ducts and a biliary stricture or mass are often identified by abdominal ultrasonography or MRCP. Endoscopic ultrasound examination provides additional information and allows fine-needle aspiration for histology to be carried out. CT is required for tumour staging by the TNM classification.

> **Occasionally raised CA19-9 is due to cholestasis alone and does not indicate an underlying malignancy**. It must therefore be interpreted alongside other investigations, particularly imaging.

Management

Most tumours present late and are not amenable to surgery. A palliative approach is taken and focuses on relieving biliary obstruction.

Medication

Chemotherapy has only a small benefit. Colestyramine and ursodeoxycholic acid are prescribed to relieve pruritus.

Endoscopy

ERCP allows biliary strictures to be identified and brushings to be obtained for cytology. Stents are inserted to treat bile duct obstruction. Cholangioscopy involves inserting a very thin endoscope directly into the bile ducts. This provides direct visualisation and biopsy of strictures.

Percutaneous transhepatic cholangiography (PTC) is used when ERCP is not possible. Like ERCP, a stent is inserted to relieve biliary obstruction (see page 304).

Surgery

Surgery is the only curative treatment for early cancer. A partial hepatectomy (liver resection) is performed for intrahepatic disease. Whipple's procedure (see Figure 8.6) is used to treat distal cholangiocarcinoma.

Prognosis

The 5-year survival if metastatic disease is present is less than 2%.

Gallbladder polyps

Gallbladder polyps are polypoidal growths in the wall of the gallbladder. Benign causes include cholesterol polyps, adenomas, lipomas, haemangiomas and adenomyomatosis. They are usually asymptomatic and detected as a coincidental finding on imaging (e.g. ultrasound or CT) performed to investigate abdominal symptoms such as pain. Cholecystectomy is performed if polyps have a diameter of >10 mm or are fast growing, or if patients are over 50 years old and have co-existing gallstones, because these all increase the risk of gallbladder cancer. Patients with polyps < 10 mm in size and without these other risk factors are monitored through 6- to 12-monthly ultrasound scans.

Answers to starter questions

1. Biliary obstruction causes increased levels of bile acid in the blood, which stimulates skin nerve receptors resulting in itch, or pruritus. This cholestatic pruritus can be relieved with bile acid sequestrants, such as colestyramine, which bind the bile acids in the intestine increasing their excretion in the stool and reducing levels in the blood stream. Symptoms also improve with treatment of the underlying cause, e.g. bile duct stent insertion for biliary strictures.

2. After a cholecystectomy, gallstones can still form, rarely, in the extrahepatic bile ducts via the same mechanisms: bile stasis and elevated bile cholesterol levels. These cause similar symptoms and complications to gallstones in the gallbladder. They are extracted from the bile ducts by endoscopic retrograde cholangiopancreatography (ERCP).

3. The gallbladder is a storage sac for bile. Whilst it can be removed without any effect on mortality, some patients develop symptoms from bile salt malabsorption, e.g. diarrhoea. Malabsorption occurs due to removal of this bile reservoir, interrupting the enterohepatic circulation of bile salts. It is treated with bile acid sequestrants such as colestyramine and a low-fat diet.

4. Biliary neoplasia are usually asymptomatic until the point of causing biliary obstruction and jaundice. By this time, treatment is usually palliative and includes insertion of a stent at ERCP or PTC to relieve the obstruction. Biliary neoplasia are rarely detected co-incidentally on imaging due to the small size of the bile ducts.

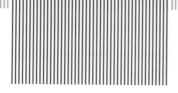

Chapter 10
Emergencies

Starter questions

Reading this chapter will enable you to answer the following questions. Answers are on page 328.

1. How do you assess the severity of an upper GI bleed?
2. What are the indications for transplantation in liver failure?
3. How is small bowel obstruction distinguishable from large bowel obstruction?

Introduction

Some emergency presentations of gastrointestinal (GI) and liver disease have characteristic features, for example jaundice in liver failure. Others are less specific, such as collapse secondary to hypovolaemic shock, which often follows haematemesis or melaena after a significant upper GI bleed. As with any emergency admission, initial management of GI emergencies is resuscitation with an emphasis on airway, breathing and circulation, including fluid status. Patients must be managed in an environment with prompt access to other specialties, including surgery and critical care. Diagnostic and therapeutic modalities, such as endoscopy and radiology, must also be easily available.

This chapter discusses the clinical features, differential diagnoses and management of three common and potentially life-threatening scenarios – upper GI bleeding, acute liver failure and significant abdominal pain.

Upper GI bleeding

Case 13 Collapse after black stool and abdominal pain

Presentation

Aruna Ranasinghe, aged 78 years, is admitted to the emergency department after collapsing at home. Over the past few days, he has been passing black tarry stool and complaining of upper abdominal pain. En route to hospital he vomits a small amount of fresh blood seen by the paramedic crew. He is pale and has clammy skin. His blood pressure is 85/60 mmHg and he has a heart rate of 120 beats per minute.

> **'Coffee-ground vomit' has the appearance of coffee grounds due to the presence of blood from the upper GI tract**: gastric acid oxidises the iron in haemoglobin, turning it brown. A similar presentation is sometimes seen with small bowel obstruction, diagnosed on an abdominal radiograph.

Initial interpretation

Mr Ranasinghe has haematemesis and melaena, indicative of an upper GI bleed. His tachycardia and hypotension suggest a significant bleed with hypovolaemic shock. He requires prompt resuscitation.

> **Patients taking beta-blockers do not mount the same tachycardic response after a significant bleed and often have a normal heart rate.**

Further history and examination

Mr Ranasinghe has had long-standing indigestion. This has been worse over the last few weeks after he started taking regular non-steroidal anti-inflammatory drugs (NSAIDs) for back pain. He has a history of hypertension but is otherwise in good health. He is not taking any anti-platelet or anticoagulant medication.

On examination, there is tenderness in the epigastric region on palpation. There are no signs of chronic liver disease, e.g. palmer erythema, spider naevi or ascites. Rectal examination reveals liquid, jet-black stool with a distinctive offensive smell.

Working diagnosis

Mr Ranasinghe is having an upper GI bleed. The most common cause of this is a peptic ulcer. His symptoms and recent use of NSAIDs support this.

Immediate intervention

Urgent resuscitation is essential. Two wide-bore cannulas are inserted and 1 litre of intravenous fluid is administered over 15 minutes to stabilise Mr Ranasinghe's blood pressure. Urgent blood tests are taken:

- Full blood count – to check for anaemia, although haemoglobin is often normal immediately after a GI bleed
- Clotting factors – to exclude abnormal clotting which may exacerbate the bleeding
- Urea and electrolytes – the plasma urea level is elevated in patients with upper GI bleeding; this is thought to be due to the haemoglobin protein component of blood being digested in the GI tract or poor perfusion of the kidneys due to blood loss (see page 108)

Case 13 *continued*

- Cross-match – so that blood is available for transfusion

He is attached to a cardiac monitor to observe his heart rate. An erect chest radiograph shows no evidence of subdiaphragmatic gas, which would usually be seen with perforation of the stomach or small intestine.

The laboratory telephones to deliver the blood test results because they are significantly abnormal: haemoglobin 68 g/L (normal 130–180 g/L), plasma urea 22 mmol/L (normal 2.5–7.0 mmol/L). A transfusion is set up to deliver 2 units of cross-matched blood.

Once Mr Ranasinghe has been resuscitated and is more stable, an upper GI endoscopy is arranged. This reveals an actively bleeding duodenal ulcer (**Figure 10.1**).

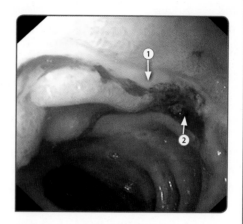

Figure 10.1 Duodenal peptic ulcer ① with visible oozing blood vessel ②.

The most common cause of upper GI bleeding is peptic ulcer disease, followed by oesophagitis, gastritis or duodenitis. Bleeding from gastro-oesophageal varices only accounts for approximately 10% of cases but confers a high mortality rate. Varices are rare if there are no features of chronic liver disease. Other causes of GI bleeding, and their treatment, are outlined in **Table 10.1**.

Patients presenting with GI bleeding are stratified using two scoring systems:

- **Glasgow–Blatchford score** – this scores according to the presence of melaena, syncope, hepatic and cardiac disease, hypotension, tachycardia, low haemoglobin concentrations and a raised plasma urea level. It is used to determine the need for medical intervention, e.g. blood transfusion and whether endoscopy is required in the inpatient setting or as an urgent outpatient
- **Rockall score** – this uses the age, presence of organ failure or disseminated malignancy, tachycardia and hypotension. A score is calculated pre-endoscopy and with the endoscopy findings to calculate the risk of an adverse outcome.

After initial resuscitation and stabilisation of the patient's condition, upper GI endoscopy is almost always performed. It has both a diagnostic and a therapeutic role:

- Endoscopy allows the cause and site of the bleeding to be identified: features of recent or active bleeding include fresh blood, adherent clot and a visible vessel in the ulcer base
- Endoscopic techniques are used to stop the bleeding: adrenaline (epinephrine) injection is combined with thermal cautery, small metal clips or a banding device. Haemostatic sprays are also used, which form a mechanical barrier over the site of bleeding and enhance clot formation.

If the bleeding cannot be controlled endoscopically, interventional radiology or surgery is used. Blood vessels are sometimes embolised (occluded) using small metal coils that induce clotting.

Upper GI bleeding: causes and treatment		
Site	Cause	Treatment
Oesophagus	Oesophagitis (inflammation)	PPI
	Ulcer	PPI Adrenaline (epinephrine) ± clips ± thermal cautery ± haemostatic spray
	Varices	Band ligation Sengstaken–Blakemore tube (for uncontrolled bleeding) TIPS (for refractory bleeding)
	Carcinoma	Radiotherapy
	Mallory Weiss tear (tear in mucosal lining)	Conservative treatment or PPI Adrenaline ± clips
Stomach	Ulcer	PPI ± *Helicobacter pylori* eradication therapy Adrenaline ± clips ± thermal cautery ± haemostatic spray
	Malignant tumour, e.g. carcinoma, lymphoma	Chemotherapy or radiotherapy *H. pylori* eradication (in MALT lymphoma*) Surgical resection
	Gastrointestinal stromal tumour (benign tumour with malignant potential)	Surgical resection
	Dieulafoy's lesion (arteriole eroding through stomach wall)	Adrenaline ± clips ± thermal cautery ± band ligation ± haemostatic spray
	Gastric antral vascular ectasia (see page 260)	Argon photocoagulation
	Varices	Cyanoacrylate glue injection Sengstaken–Blakemore tube (for uncontrolled bleeding) TIPS (for refractory bleeding)
	Angioectasia (small dilated vessels)	Adrenaline injection ± APC
Small intestine	Ulcer	PPI ± *H. pylori* eradication therapy Adrenaline ± clips ± thermal cautery ± haemostatic spray
	Angioectasia	Adrenaline injection ± APC
	Malignancy (rare), e.g. carcinoma, metastatic melanoma	Surgical resection Chemotherapy or radiotherapy
	Diverticulum (rare) or Meckel's diverticulum	Adrenaline injection ± clips Surgical resection

PPI, proton pump inhibitor; TIPS, transjugular intrahepatic portosystemic shunt.

*MALT lymphoma, lymphoma in mucosal-associated lymphoid tissue; see Table 4.6.

Table 10.1 Upper GI bleeding: causes and treatment

Peptic ulcer disease

Peptic ulcers are more common with increasing age and in patients taking NSAIDs (see Chapter 4, page 186). As well as bleeding, ulcers occasionally present as an emergency with signs of perforation (guarding on examination and subphrenic gas on an erect chest radiograph; see Figure 4.3). Endoscopic investigation and treatment is as outlined above. Peptic ulcers at high risk of further bleeding include those with a visible blood vessel, active bleeding or adherent clot at the time of endoscopy. After endoscopy, a proton pump inhibitor is given intravenously to reduce gastric acid secretion; this helps ulcer healing by assisting formation of an overlying clot.

A *Campylobacter*-like organism test (Figure 4.5) is performed to confirm whether *Helicobacter pylori* infection is present as a cause for the ulcer. If it is, eradication treatment is started (see Table 4.4).

Patients whose bleeding cannot be controlled and those who re-bleed after endoscopic intervention usually require radiological embolisation, or surgery to oversew the ulcer (stitches inserted to compress the bleeding vessels).

Gastro-oesophageal varices

A varix (plural varices) is a dilated submucosal vein, which most commonly occurs in the oesophagus as a result of portal hypertension. They also arise in the stomach, rectum and as distended veins seen on the abdominal wall called caput medusa (Figure 7.3). Variceal bleeds are a major cause of significant morbidity and mortality in those with chronic liver disease. After initial resuscitation with intravenous fluids and blood products, early endoscopy is performed to provide treatment.

Antibiotics are given to reduce the risk of infection. The vasoconstrictor Terlipressin is also started to reduce the portal pressure and blood flow to the varices, until endoscopic treatment is undertaken.

In 80% of patients, band ligation (use of a tight rubber band to occlude the varix) controls the bleeding (Figure 7.4). If this is unsuccessful, balloon tamponade using a Sengstaken–Blakemore tube is used to compress the varices (**Figure 10.2**). However, this is a temporary measure until further attempts at banding or a TIPS (transjugular intrahepatic portosystemic shunt) procedure is undertaken (Figure 7.5).

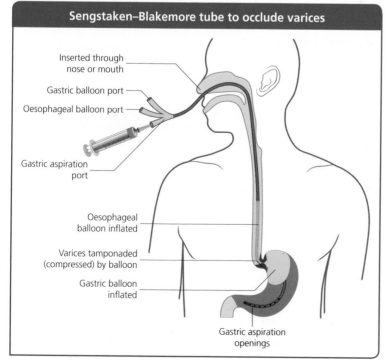

Sengstaken–Blakemore tube to occlude varices

Inserted through nose or mouth

Gastric balloon port

Oesophageal balloon port

Gastric aspiration port

Oesophageal balloon inflated

Varices tamponaded (compressed) by balloon

Gastric balloon inflated

Gastric aspiration openings

Figure 10.2
Positioning of a Sengstaken–Blakemore tube to occlude bleeding varices.

Mallory–Weiss tear

These are tears in the mucosal lining of the oesophagus. Patients often give a history of repeated retching or vomiting prior to the onset of haematemesis. The vast majority of tears heal spontaneously without intervention. The endoscopic treatment of those with active bleeding is outlined in **Table 10.1.**

Acute liver failure

Case 14 Confusion and jaundice

Laura Bennett is a 19-year-old woman, admitted to the hospital emergency unit after her flatmate finds her on a Monday morning, when she had not shown up for lectures. Laura is drowsy, confused and jaundiced. Her pulse rate is 125 beats per minute and her blood pressure 85/60 mmHg.

Initial interpretation

The altered level of consciousness with confusion in the presence of jaundice suggests hepatic encephalopathy. The combination of altered mental function, jaundice and haemodynamic instability indicate significant liver dysfunction.

History and examination

Laura's flatmate reports that she had not been seen since Friday evening after an argument with her boyfriend. She says that Laura has a history of low mood for which she has been taking citalopram for the last year, but she is not aware that Laura has any history of other illnesses. Laura has otherwise been well. They drink approximately two bottles of wine between them a week.

On examination, Laura is deeply jaundiced, but there are no stigmata of chronic liver disease.

Immediate interventions

The presence of jaundice and confusion indicates acute liver failure. The fact that Laura has depression makes an overdose of medication such as paracetamol a possible cause of the liver failure. An elevated paracetamol level is confirmed on blood testing. Given that it takes over 24 hours for jaundice to develop after paracetamol overdose, Laura's presentation clearly is delayed. Nevertheless, the antidote N-acetylcysteine is given because even at this late stage it can still have some benefit.

Liver and renal function, prothrombin time and arterial blood gases must be measured. In addition, intravenous fluids are given, as she is unable to drink fluids due to drowsiness. Laura is admitted to the high-dependency unit for close observation, where they have the facilities to provide ventilation to support her breathing and intracranial pressure monitoring, should she deteriorate further. Her glucose

Indications for liver transplantation	
Acute liver failure	Chronic liver disease
Encephalopathy	Recurrent encephalopathy
Metabolic acidosis	Refractory variceal bleeding
Raised creatinine	Recurrent or persistent ascites
Significant coagulopathy	Hepatocellular carcinoma (see Table 7.11)
	Significant impairment in quality of life (e.g. intractable itching in primary biliary cholangitis)

Table 10.2 Main indications for consideration of liver transplantation

Case 14 *continued*

level is closely monitored as low blood glucose (hypoglycaemia) often occurs with acute liver failure and sometimes results in neurological deterioration, or occasionally death.

The local tertiary liver centre should be contacted to discuss Laura's further management if the test results demonstrate any of the indications for consideration of liver transplantation (**Table 10.2**).

The majority of patients who present with jaundice and encephalopathy have decompensated chronic liver disease (see Chapter 7, page 257). This is apparent from the history, physical examination and results of radiology, which show features of cirrhosis (e.g. nodular appearance to the liver). Whereas patients with acute liver failure have rapidly developing liver dysfunction often in association with deranged clotting (coagulopathy) and encephalopathy, in a previously normal liver (see Chapter 7, page 255). Acute liver failure is far more common in the developing world, where viral causes are commonest. This compares with Europe, where drugs are the most common cause of acute liver failure (**Table 10.3**).

Paracetamol overdose

The damage caused by paracetamol is dose related and occurs at a lower dose in individuals with underlying liver disease.

For all patients who present within 24 hours of ingesting a paracetamol overdose a nomogram chart is used to determine the need for *N*-acetylcysteine (NAC) treatment (**Figure 10.3**). Plasma paracetamol concentration is plotted against the number of hours since ingestion. Anybody falling on or above the predefined treatment line is commenced on an NAC infusion. This prevents severe liver damage and death in nearly all cases when commenced within 8–10 hours of paracetamol ingestion, following which time its benefit falls significantly.

N-acetylcysteine is also given if the timing of paracetamol overdose is uncertain or staggered (i.e. tablets taken over a period of more than 1 hour) or in patients presenting more than 24 hours after ingestion, where there is liver or renal impairment.

Other drugs

Idiosyncratic reactions to many prescribed medications can damage the liver, as can recreational drugs such as cocaine, ecstasy and magic mushrooms.

Viruses

Worldwide, the predominant cause of acute liver failure is viral infection e.g. Hepatitis A, C and E. In Europe and North America, public health measures have reduced their incidence.

Causes of acute liver failure			
Cause	United Kingdom	Japan	India
Paracetamol overdose	56%	0%	0%
Other drugs	12%	10%	2%
Unknown	17%	32%	31%
Hepatitis A	2%	6%	2%
Hepatitis B	5%	43%	14%
Hepatitis E	1%	1%	44%
Other	7%	8%	7%

Table 10.3 Causes of acute liver failure vary worldwide, as shown in these contrasting examples of developed Western and Eastern countries and a developing country

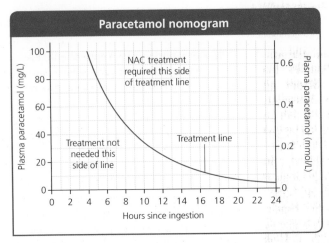

Figure 10.3 Paracetamol nomogram

Other viruses also occasionally cause liver failure, for example Epstein–Barr virus (which causes glandular fever), cytomegalovirus and herpes simplex.

Other causes of acute liver failure

A range of other conditions occasionally cause acute liver failure, including malignant infiltration of the liver, Wilson's disease, autoimmune hepatitis, Budd–Chiari syndrome and rarely pregnancy. Ischaemic necrosis sometimes occurs in critically ill patients with hypoperfusion of the liver, such as following cardiac arrest or low blood pressure due to significant blood loss (e.g. following a road traffic accident).

Unknown

In a significant number of patients the cause of acute liver failure cannot be determined despite a thorough review of the history and appropriate investigations. The outcome in these patients is relatively poor. It is believed that in some cases there is an unidentified viral aetiology.

Intestinal obstruction

Case 15 Abdominal pain and persistent vomiting

Presentation

Martina Olsson, aged 31 years, presents to the emergency department with an acute-onset abdominal pain, abdominal distension and persistent vomiting of a pale brown fluid. She has dry mucus membranes due to dehydration and is clutching a vomit bowl. Her pulse is 110 beats per minute and her blood pressure is 90/55 mmHg.

Initial interpretation

The rapid onset of symptoms is suggestive of small bowel obstruction. Gastroenteritis is unlikely in the absence of diarrhoea. The tachycardia and hypotension suggest hypovolaemia due to fluid loss from vomiting.

History and examination

Martina was feeling well until 2 hours before her admission, when she developed

Case 15 *continued*

severe colicky abdominal pain and progressive distension of her abdomen. The vomiting is uncontrollable despite an injection of an intravenous antiemetic medication given by the nursing staff on arrival in the department. Martina reports that she has no other medical complaints.

Her abdomen is grossly distended, with a visible scar in the right lower quadrant of her abdomen. This is from an appendectomy 10 years ago for a perforated appendix with peritonitis. Percussion is tympanic throughout, and high-pitched, tinkling bowel sounds are heard on auscultation. No hernias are identified.

Immediate intervention

The examination findings, along with the history of previous surgery and peritonitis, suggest a diagnosis of intestinal obstruction secondary to adhesions. This is one of the most common causes of small bowel obstruction in the absence of a hernia. The differential diagnoses of intestinal obstruction are described in **Table 10.4**.

An abdominal radiograph shows dilated loops of small bowel (**Figure 10.4**). A nasogastric tube is inserted into the stomach

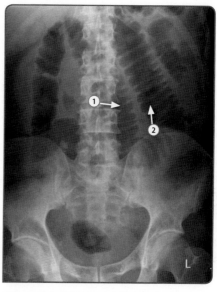

Figure 10.4 Abdominal radiograph demonstrating dilated loops of bowel in the central abdomen ①. The presence of valvulae conniventes ② confirms this is small bowel obstruction.

Key features and causes of intestinal obstruction		
Site	**Features**	**Causes**
Small intestine	Colicky abdominal pain	Adhesions or bands
	Abdominal distension	Hernia
	Vomiting (often the only feature in high jejunal obstruction)	Intussusception
		Strictures (due to Crohn's disease, NSAIDs, radiation)
		Gallstone ileus
		Foreign body
		Primary or secondary tumours
Large intestine	Colicky abdominal pain	Colorectal carcinoma
	Abdominal distension	Sigmoid or caecal volvulus
	Absolute constipation	Adhesions
	Vomiting (late sign if Ileocaecal valve incompetent)	Diverticular disease
NSAID, non-steroidal anti-inflammatory drug.		

Table 10.4 Key features and causes of intestinal obstruction

Case 15 *continued*

to remove fluid from above the level of the obstruction and to decompress the small intestine. Intravenous fluids and potassium replacement are given to treat the losses caused by the vomiting. Urine output and plasma urea and electrolytes are monitored carefully.

Intestinal obstruction is caused by mechanical factors or by a paralytic ileus. In the latter, there is no fixed occlusion of the intestine but the patient presents with similar symptoms to a mechanical obstruction, due to reduced mobility of the intestine. Paralytic ileus usually resolves with conservative treatment involving insertion of a nasogastric tube, aspiration and intravenous fluids ('drip and suck').

> **Postoperative paralytic ileus** sometimes occurs due to medications (e.g. opiates, anticholinergic agents) or metabolic factors (e.g. hypokalaemia, diabetic ketoacidosis).

Adhesions

Adhesions are the most common cause of small bowel obstruction, accounting for 50–75% of cases. They usually occur after abdominal surgery. The diagnosis is suggested on CT imaging by an abrupt transition point in the small intestine in the absence of an alternative underlying cause on the scan, such as a tumour. Symptoms sometimes settle with conservative treatment or require surgical division of the adhesions.

Strictures

Strictures of the small or large intestine occur secondary to Crohn's disease, tumours, NSAIDs or previous radiotherapy (when this affects the small intestine it is called radiation enteritis). Inflammatory Crohn's strictures often improve by increasing medical therapy, for example corticosteroids, whereas chronic fibrotic Crohn's strictures require dilatation or surgical treatment.

Hernias

An abdominal hernia is defined as protrusion of part of the small or large intestine from the abdominal cavity through the abdominal wall at one of several potential sites (**Figure 10.5**). Hernial orifices (for inguinal, femoral, paraumbilical and umbilical hernias) are examined in all patients with intestinal obstruction. Incisional hernias occur at the site of abdominal scars. Surgical repair of a hernia is undertaken for symptomatic patients or cosmetic reasons, such as those with pain or deformity of the abdominal wall.

A strangulated hernia occurs when the blood supply to the intestine becomes compromised, causing ischaemia and eventually necrosis of the bowel. Tachycardia, pyrexia and an elevated white cell count are features.

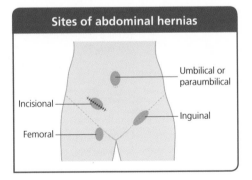

Figure 10.5 Sites of abdominal hernias.

Surgery is required to treat the hernia and resect ischaemic bowel.

Volvulus

The intestine and its mesentery twist around a focal point, resulting in bowel obstruction and sometimes ischaemia. Volvulus most frequently occurs in the sigmoid colon and is more common in men and elderly individuals. An abdominal radiograph shows a characteristic 'coffee-bean' sign (the twisted and dilated sigmoid colon resembles a coffee-bean shape).

The initial treatment of a sigmoid volvulus is by insertion of a sigmoidoscope into the lower large intestine, which is used to untwist the sigmoid colon. If the volvulus is recurrent or is accompanied by ischaemia (identified through symptoms of abdominal pain and a metabolic acidosis and raised white cell count on blood tests), a sigmoid colectomy is required (see page 238). In frail elderly patients who are not fit enough for surgery or an anaesthetic, percutaneous endoscopic colostomy (PEC) tubes are an alternative treatment. PEC tubes are percutaneous endoscopic gastrostomy tubes that are inserted through the abdominal wall into the left colon (rather than the stomach where they are usually used for feeding). Two tubes are inserted to fix the large intestine to the abdominal wall and prevent the bowel from twisting.

Volvulus of the caecum or small intestine occurs less frequently and is treated surgically.

Tumours

Caecal carcinoma occasionally presents with small bowel obstruction, whereas all other obstructing colorectal tumours present with large bowel obstruction. Urgent CT staging is performed to assess for metastatic disease.

Primary surgical resection of the tumour is considered if there is localised or limited metastatic disease. A defunctioning ileostomy or colostomy is undertaken if there are widespread metastases. Insertion of a self-expanding metal stent is an alternative palliative treatment to surgery and is mainly used for obstructing cancers in the left colon.

Small bowel tumours are rare. However, they can result in obstruction due to occlusion of the lumen or intussusception (the prolapse of one section of intestine into an adjacent section).

Gallstone ileus

This occurs when a gallstone erodes through the gallbladder wall into the small intestine, usually the distal ileum (Table 9.4). This causes a mechanical obstruction. Treatment includes surgical removal of the stone and cholecystectomy to reduce the risk of further gallstone related complications.

Answers to starter questions

1. Patients presenting with upper GI bleeding are initially assessed using the Glasgow–Blatchford score (GBS) and the Rockall score. GBS is used to determine the need for inpatient versus outpatient endoscopy, based on clinical features including heart rate, blood pressure and the presence of maelena. A pre- and post-endoscopy Rockall score can be calculated to determine mortality rates. This takes into account the endoscopic diagnosis and the presence of the stigmata of recent haemorrhage, i.e. endoscopic signs of recent, or at risk of, bleeding.

2. Patients with significantly impaired liver function (e.g. severe coagulopathy or encephalopathy) due to acute liver failure or cirrhosis and its complications, should be considered and assessed for liver transplantation. Other factors influencing the decision include the prognosis, the impact of the illness on their quality of life, comorbidities, compliance with treatment and follow-up medical appointments.

3. Both small bowel obstruction (SBO) and large bowel obstruction (LBO) present with symptoms of colicky abdominal pain and distension. Vomiting tends to be an earlier sign in SBO and can be absent in LBO; whereas constipation is a main feature of LBO and may not be evident with proximal SBO. SBO may be distinguished from LBO on abdominal X-ray due to the central position of the distended bowel loops and presence of visible valvulae conniventes. In LBO the dilated intestine is more peripheral, with visible haustra.

Chapter 11
Integrated care

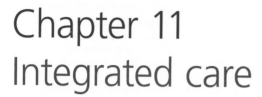

Starter questions

Reading this chapter will enable you to answer the following questions. Answers are on page 340–341.

1. How do you know when bowel function is abnormal?
2. Does iron deficiency anaemia need to be investigated in all patients?
3. How do you distinguish between malaena and black stool secondary to iron supplements?
4. What lifestyle changes should patients with GI and liver disorders make?

Introduction

Gastrointestinal symptoms are common and often self-managed without medical advice being sought or needed. A person makes dietary changes or buys over-the-counter medications from a supermarket or chemist, sometimes with advice from the pharmacist. When people do seek medical attention for GI problems, this is most commonly from their general practitioner (GP). More rarely their symptoms are sufficiently acute or severe to present to secondary care services such as the emergency department, for example if there is GI haemorrhage.

Irritable bowel syndrome affects 10–20% of people in the UK. About half of those affected seek help from their GP, and about 20% of these are referred to gastroenterology services.

Many conditions such as dyspepsia or functional gut disorders are managed effectively in primary care by treating the symptoms, without the need for invasive investigations or referral to secondary care. Such treatment is GP led but other healthcare professionals are often involved, for example a community dietician. Patients with 'alarm' features or whose diagnosis is uncertain require further assessment to obtain a diagnosis and formulate a management plan. This usually requires referral either for review by a gastroenterologist in a hospital outpatient clinic or directly to the endoscopy department. Similarly, acutely unwell inpatients are referred for inpatient gastroenterology assessment. Other healthcare professionals are commonly brought in at this stage – specialist nurses, dieticians, radiologists, surgeons, oncologists and palliative care physicians.

> **All healthcare practitioners have a role in prevention of GI disease via patient education and promotion of a healthy lifestyle.** This has become more important with changes in the Western diet which have raised the prevalence of alcohol- and obesity-related GI conditions, and with wider adoption of this diet in other parts of the world.

Gastrointestinal multidisciplinary teams

Team (indications)	Gastroenterologist	Hepatologist	Oncologist	Surgeon	Radiologist	Pathologist	Specialist nurse	Nurse endoscopist	Palliative care team	Dietician	Pharmacist
Upper GI tract (malignancy, complex benign disease)	✓		✓ (UGI)	✓ (UGI)	✓	✓	✓ (UGI)	✓	✓		
Hepatobiliary (malignancy, complex benign disease)	✓	✓	✓	✓ (H)	✓	✓	✓ (H)		✓		
Pancreatic (malignancy, complex benign disease)	✓		✓	✓ (P)	✓	✓	✓ (P)		✓		
Lower GI (malignancy, complex benign disease)	✓		✓	✓ (C)	✓	✓	✓ (C)	✓	✓		
Endotherapy (endoscopically removable lesions)*	✓			✓ (C & UGI	✓	✓		✓			
IBD (complex disease or treatment with biological agents)	✓			✓ (C)	✓	✓	✓ (IBD)				
Nutrition (complex nutrition, home parenteral nutrition)	✓			✓ (C & UGI)			✓ (N)			✓	✓

C, colorectal; GI, gastrointestinal; H, hepatobiliary; IBD, inflammatory bowel disease; LGI, lower GI; N, nutrition; P, pancreatic; UGI, upper GI.

*Benign lesions and early cancers in upper or lower GI tract.

Table 11.1 Gastrointestinal multidisciplinary teams. Some of these specialists are directly involved in the patient's care, for example in clinics, whilst others such as the pathologist and radiologist, participate in multidisciplinary team meetings to review clinical information and results to inform optimal patient management

For the health and wellbeing of patients with chronic disease or GI malignancies, it is especially important that care provided by different healthcare professionals is integrated. This is done by taking a multidisciplinary team approach (**Table 11.1**), in which care is coordinated between professionals in the hospital and community. In this chapter, we discuss common GI conditions – constipation, abnormal liver function tests and iron deficiency anaemia – to demonstrate this and show the key role of the patient in self-management.

Chronic disease management

In all parts of the GI tract there are disorders that are treatable but cannot be cured. As a result, many people live with chronic GI disease that is lifelong after diagnosis and usually has a variable course, with episodes of remission where there are no symptoms and then relapse.

> **Examples of chronic GI disease that begin at a young age and require lifelong management** are inflammatory bowel disease and autoimmune hepatitis.

In chronic disease the aim of treatment is to control symptoms and provide a better quality of life so that normal daily activities can be fulfilled. This is achieved by ensuring the treatment is effective, tailored to the patient's needs, well tolerated and safe. A small number of medications require monitoring for significant side effects, for example azathioprine used for IBD requires a full blood count to be checked every 2–3 months for neutropaenia. In certain disorders surveillance for common or serious complications is required, for example cancer in Barrett's oesophagus, diabetes in chronic pancreatitis, and osteoporosis in coeliac disease and in patients who have been treated with long-term or high-dose corticosteroids.

> **Patients may not always be able to use optimal treatments because of other health problems.** For example, patients with severe arthritis and left-sided colitis are often physically unable to self-administer topical 5-ASA enemas. An oral preparation is usually more suitable.

Thus in chronic disease an integrated approach to care is particularly necessary. Who leads this approach depends on the nature of the disease, and there are several strategies:

- **Primary care management** – many conditions are effectively treated in primary care e.g. gastro-oesophageal reflux and irritable bowel syndrome. Patients either don't need gastroenterology referral at any stage or are quickly discharged back to the GP with a management plan after investigation and diagnosis, or initiation of treatment in hospital. When the GP judges appropriate – if the condition worsens or new symptoms arise – the patient is referred back to secondary care
- **Secondary care management** – monitoring and treatment are directed by the consultant, periodically reviewing the patient in the gastroenterology clinic. When appropriate, the patient is referred to or reviewed jointly with other members of a multidisciplinary team, for example the colorectal surgeon for poorly controlled Crohn's disease. Often the GP is asked to monitor with regular blood tests and to provide prescriptions for long-term medications between hospital appointments, in a 'shared care' approach. This has been the traditional model of care for many chronic disorders but other options can supplement or replace it, for example management by specialist nurses and self-directed care
- **Management by specialist nurses** – usually working within the gastroenterology clinic, specialist nurses manage care for patients with stable and more straightforward disorders, for

example coeliac disease, inflammatory bowel disease (IBD) and chronic liver diseases. In addition, they provide easily accessible advice via the telephone, text messaging and e-mail, for example giving telephone advice on management of an IBD flare or texting a reminder when monitoring blood tests are due

■ **Patient self-directed care** – provision of information about their disease and long-term treatment allows patients to play a significant role in management of their condition, improving adherence to medication and lifestyle advice. They should be empowered to take control of

their illness, for example to use antacids to treat the symptoms of gastro-oesophageal reflux when these occur or to increase the dosage of oral mesalazine during ulcerative colitis flares

> **A well informed patient is more likely to adopt appropriate lifestyle changes,** for example alcohol cessation in chronic pancreatitis or cirrhosis and avoidance of all gluten products in coeliac disease. Online patient groups provide excellent resources for chronic GI disorders.

Case 16 Chronic constipation

Presentation

Clare Pinto, aged 32 years, has had symptoms of constipation since a teenager. She takes intermittent over-the-counter laxatives (see page 136) that she buys from her local supermarket. Clare develops severe colicky abdominal pain and distension shortly after getting off an aeroplane from Australia. She has not opened her bowels for over two weeks despite taking her usual laxative treatments. Due to the severity of her symptoms she goes straight from the airport to her local emergency department at 2 o'clock in the morning.

Initial interpretation

Clare has symptoms of chronic constipation that have worsened despite her normal self-management, resulting in an acute presentation to secondary care due to their severity at a time when her GP surgery is closed.

Further history

A junior doctor in the emergency department takes a clinical history and identifies that Clare has recently started work as an

air hostess, which involves regular long-haul flights. Her work pattern is erratic and she often finds it difficult to drink enough fluids. She also relies on meals supplied by the airline. Without laxatives, her bowels are open once weekly and she strains to pass pellet-like stool. There is bloating and abdominal distension, which improve after defaecation. She says has presented now due to the abdominal pain and because she still hasn't passed any stool despite several different laxatives, though she is able to pass flatus.

Clare reports no rectal bleeding, anal discomfort or weight loss. There is no family history of colorectal cancer. She has not given birth, uses a subcutaneous implant containing progesterone as contraception and takes no other regular medication.

> **Giving birth through vaginal delivery often leads to injury of the pelvic floor and anal sphincters.** This sometimes causes symptoms of constipation and straining, a feeling of incomplete evacuation ('obstructive defaecation') or faecal incontinence.

Examination and interpretation of findings

Clare looks uncomfortable and is in pain. She is of very slim build. Her abdomen is visibly distended and rectal examination reveals hard stool. These features are consistent with constipation.

Investigations

Blood tests are performed to exclude conditions that rarely cause constipation, such as hypercalcaemia, hypothyroidism and coeliac disease (this condition is usually thought of as causing diarrhoea but sometimes causes constipation and bloating). An abdominal X-ray shows faecal loading throughout the large intestine.

Diagnosis

Clare has chronic constipation exacerbated by lifestyle factors. Her new job, with its erratic work pattern and reduced fluid intake, is the likely cause of her worsening symptoms. She has presented acutely as she has been unable to manage the symptoms herself.

> In healthy individuals, raising fluid intake to 2 L per day increases stool output; above 2 L there is no additional effect on output.

Management

Initial hospital management

Clare is treated with a phosphate enema (see Table 2.29) following which she opens her bowels with an improvement in her abdominal distension and pain. Initial blood tests reveal a normal calcium level. She is discharged from the emergency department and advised to see her GP over the next few days to review her treatment and outstanding blood test results. The junior doctor outlines the importance of drinking fluids regularly during her shifts.

GP follow up

Clare is reviewed by her GP to discuss her symptoms and recent presentation to hospital. The coeliac and thyroid function tests are noted to be normal. She describes using an over-the-counter stimulant (senna) laxative, which she has taken without effect. The GP prescribes an osmotic laxative (polyethylene glycol) as an alternative. Clare feels anxious as her sister has said she should be opening her bowels at least once a day. To help allay Clare's anxieties and manage her expectations, the GP explains that each individual's stool frequency is different and that defaecation on a daily basis is not required for health. He describes the optimal position to take on the toilet for defaecation and also suggests Clare discusses the possibility of alternative work patterns with her employer.

Clare follows the advice of her GP over the next 4 weeks including increasing the oral polyethylene glycol laxative dose. At a follow-up appointment she reports that her symptoms have not improved and so a referral to the gastroenterology outpatient clinic is made.

Further review

A specialist nurse reviews Clare in the gastroenterology clinic. Due to the chronic nature of her symptoms and in the absence of any alarm features such as weight loss or persistent rectal bleeding, she is advised that no invasive investigations such as colonoscopy are required. She is diagnosed with functional constipation (**Table 11.2**). Because the symptoms have failed to respond to two different classes of laxative, Clare is

Case 16 *continued*

Rome IV criteria for functional constipation

Symptom onset ≥6 months prior to diagnosis, with ≥2 criteria fulfilled for ≥ 3 months:

- Straining during at least 25% of defaecations
- Lumpy or hard stool in at least 25% of defaecations
- Sensation of incomplete evacuation for at least 25% of defaecations
- Sensation of anorectal blockage for at least 25% of defaecations
- Manual manoeuvres to facilitate at least 25% of defaecations (e.g. digital evacuation)
- Fewer than three spontaneous bowel movements per week

Plus:

- Loose stools rarely present without the use of laxatives
- Insufficient criteria for irritable bowel syndrome

Table 11.2 The Rome IV criteria for diagnosis of functional constipation

given a prescription for lubiprostone (see Table 2.30). The specialist nurse advises her that if this does not help then several other newer constipation medications or trans-anal rectal irrigation can be considered. During the same clinic visit the dietician also reviews Clare and advises an increase in dietary fibre, providing her with an information sheet about high fibre foods.

The specialist nurse contacts Clare by telephone 3 weeks later. She reports that her symptoms are a lot better and she is now opening her bowels every day with no bloating. Clare is therefore discharged back to the care of her GP, with advice to continue lubiprostone as required in the future.

Constipation

Constipation is an example of a common GI complaint usually either self-managed by patients or managed by their GP. The causes are outlined in **Table 11.3**. At initial presentation to the GP, a detailed clinical history is needed from the patient and blood tests are required to ascertain the probable cause and determine whether secondary care referral or further investigation is needed.

When a patient first presents with constipation the following blood tests are done: FBC to exclude an iron deficiency anaemia (men or post-menopausal women); TFT to exclude hypothyroidism, coeliac serology and bone profile to exclude hypercalcaemia.

The patient whose diagnosis is straightforward receives lifestyle advice from the GP, in particular on adequate fluid intake, regular exercise and optimal seating position for defaecation. His or her medications are reviewed for potential precipitants, for example codeine phosphate. If dietary triggers are identified the patient is instructed on keeping a food diary for several weeks prior to an appointment with a community dietician. Advice is given on ensuring adequate intake of fibre (e.g. fruit and vegetables) or bulking agents (e.g. wheat bran) (see Table 2.37). If symptoms are ongoing, a laxative or one of the newer agents is prescribed (see page 137).

Patients occasionally present to the emergency department with symptoms of abdominal pain due to severe constipation. After treatment with high dose laxatives and enemas most patients are discharged to their GP for ongoing long-term management.

Causes of constipation	
Primary causes	**Secondary causes**
■ Functional constipation according to Rome IV criteria (see Table 11.2) ■ Irritable bowel syndrome with chronic constipation ■ Pelvic floor disorders (structural, e.g. obstetric injury, and functional, e.g. failure to coordinate pelvic or anal muscles) or obstructive defaecation (also called dyssynergic defaecation). Patients may describe a need to digitate (manually expel stool) ■ Idiopathic megacolon and megarectum ■ Hirschsprung's disease (megacolon caused by absence of ganglion cells) ■ Chronic pseudo-obstruction (luminal pathology absent) ■ Anorectal disorders: anal fissures, haemorrhoids, fistulae	■ Medications: opiates, iron supplements, tricyclic antidepressants, antipsychotic agents, diuretics ■ Intrinsic: colorectal cancer, diverticular disease ■ Metabolic or endocrine: hypothyroidism, hypercalcaemia, coeliac disease, hypokalaemia ■ Neurological: Parkinson's disease, multiple sclerosis, spinal cord injury ■ Psychological: depression, eating disorders

Table 11.3 Causes of constipation

Constipation as a change in bowel habit

Older patients whose constipation is a new and persistent change in bowel habit may have bowel cancer. They require urgent referral to secondary care for investigation. Referral is either to a gastroenterologist or colorectal surgeon for lower GI endoscopy or to the radiology department for CT imaging.

Constipation due to dyssynergic defaecation

Ideally, a patient with symptoms of dyssynergic (obstructive) defaecation (e.g. constipation, feeling of incomplete evacuation and/or digitation to evacuate stool) is referred to a specialist multidisciplinary pelvic floor clinic for investigation and advice. Here colorectal surgeons and specialist nurses work in conjunction to provide:

■ consultant assessment of the underlying cause and any need for further investigation (e.g. defaecating proctogram)
■ surgical correction of identified underlying causes such as a rectocoele (herniation of the rectal wall into the wall of the vagina)
■ specialist nurse advice and treatment, including pelvic floor retraining and use of rectal irrigation devices (see page 156)

Case 17 Abnormal liver function tests

Presentation

Mrs Leela Gupta, aged 58 years, has type 2 diabetes and attends the hospital diabetes outpatient clinic for annual review. Routine blood tests performed during the visit reveal an elevated alanine transaminase (ALT) level of 68 U/L (normal range 5–35 U/L) and cholesterol level of 7.0 mmol/L (normal range 3.5–6.5 mmol/L) but are otherwise normal.

Initial interpretation

Mildly elevated liver function test results are common and often found incidentally in asymptomatic individuals.

Further history

The diabetes specialist nurse contacts Mrs Gupta by telephone to discuss the test results. Apart from the diabetes she is

Case 17 *continued*

otherwise fit and well. She has not taken any new prescribed or over-the-counter medications or herbal remedies. Her alcohol intake is 10 units per week. There is no personal or family history of liver disease, no risk factors for hepatitis B or C and no recent foreign travel.

Examination

The diabetes clinic records show Mrs Gupta to be overweight with a body mass index of 29 kg/m². Her blood pressure was normal. Abdominal examination was normal, with no stigmata of chronic liver disease such as spider naevi or Dupytren's contracture.

Investigations

After discussion with a diabetes consultant, the specialist nurse requests the set of blood tests known as a 'liver screen' (see Table 7.2) to try to determine an underlying cause for the raised ALT. Mrs Gupta is sent the blood test forms through the post, following which she makes an appointment with her GP practice nurse to have them performed.

A referral for an abdominal ultrasound scan is also sent by the nurse to the radiology department. Four weeks later the specialist nurse receives the ultrasonographer's report that Clare has a 'bright' liver appearance due to a fatty liver (Ch 7, page 270).

Interpretation of findings

Non-alcoholic fatty liver disease is a common cause of mildly abnormal liver function tests and is associated with conditions such as diabetes and elevated cholesterol levels (hypercholesterolaemia). Clinical examination is usually normal.

Management

After review of Mrs Gupta's investigation results, the diabetes consultant refers her to the hepatology outpatient clinic. The consultant hepatologist jointly reviews her with a specialist nurse. They advise her to lose weight and increase her exercise level. These lifestyle modifications help to address her risk factors for developing chronic liver disease. A NAFLD fibrosis score is calculated for Mrs Gupta and predicts the absence of significant fibrosis. The hepatologist asks the GP to prescribe a statin to treat the elevated cholesterol level and to refer Mrs Gupta to the community dietician for advice regarding hypercholesterolaemia and weight reduction (e.g. calorie reduction).

Mrs Gupta loses over 12 kg in weight over the next 6 months by modifying her diet and taking regular exercise; her GP referred her to a local gym to aid this. The hepatology specialist nurse reviews her in the hospital outpatient clinic 6 months later. Repeat blood tests at this point show that her alanine transaminase levels have returned to normal and her cholesterol level has fallen to 6.1 mmol/L. The specialist nurse congratulates her on her weight loss and reassures her that no further intervention is required. Mrs Gupta is discharged back to the care of her GP and the diabetes clinic for long-term follow up.

Abnormal liver function tests

Most patients with abnormal liver function test (LFT) results are asymptomatic; the abnormality is detected during monitoring of other medical conditions by their GP, for example diabetes. Patients who have features of liver disease or impairment require prompt referral to a hepatologist. The rest require further review, as shown in **Figure 11.1**. Referral to secondary care is not required unless the abnormalities persist despite modification of risk factors or features of chronic liver disease are present.

Chronic LFT abnormalities are most commonly the result of alcohol misuse or non-alcoholic fatty liver disease.

Alcohol misuse

Chronic alcohol misuse requires an integrated approach to management by community alcohol support services, which include a multi-disciplinary team of specialists. A psychiatrist, psychologist and specialist nurses provide counselling and drug treatments

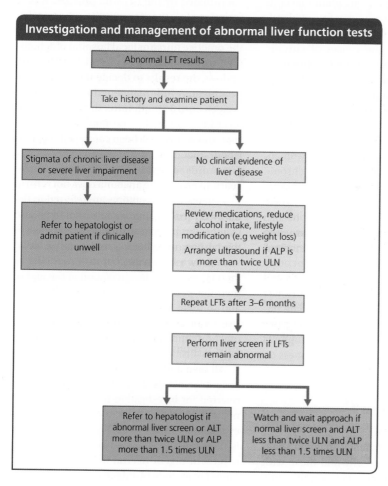

Figure 11.1 Investigation and management of abnormal liver function tests (LFTs). ULN, upper limit of normal. ALT, alanine transaminase; ALP, alkaline phosphatase.

such as acamprosate (see page 149). Advice from a social worker may also be needed because alcohol misuse can also negatively impact patient's employment and financial situation.

Non-alcoholic fatty liver disease (NAFLD)

This is treated through the modification of risk factors (see page 270). Verbal advice is usually provided by the GP or reviewing specialist, e.g. weight reduction and regular exercise, with medications such as statins prescribed for high cholesterol. The patient's weight needs to be monitored; often this is done by the nurse in the GP practice. All patients require detailed dietary advice and this is best provided by referral to a community dietician for help instituting a calorie restricted and/or reduced fat diet.

Iron deficiency anaemia

Anaemia is a reduced haemoglobin level. It occurs acutely due to a sudden loss of blood, for example with GI bleeding, but it is more commonly chronic. The causes of chronic anaemia are numerous; the most common is a deficiency in iron, which is required for the production of haemoglobin. Iron deficiency causes a microcytic anaemia (where the red cells are smaller). This most commonly occurs due to menstruation, but also affects 1 in 20 men and postmenopausal women, in who it is usually due to slow and chronic blood loss. Iron deficiency anaemia (IDA) is occasionally due to dietary deficiency (rare in the Western world) or malabsorption.

In many patients iron deficiency anaemia is asymptomatic and is detected coincidentally when blood tests are performed for other reasons, for example during a diabetes annual review or during a screening finger prick test prior to blood donation. However, some patients present to their GP or the emergency department with chronic or acute symptoms such as persistent lethargy, breathlessness on exertion and collapse.

Investigation and management

Patients with iron deficiency anaemia anaemia detected coincidentally and those with symptoms of anaemia not significantly impacting their activities of daily living are usually commenced on oral iron supplements (e.g. ferrous fumarate or ferrous sulphate). Management and monitoring are coordinated by the GP, who provides a prescription for the community pharmacist, arranges for blood samples to be taken by the practice nurse or local hospital phlebotomist to test haemoglobin and ferritin, and reviews the results to decide the duration of treatment. A full treatment dose of oral iron is given until 3 months after the haemoglobin level has returned to normal. This ensures that iron stores have been completely replenished. Blood tests are taken periodically afterwards, every 3–6 months over several years, to ensure the anaemia does not return.

Patients with symptoms are referred to the hospital medical admissions unit or day-case facilities for blood transfusion. This increases the number of red cells present in the blood stream for a few weeks, but as these cells are then taken out of the circulation at the end of their lifespan, the iron stores will still be low and so there is a reduced capacity to synthesise more normal haemoglobin. As a result, oral iron supplements are still required following transfusion.

All men and postmenopausal women who have anaemia as defined in **Figure 11.2** are referred for investigation to rule out GI tract malignancy, which is a cause of iron deficiency anaemia. In addition, a urine dipstick test is performed to exclude haematuria – if this is present urgent referral to a urologist is required to exclude bladder cancer.

Patients whose GI investigation results are normal are discharged to their GP for long-term monitoring of haemoglobin and ferritin levels and treatment with iron supplements.

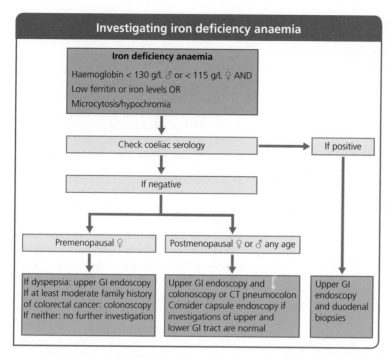

Figure 11.2
Investigation of a new finding of iron deficiency anaemia.

For those whose anaemia is found to have been the result of GI haemorrhage due to an underlying GI condition that can be managed within primary care, treatment recommendations are usually made by the hospital specialist, for example a proton pump inhibitor for a duodenal ulcer. If significant pathology is detected, such as colorectal cancer or coeliac disease, management usually continues within the secondary care setting, as outlined in the appropriate chapter.

NSAIDs are a common cause of GI symptoms and iron deficiency anaemia. However, be careful to carry out GI investigations before attributing symptoms to these drugs. This is especially true for older patients: many take daily low-dose aspirin, e.g. for ischaemic heart disease, but older people are also more likely to have a GI tract malignancy.

Palliative care

GI malignancies have a higher rate of cure if they are detected early on, i.e. before they are symptomatic. An example is bowel cancer, often identified at an early stage via a community-based cancer screening programme. However, a high proportion of GI cancers tend to be asymptomatic until their later stages, for example oesophageal and pancreatic cancers. Their late presentation makes prognosis very poor and the focus of treatment is therefore supportive – symptom based or palliative – rather than curative.

The palliative care team provides holistic care to patients with advanced progressive diseases. Within gastroenterology this includes end-stage decompensated liver disease as well as malignancy. The team consists of a consultant in palliative medicine and clinical nurse specialists. They are usually supported by a physiotherapist who helps the patient with movement, an occupational therapist who helps the patient carry out everyday activities, a social worker who acts as an advocate to organise services or direct the patient and carers to the services they require, a dietician and a psychologist. The roles of this team include:

■ Psychological support to the patient and their family
■ Management of symptoms, for example pain and vomiting
■ Provision of advice to other healthcare professionals involved in the patient's care
■ Supporting the patient in planning end-of-life and resuscitation decisions
■ Support with financial planning
■ Advice and support to enable the patient to stay in their own home
■ Bereavement support for those who have been involved in care, following the patient's death

Care is provided in hospital, outpatient clinics, the patient's home and the hospice, a dedicated unit that treats patients who are terminally ill. Alternative therapies including reflexology, acupuncture, aromatherapy and massage are also made available.

> **A patient receiving palliative care often moves between different care settings,** for example from their own home into hospital with acute symptoms and then to a hospice, sometimes alternating between these depending on their symptoms. This makes good communication between different professionals even more essential.

Another role of the palliative care team is the education and training of medical and nursing staff who care for patients with advanced diseases. This includes the management of complications of disease, such as spinal cord compression or hypercalcaemia due to bone metastases, as well as the management of pain killers, e.g. conversion of oral medication to a subcutaneous syringe driver for patients with a blocked oesophageal stent. The goal always is to maintain patient comfort, right to the end of life.

Answers to starter questions

1. There are guidelines defining constipation and diarrhoea; however, 'normal' stool frequency and consistency vary significantly between individuals. The key factor is to establish whether there has been a new change in bowel habit, as this may indicate underlying pathology. An individual's expectation to defaecate on a regular (i.e. daily) basis can lead to significant anxiety, but there is no evidence that long residence of stool causes autointoxication (self-poisoning resulting from the absorption of toxins from intestinal matter).

2. Menstrual blood loss is the commonest cause of iron deficiency anaemia (IDA) in pre-menopausal women. In this patient group, investigation is not required in the absence of any specific gastrointestinal symptoms, significant family history of colorectal cancer or positive coeliac serology. All male patients and postmenopausal women with IDA should be referred for urgent investigation of the GI tract. Other factors, including patient choice, age and comorbidity, should also be considered.

3. Stool that appears black due to iron supplements is usually a matt black colour, whereas in malaena stool is typically more glossy black with an offensive smell. Blood has a laxative effect on the bowel, also causing the stool to be loose.

4. Patients who have a GI or liver condition on a background of alcohol excess, obesity or other high-risk behaviours, such as intravenous drug misuse, need to be made aware of the close association of these factors with chronic disease and advised that this means there are lifestyle changes they can make that potentially will help

Answers *continued*

to improve their condition or to prevent or slow further deterioration. Community support groups are available for alcohol and substance misuse, and there are weight reduction programmes that combine dietetic and exercise support. It is essential that doctors initiate discussions, educate and engage the patient, and offer all means of support available to allow change in unhealthy lifestyles.

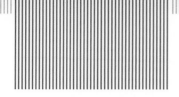

Chapter 12
Self-assessment

SBA questions

Oesophagus

1. A 24-year-old man has a 2-year history of dysphagia to solids and liquids, with episodes in which he regurgitates undigested food. He has been prescribed several courses of antibiotics for chest infections. He has lost 4 kg in weight since the onset of these symptoms.
   What is the single most likely diagnosis?

   A Achalasia
   B Adenocarcinoma of the oesophagus
   C Globus pharyngeus
   D Peptic oesophageal stricture
   E Pharyngeal pouch

2. A 56-year-old man has a long history of heartburn partly controlled by omeprazole. An upper GI endoscopy shows Barrett's oesophagus. Samples of oesophageal tissue are taken from this region for biopsy.
   What is the single most likely histological feature present?

   A Adenocarcinoma
   B Eosinophilic infiltration
   C Intestinal metaplasia
   D Reflux oesophagitis
   E Squamous hypertrophy

3. A 61-year-old woman consults her general practitioner (GP) with recurrent pain in the centre of her chest on swallowing. This is particularly severe on swallowing hot fluids.
   What is the single best term to describe this symptom?

   A Aerophagia
   B Dyspepsia
   C Dysphagia

D Dysphasia
E Odynophagia

4. A 78-year-old woman has progressive dysphagia to solids. She has a 40-year-pack history of smoking. A stricture is found in the upper oesophagus during upper GI endoscopy.
   What is the single most likely diagnosis?

   A Adenocarcinoma
   B Barrett's oesophagus
   C Eosinophilic oesophagitis
   D Reflux oesophagitis
   E Squamous cell cancer

5. A 38-year-old man gets a burning pain that rises from the low chest to the back of his throat. It is worse at night and after eating rich foods and drinking alcohol.
   Which single treatment is most likely to alleviate his symptoms?

   A Aluminium hydroxide
   B Domperidone
   C *Helicobacter pylori* eradication therapy
   D Lansoprazole
   E Ranitidine

6. A 46-year-old woman has significant heartburn despite medication. To decide further treatment, the consultant wants to quantify how much gastro-oesophageal reflux is occurring.
   What is the single best investigation to perform?

   A Barium swallow
   B Manometry
   C Oesophageal biopsy
   D pH studies
   E Upper GI endoscopy

7. A 68-year-old man receives a diagnosis of oesophageal adenocarcinoma on OGD. He undergoes investigations to determine the stage of the tumour.
Which single investigation is best for determining the 'T' stage of the cancer?

A CT scan
B Endoscopic US
C Oesophageal biopsy
D PET scan
E Upper GI endoscopy

8. An 84-year-old woman has a 4-month history of progressive dysphagia. A T3N1M1 cancer of the distal oesophagus is diagnosed. She has a past history of severe chronic obstructive pulmonary disease and angina, with an exercise tolerance of less than 20 m. She can swallow only liquids and is losing weight.
What is the single most appropriate treatment to alleviate her symptoms?

A Chemotherapy
B IV fluids
C Radiotherapy
D Stent
E Surgery

9. A 60-year-old woman has recently completed chemoradiotherapy for breast cancer. She has retrosternal pain on swallowing.
What is the single most likely diagnosis?

A Candidiasis
B Cytomegalovirus infection
C Eosinophilic oesophagitis
D Herpes simplex infection
E Reflux oesophagitis

10. A 79-year-old man has intermittent episodes in which he finds that food sticks at the back of his throat. A barium swallow shows 'spasm of the cricopharyngeus muscle'.
What is the single most likely diagnosis?

A Globus pharyngeus
B Oesophageal web
C Pharyngeal pouch
D Presbyoesophagus
E Schatzki's ring

Stomach

1. A 35-year-old woman has epigastric pain but describes no 'alarm symptoms'. Several years ago, she was given *H. pylori* eradication therapy. Her GP wants to see if this treatment was successful.
What is the single most appropriate test to request?

A Carbon urea breath test
B *H. pylori* serology
C OGD and histology
D OGD and rapid urease test
E Stool antibody

2. A 44-year-old man has persistent dyspeptic symptoms, which include bloating, belching and nausea. Blood tests were normal except for a low ferritin level.
What single aspect of this presentation suggests the need for further investigation?

A Age
B Belching
C Bloating
D Iron deficiency
E Nausea

3. An 82-year-old man has a long-standing problem with upper abdominal cramps, nausea, diarrhoea and malaise that come on soon after meals. He had a Billroth type I gastrectomy for a peptic ulcer when he was 23.
What is the single most likely diagnosis?

A Dumping syndrome
B Functional dyspepsia
C Gastro-oesophageal reflux
D Gastroparesis
E Recurrent peptic ulcer

4. A 66-year-old man vomits undigested food an hour or more after meals.
What single complication of a gastric ulcer is most likely to have occurred?

A Erosion through a blood vessel
B Fistula formation with the small intestine
C Gastric outlet obstruction
D Malignant transformation
E Perforation through the gastric wall

5. A 47-year-old man has diarrhoea and 5 kg of weight loss. OGD shows multiple gastric and duodenal ulcers. He takes no medications, and a recent carbon urea breath test was negative.
What single blood test is most appropriate to request next?

A Anti-endomysial antibodies
B Chromogranin A
C Gastrin
D *H. pylori* serology
E Vasoactive intestinal peptide

6. A 57-year-old woman has a 2 cm gastric ulcer at endoscopy. The rapid urease test is positive, and she is prescribed *H. pylori* eradication therapy and a proton pump inhibitor (PPI) for 2 months.
What is the single most important follow-up plan?

A   Carbon urea breath test
B   Continue PPI long term
C   Reassurance; the PPI can be stopped
D   Repeat OGD
E   Stool antigen test for *H. pylori*

7. A 27-year-old man has intermittent epigastric pain and positive *H. pylori* serology. He is allergic to penicillin.
What is the single most appropriate treatment regimen?

A   Omeprazole alone
B   Omeprazole, amoxicillin and clarithromycin
C   Omeprazole, amoxicillin and metronidazole
D   Omeprazole, clarithromycin and metronidazole
E   Ranitidine, bismuth, clarithromycin and metronidazole

8. A 71-year-old woman has recurrent bouts of dyspepsia and recent loss of appetite. Her medications include metformin, alendronic acid, naproxen, amlodipine and ramipril. OGD shows multiple erosions in the stomach with diffuse gastritis.
Which single one of these drugs is most likely to have caused these findings?

A   Alendronic acid
B   Amlodipine
C   Metformin
D   Naproxen
E   Ramipril

9. A 25-year-old man has symptoms of epigastric discomfort, bloating and belching. His weight is stable.
Which single investigation is most appropriate to perform?

A   Abdominal US
B   Carbon urea breath test
C   Faecal calprotectin
D   *H. pylori* serology
E   OGD

10. An 82-year-old woman is admitted to hospital from a nursing home because of a gradual reduction in oral intake over the past 6 months. She has significant cognitive impairment because of Alzheimer's disease and is very confused and restless. Whenever she takes oral fluids and food, she coughs.
What is the single most appropriate form of long-term nutritional support?

A   At-risk oral feeding
B   IV fluids
C   IV nutrition (total parenteral nutrition)
D   Nasogastric tube
E   Percutaneous endoscopic gastrostomy feeding

Small intestine

1. A 23-year-old woman is reviewed by her GP with symptoms of diarrhoea, bloating and weight loss. Her sister has a history of coeliac disease.
Which single blood test is most appropriate to perform?

A   Anti-endomysial antibody
B   Anti-gliadin antibody
C   Anti-mitochondrial antibody
D   Anti-tissue transglutaminase antibody
E   Human leukocyte antigen (HLA) DQ2/ DQ8

2. A 48-year-old man is admitted to hospital with recurrent melaena. Blood pressure and heart rate are stable. Upper GI endoscopy and colonoscopy are normal.
Which single investigation would be most appropriate to perform next?

A   Barium follow-through
B   CT enterogram
C   Enteroscopy
D   MRI enterogram
E   Small bowel capsule

3. A 32-year-old woman has small bowel Crohn's disease, with symptoms of diarrhoea and abdominal pain.
Which single lifestyle change is most likely to improve her symptoms?

A   Exercise regularly
B   Increase dietary fibre
C   Lose weight
D   Reduce alcohol intake
E   Stop smoking

4. A 23-year-old man has a diagnosis of small bowel Crohn's disease.
Which single section of small intestine is most likely to be abnormal on radiological imaging?

A   Distal duodenum
B   Distal ileum
C   Distal jejunum
D   Proximal ileum
E   Proximal jejunum

5. A 25-year-old man has an ileocaecal resection for small bowel Crohn's disease. His haemoglobin concentration is 101 g/L and his mean corpuscular volume is 101 fL.
A deficiency of which single vitamin is most likely?

A   Vitamin A
B   Vitamin B_9
C   Vitamin B_{12}
D   Vitamin C
E   Vitamin D

6. A 43-year-old woman has symptoms of diarrhoea occurring after eating, which started following a cholecystectomy.
What is the single most likely cause of her symptoms?

A Bacterial overgrowth
B Bile salt malabsorption
C Coeliac disease
D Lactose intolerance
E Pancreatic insufficiency

7. A 64-year-old man has diarrhoea, abdominal pain and flushing. An abdominal CT scan shows a mass in the small intestine, with multiple liver lesions.
Which single one of the following tumours is most likely?

A Adenocarcinoma
B Angiosarcoma
C B-cell lymphoma
D Carcinoid
E T-cell lymphoma

8. A 28-year-old woman has a history of small bowel Crohn's disease affecting the jejunum and ileum. Her symptoms of diarrhoea recur soon after completing a course of steroids. She takes no regular medication. Her faecal calprotectin result is 324 µg/g.
What is the single most appropriate initial long-term medical treatment?

A Azathioprine
B Infliximab
C Mesalazine
D Methotrexate
E Prednisolone

9. A 19-year-old woman has symptoms of diarrhoea and positive coeliac serology. She is referred for upper GI endoscopy.
What is the single most appropriate part of the upper GI tract from which to take tissue samples for biopsy?

A Antrum
B Duodenum
C Gastric body
D Jejunum
E Pylorus

10. A 39-year-old man has diarrhoea, weight loss and joint pains. Periodic acid–Schiff–positive macrophages containing Gram-positive bacilli are visible on duodenal biopsy.
What is the single most likely causative pathogen?

A Cholera
B Giardiasis
C Intestinal tuberculosis
D Tropical sprue
E Whipple's disease

Large intestine

1. An 83-year-old man is admitted to hospital with offensive diarrhoea. He has recently completed a 1-week course of antibiotics for pneumonia. His only medication is omeprazole.
Which bacterial infection is the single most likely cause of his symptoms?

A *Campylobacter jejuni*
B *Clostridium difficile*
C *Escherichia coli*
D *Salmonella* Typhi
E *Shigella dysenteriae*

2. A 41-year-old man has a 7-week history of alternating bowel habit, weight loss and rectal bleeding. His brother received a diagnosis of colorectal cancer at the age of 40 years.
Which single investigation would be most appropriate to perform?

A Barium enema
B Colonoscopy
C CT pneumocolon
D Minimal preparation CT abdomen
E Sigmoidoscopy

3. A 30-year-old man has a diagnosis of an ascending colon adenocarcinoma and a caecal adenoma at colonoscopy. His mother and maternal grandmother died of colorectal cancer.
Which single hereditary condition is he most likely to have?

A Attenuated familial adenomatous polyposis
B Familial adenomatous polyposis
C Hereditary intestinal polyposis syndrome (Peutz–Jeghers syndrome)
D Hereditary non-polyposis colorectal cancer (Lynch's syndrome)
E MUTYH polyposis

4. A 72-year-old man is admitted to hospital with severe abdominal pain. A chest radiograph shows subphrenic gas. There is a known history of diverticular disease.
Which single complications of this disease is most likely?

A Abscess
B Fistula
C Haemorrhage
D Inflammation
E Perforation

5. A 43-year-old woman has profuse diarrhoea and vomiting shortly after visiting a friend in hospital. She has no medical history of note. Parts of the ward were shut at the time in response to an outbreak of similar symptoms.
Which single following infective cause is most likely?

A *Campylobacter jejuni*
B *Clostridium difficile*
C *Escherichia coli*
D Norovirus
E *Salmonella typhi*

6. An 87-year-old man has iron deficiency anaemia. A previous stroke resulted in a dense right-sided weakness, making it very difficult for him to move, including rolling on to his side or front.
Which single test would be most appropriate to investigate his lower GI tract?

A Barium enema
B Colonoscopy
C CT pneumocolon
D Minimal preparation CT of the abdomen and pelvis
E Sigmoidoscopy

7. A 67-year-old man has diarrhoeal symptoms following a 9-month admission to hospital. His bowels are open three times per day. There is no history of abdominal pain. Tests on samples of his stool give glutamate dehydrogenase–positive and toxin-positive results. He is apyrexial, with normal blood test results for full blood count and urea and electrolytes.
What is the single most appropriate first-line treatment?

A Amoxicillin
B Ciprofloxacin
C Metronidazole
D Rifampicin
E Vancomycin

8. A 65-year-old woman undergoes colonoscopy for a 3-month history of persistent non-bloody diarrhoea. This is reported as normal. However, colonic biopsy shows a thickened subepithelial collagenous plate.
Which single treatment would be most appropriate?

A Azathioprine
B Budesonide
C Infliximab
D Mesalazine
E Methotrexate

9. A 73-year-old man has a history of rectal bleeding and altered bowel habit. Colonoscopy shows a mid-rectal cancer but is otherwise normal. Radiological staging shows a T2N0M0 tumour.
Which single surgical operation would be most appropriate?

A Abdominoperineal resection
B Anterior resection

C Left hemicolectomy
D Proctocolectomy
E Right hemicolectomy

10. A 28-year-old man is admitted to hospital with diarrhoea and abdominal pain. His bowels are open 20 times a day with the passage of fresh blood. His temperature is 38°C and his heart rate is 120 bpm. The results of his sigmoidoscopy are consistent with ulcerative colitis.
What is the single most appropriate initial medical treatment?

A Ciclosporin
B Hydrocortisone
C Infliximab
D Mesalazine
E Prednisolone

11. A 61-year-old man attends the endoscopy unit for a diagnostic colonoscopy to investigate symptoms of diarrhoea and weight loss. As part of the consent process, the risk of complications is discussed.
What is the single most accurate risk of perforation associated with this procedure?

A 1 in 100
B 1 in 250
C 1 in 500
D 1 in 1000
E 1 in 5000

12. A 33-year-old woman presents with an 18-month history of abdominal bloating. It is worse towards the end of the day. She has a daily bowel motion and is otherwise well.
What is the single most appropriate next step in her management?

A Dietary modification
B Laxative
C Omeprazole
D Pregnancy test
E Prokinetics

Liver disease

1. A 63-year-old man has a large-volume haematemesis. Endoscopy reveals oesophageal varices, which are treated with banding. Which single medical treatment is most appropriate as secondary prevention to avoid further variceal bleeding?

A Carvedilol
B Disulfiram
C Omeprazole
D Spironolactone
E Sucralfate

2. A 19-year-old student is admitted to the medical assessment unit with a 2-day history of jaundice. She has been feeling generally unwell, with flu like symptoms, nausea and diarrhoea. Her temperature is 38.7°C. She has recently returned home after volunteering in rural India. What is the single most likely diagnosis?

A Acute hepatitis B
B Chronic hepatitis B
C Hepatitis A
D Hepatitis C
E Hepatitis D

3. A 73-year-old man with a long-standing history of excessive alcohol consumption is brought to hospital by relatives after being found confused and unsteady at home. His gait is broad-based. On examination of his cranial nerves, he is unable to abduct his right eye. What is the single most likely diagnosis?

A Alcohol withdrawal
B Hepatic encephalopathy
C Hypoglycaemia
D Korsakoff's psychosis
E Wernicke's encephalopathy

4. A 69-year-old man attends the diabetes clinic for his annual review. The results of his liver function tests (LFTs) are found to be abnormal. He is noted to appear quite tanned. He has a history of heart problems, and his grandfather died of liver cancer. Which single blood test is most likely to diagnose the cause of his abnormal liver function?

A Anti-mitochondrial antibody
B Anti-neutrophil cytoplasmic antibody (ANCA)
C Ferritin
D Haemoglobin A1C
E Hepatitis C serology

5. A 57-year-old woman has symptoms of lethargy and nausea. She drinks 8 units of alcohol per week, and her body mass index (BMI) is 37 kg/m². She had a course of flucloxacillin 2 weeks ago to treat a skin infection but is otherwise fit and well. Her alanine transaminase (ALT) concentration is 95 U/L, and her alkaline phosphatase (ALP) concentration is 344 U/L. What is the single most likely cause of her abnormal LFT results?

A Alcohol-related liver disease
B Autoimmune hepatitis
C Drug-induced liver injury
D Haemochromatosis
E Non-alcoholic fatty liver disease

6. A 65-year-old man with diabetes is seen in the gastroenterology clinic because of abnormal LFT results. Investigations show ferritin concentration, 2400 µg/L; transferrin saturation, 89%; and HFE gene C282Y mutation. What is the single most appropriate treatment?

A Desferrioxamine
B Low-iron diet
C Oral iron supplements
D Transfuse 2 units of blood
E Venesection

7. A 59-year-old woman has had symptoms of itching and tiredness for the past few months. She drinks 6 units of alcohol per week. Her BMI is 21 kg/m². Test results show ALT, 45 U/L; bilirubin, 24 µmol/L; ALP, 483 U/L; and immunoglobulin (Ig) M, 5g/L. What single condition is most likely?

A Alcoholic liver disease
B Autoimmune hepatitis
C Non-alcoholic fatty liver disease
D Primary biliary cholangitis
E Primary sclerosing cholangitis

8. A 48-year-old businessman returns from a trip to Thailand feeling generally unwell. He is noted to be jaundiced. Investigation results are hepatitis A IgM-negative, hepatitis A IgG-positive, hepatitis B surface antigen-positive, hepatitis B antigen-positive, hepatitis B IgM-positive and hepatitis B IgG-negative. What is the single most likely diagnosis?

A Acute hepatitis A
B Acute hepatitis B
C Chronic hepatitis A
D Chronic hepatitis B carrier
E Previous hepatitis B vaccination

9. A 38-year-old man has abdominal pain and jaundice. He has a history of ulcerative colitis. Test results show ALT, 65 U/L, and ALP, 364 U/L. The perinuclear ANCA test result is positive. Which single investigation is most appropriate to help identify the underlying diagnosis?

A Abdominal US
B Colonoscopy
C CT abdomen
D Endoscopic retrograde cholangiopancreatography (ERCP)
E Magnetic resonance cholangiopancreatography (MRCP)

10. A 68-year-old man is seen in the gastroenterology clinic because of abnormal blood tests. They include an α-fetoprotein concentration of 480 kU/L. CT of the abdomen

reveals a 4-cm hypervascular area with washout within the liver.
What is the single most likely diagnosis?

A Adenoma
B Cirrhosis with a regenerative nodule
C Colorectal cancer with liver metastases
D Haemangioma
E Hepatocellular carcinoma

11. A 37-year-old woman is referred to the gastroenterology clinic because of abnormal blood test results. They show ALT, 435 U/L; ALP, 110 U/L; bilirubin, 56 µmol/L; albumin, 38 g/L; and IgG, 17 g/L. The smooth muscle antibody test result is positive.
What is the single most appropriate initial treatment?

A Ciclosporin
B Methotrexate
C Mycophenolate mofetil
D Prednisolone
E Ursodeoxycholic acid

12. A 67-year-old woman visits her GP feeling generally unwell. Tests on blood samples taken by the phlebotomist show an ALP concentration of 231 U/L and a γ-glutamyl transferase (GGT) concentration of 30 U/L.
What is the single most likely source of the increased ALP?

A Biliary tree
B Bones
C Hepatocytes
D Placenta
E Skeletal muscle

13. A 55-year-old man is admitted to hospital with jaundice, ascites and peripheral oedema. He has a long history of heavy alcohol intake. During admission, he becomes drowsy and confused for the first time. His stool colour is normal, and blood test results for urea and electrolytes are in the normal range.
What is the single most appropriate additional investigation at this stage?

A Abdominal US
B Ascitic tap
C Digital rectal examination
D Prothrombin time
E Upper GI endoscopy

Pancreatic disease

1. A 53-year-old man with long-standing excessive alcohol consumption is seen in the outpatient clinic, complaining of loose fatty stools that are difficult to flush.

What is the single most appropriate initial investigation?

A Abdominal ultrasound
B Colonoscopy
C CT of the pancreas
D Faecal calprotectin
E Faecal elastase

2. An 89-year-old man has a 3-week history of painless jaundice and significant weight loss. He has dark urine and pale stool but no other symptoms. His test results show ALT, 65 U/L; ALP, 1056 U/L; bilirubin, 240 µmol/L; albumin, 34 g/L; and amylase 100 U/L.
What is the single most likely diagnosis?

A Common bile duct stone
B Chronic pancreatitis
C Hepatocellular carcinoma
D Oesophageal cancer with liver metastases
E Pancreatic cancer

3. A 34-year-old woman is admitted to the surgical admissions unit with severe epigastric pain, which radiates through to the back. Her amylase concentration is 2100 U/L.
Which single initial radiological investigation is the most helpful for further assessment?

A Abdominal US
B Abdominal radiograph
C CT of the abdomen
D Erect chest radiograph
E MRCP

4. A 76-year-old woman is brought to the emergency department with a 48-h history of epigastric pain and vomiting. She is on the waiting list for a cholecystectomy. Her temperature is 38.8°C, her heart rate is 120 bpm and her blood pressure is 100/65 mmHg. There is marked epigastric tenderness on examination. Test results show amylase, 954 U/L; lactate dehydrogenase (LDH), 700 U/L (reference range 10–250 U/L); and corrected calcium, 1.94 mmol/L.
What is the single most likely diagnosis?

A Acute cholecystitis
B Acute pancreatitis
C Chronic pancreatitis
D Common bile duct stone
E Peptic ulcer disease

5. A 44-year-old mother of five is admitted with severe central abdominal pain. Her BMI is 39 kg/m². She drinks 4 units of alcohol per week and is not on any regular medication. Her amylase concentration is 635 U/L.
What is the single most likely underlying cause of her presentation?

A Alcohol
B Drug-induced
C Gallstones
D Hereditary
E Idiopathic

6. An 87-year-old man has painless jaundice and has lost almost 13 kg. An abdominal CT scan shows a mass within the head of the pancreas and multiple liver metastases.
What is the single most appropriate treatment?

A Cholestyramine
B ERCP and stent insertion
C Liver resection
D Percutaneous transhepatic cholangiogram
E Whipple's operation

7. An underweight 52-year-old man has abdominal pain and fatty stools that are difficult to flush. He drinks 10 cans of lager a day. His faecal elastase level is 95 µg/g. On abdominal CT scan, his pancreas is found to be atrophic. He has previously been admitted to hospital with acute pancreatitis.
Which single treatment is most likely to help his symptoms?

A Alcohol cessation
B Insulin
C Low-fat diet
D Opioid analgesia
E Pancreatic enzyme supplements

Biliary disease

1. A 53-year-old woman is admitted to the surgical assessment unit with right upper quadrant pain and jaundice. Her temperature is 38.7°C and her blood pressure is 95/40 mmHg. Her white cell count is 14 × 10⁹/L. US shows stones within the gallbladder and a common bile duct stone of 12 mm containing echogenic material. She is started on intravenous antibiotics.
What is the single most appropriate next step?

A Cholecystectomy
B CT of the abdomen
C Endoscopic retrograde cholangio-pancreatography (ERCP)
D Hepatobiliary iminodiacetic acid (HIDA) scan
E Magnetic resonance cholangio-pancreatography (MRCP)

2. A 68-year-old man has a 3-day history of right upper abdominal pain, rigors and jaundice. His temperature is 39.4°C and his blood pressure is 125/76 mmHg. An US scan shows gallstones. Which is the single most likely site of gallstones causing his symptoms?

A Common bile duct

B Cystic duct
C Gallbladder
D Hepatic duct
E Pancreatic duct

3. A 42-year-old woman visits her GP with a 12-month history of intermittent right upper quadrant pain after eating fatty foods. It lasts about 1 h and radiates to the right shoulder. Her BMI is 37 kg/m². She is otherwise well. Her LFT results are normal.
What is the most likely diagnosis?

A Acute cholecystitis
B Biliary colic
C Chronic cholecystitis
D Cholangitis
E Peptic ulcer

4. A 54-year-old woman is admitted to the emergency department with abdominal pain and rigors. There is no history or recent travel, and she is otherwise fit and well. Her temperature is 39.2°C, her blood pressure is 90/40 mmHg and her heart rate is 120 bpm. A tender mass is felt in the right upper quadrant.
What is the single most likely diagnosis?

A Cholangiocarcinoma
B Cholangitis
C Gallbladder cancer
D Gallbladder empyema
E Pyogenic liver abscess

5. A 41-year-old man is admitted to hospital with right upper quadrant pain. He is haemodynamically stable. Test results show an ALP concentration of 325 U/L and a bilirubin concentration of 20 µmol/L. Abdominal US reveals gallstones within the gallbladder, with the suspicion of a slightly dilated common bile duct.
What is the single most appropriate next step?

A Cholecystectomy
B Percutaneous drainage
C MRCP
D ERCP
E CT abdomen

6. An 81-year-old man has jaundice and has lost 19 kg. On examination, he has hepatomegaly. Test results show ALT concentration, 125 U/L; ALP concentration, 1066 U/L; and bilirubin concentration, 344 µmol/L. A CT scan reveals an irregular stricture of the distal common bile duct and multiple hypoattenuating (low density) liver lesions.
What is the single most likely diagnosis?

A Cholangiocarcinoma
B Cholangitis
C Cholecystitis
D Hepatocellular carcinoma
E Primary sclerosing cholangitis

Emergencies

1. A 58-year-old man with a long history of alcohol misuse is seen in the emergency admission department. He presents with a large-volume haematemesis. On examination, he is jaundiced, he has multiple spider naevi and his abdomen is markedly distended. He is receiving fluid resuscitation.
   What single additional treatment is most likely to reduce the chance of further bleeding before endoscopy?

   A Adrenaline (epinephrine)
   B Cefotaxime
   C Omeprazole
   D Terlipressin
   E Tranexamic acid

2. An 80-year-old woman has an endoscopy for melaena. An ulcer is seen on the posterior wall of the duodenum, but haemostasis cannot be achieved. She is referred for an urgent angiogram and embolisation.
   What single artery will the interventional radiologist most need to selectively catheterise?

   A Coeliac
   B Gastroduodenal
   C Hepatic
   D Inferior mesenteric
   E Superior mesenteric

3. A 38-year-old woman is admitted to hospital with drowsiness, and on examination she is jaundiced. The admitting acute physician diagnoses acute liver failure.
   Which single blood test is the most sensitive indicator of the severity of liver disease in this setting?

   A Albumin
   B Aspartate transaminase (AST)
   C Bilirubin
   D Prothrombin time
   E Urea

4. A 19-year-old woman is assessed in the emergency department. She admits to taking more than 30 paracetamol tablets 24 h ago. Prothrombin time is 29 s.
   What is the single most appropriate treatment?

   A Charcoal
   B Fresh frozen plasma
   C Glutathione
   D N-acetyl cysteine
   E Supportive care only

5. A 65-year-old woman is admitted to hospital. The on-call surgical registrar diagnoses large bowel obstruction after reviewing an abdominal radiograph.

Which single clinical feature most suggests large rather than small bowel obstruction?

   A Absolute constipation
   B Colicky abdominal pain
   C Distension
   D High-pitched bowel sounds
   E Vomiting

6. An 81-year-old man has sudden onset, severe abdominal pain and a large volume of fresh rectal bleeding. He has atrial fibrillation but is not on warfarin. The venous lactate level is 7.4 mmol/L (reference range 0.6–1.8 mmol/L).
   What is the single most likely region of the intestine to be affected?

   A Caecum
   B Duodenum
   C Ileum
   D Rectum
   E Splenic flexure

Integrated care

1. A 31-year-old women sees her GP because of lethargy, but she has no other symptoms. Test results show haemoglobin, 96 g/L; mean corpuscular volume, 76 fL; and ferritin concentration, 4 µg/L. She is started on oral iron supplements but takes no other medication.
   What is the single next most appropriate management?

   A Coeliac serology
   B Dipstick urinalysis
   C No further investigation
   D OGD
   E OGD and colonoscopy

2. A 26-year-old woman is seen in primary care for the first time because of constipation. She opens her bowels only every 3 days, but has been like this for years. Her diet is good and she is otherwise well.
   What is the single most appropriate initial treatment?

   A Biofeedback
   B Prucalopride
   C Stimulant laxatives
   D Stool softeners
   E Transanal irrigation

3. A 57-year-old man has developed constipation over the past 2 months. He passes hard motion every 5 days. There is no weight loss or rectal bleeding. He previously opened his bowels daily and has no medical history.
   What is the single most appropriate management?

   A Barium enema

B Coeliac serology
C Colonoscopy
D Laxatives only
E Thyroid function tests

4. A 51-year-old woman has blood tests taken in primary care as part of an annual review for type 2 diabetes. She takes metformin and gliclazide. Her BMI is 32 kg/m². She drinks 10 units of alcohol per week. Test results show an AST concentration of 61 U/L and a GGT concentration of 76 U/L.
   What is the single most likely cause of these test results?

   A Alcohol
   B Fatty liver disease

C Hepatitis C
D Medications
E Primary biliary cholangitis

5. A 23-year-old man volunteers for a clinical trial to evaluate a new medication. He is fit and healthy. Blood tests show a bilirubin concentration of 34 μmol/L with otherwise normal LFT results.
   What is the single most likely cause?

   A Alcohol
   B Gilbert's syndrome
   C Haemolysis
   D Hepatitis
   E Mirizzi's syndrome

SBA answers

Oesophagus

1. A

The long duration and nature of the symptoms are characteristic of achalasia. This disorder can occur at any age. The associated recurrent chest infections result from aspiration of undigested food and drink from the dilated oesophagus. A peptic stricture caused by reflux would be the differential diagnosis, but it is less likely in a young person. C and E give 'high' dysphagia, i.e. at the back of the throat. The history is too long for B, which is also very rare at this age.

2. C

Intestinal metaplasia is the diagnostic histological feature of Barrett's oesophagus. It is possible that there will also be oesophagitis as a result of acid reflux, but this can occur without Barrett's. A is a complication arising from dysplastic change in Barrett's oesophagus. B can occur because of reflux or in eosinophilic oesophagitis. E is of no clinical significance and not associated with Barrett's.

3. E

This is odynophagia, which occurs with oesophageal ulceration or inflammation. A is swallowing air and results in excess belching. B relates to a number of symptoms from the upper GI tract, such as epigastric pain. C is difficulty in swallowing, and D is difficulty speaking.

4. E

Squamous cell cancer arises in the upper or mid-oesophagus, i.e. the parts lined by squamous mucosa, and is more common in smokers. A occurs in the distal oesophagus, usually in a segment of Barrett's oesophagus; reflux oesophagitis from gastric acid may occur in the same region. C causes dysphagia, including obstruction of the passage of food boluses. It can affect any part of the oesophagus and very rarely causes strictures.

5. D

The history suggests gastro-oesophageal reflux. The most effective medical treatments are PPIs, including lansoprazole. H_2 receptor antagonists (e.g. ranitidine) and antacids (e.g. aluminium hydroxide) can be helpful but are less potent. B is an antiemetic, which can be used for short durations. *H. pylori* infection is not associated with gastro-oesophageal reflux.

6. D

The best way of determining the amount of acid reflux is 24-h oesophageal pH monitoring, in which pH is measured by a monitor at the end of a fine tube passed through the nose. If a motility disorder is suspected, the tube can also be used to measure the contraction and relaxation of the oesophagus via manometry. E may show visible oesophagitis or the oesophagus may appear normal, even in cases of significant reflux. C is rarely carried out in simple gastro-oesophageal reflux. A is of limited value in patients with reflux or dyspepsia.

7. B

The T (or tumour) stage relates to the depth of invasion in the intestinal wall; it is determined when a surgical specimen is examined by a pathologist. During investigation, B is the most accurate. A and D are helpful in determining the N (nodal) and M (metastases) stage. E is used to diagnose the tumour but visualises only mucosal structures. C confirms the diagnosis.

8. D

An oesophageal stent will rapidly improve this patient's dysphagia. Given her age, comorbidity and tumour stage, it may be the most appropriate definitive palliative treatment. B may be indicated as temporary support while she is awaiting the stent. A with or without C may be considered as palliative treatments, possibly in addition to D. An oesophagectomy would not be indicated for this patient, given her age, significant cardiorespiratory problems and metastatic disease.

9. A

Odynophagia can be caused by any of these conditions. Because this patient is immunosuppressed due to chemotherapy, A, B and D are possible, but candidiasis ('thrush') is much more common. Patients with candidiasis usually complain of a bad taste in their mouth, and white plaques may be visible in this area on examination. It is reasonable to treat empirically with an antifungal medication (e.g. fluconazole).

10. A

This is the finding in globus pharyngeus. B, C and E are all specific structural abnormalities that may be seen on barium swallow or OGD. D is a motility disorder that is more common in the elderly when there is a diffuse dysfunction; it can also be diagnosed by these investigations.

Stomach

1. A

The patient is young and there are no 'red flag' symptoms, so she does not require OGD at this stage. It would be reasonable to determine if there is persistent infection with *H. pylori*, because she is now symptomatic. Eradication regimens are about 90% effective. B will remain positive, probably for life, even after the infection has been cleared, so it is of value only as an initial test. A is the best test to determine *H. pylori* status. Stool antigen (not antibody) testing is also of value.

2. D

Unexplained iron deficiency in a man of any age or a woman who is not menstruating requires further GI investigation. It is deemed an 'alarm feature', because it may indicate chronic occult bleeding from a cancer. This patient's young age and symptoms would on their own not necessitate referral for OGD.

3. A

These symptoms strongly suggest dumping syndrome post gastrectomy. It occurs when food enters the intestine quickly from the gastric remnant, with resultant osmotic and other effects. If the symptoms were new, then it would be necessary to exclude E. The symptoms do not suggest C or D. B can cause similar problems in someone who has not had a gastrectomy.

4. C

This presentation suggests C. Pyloric stenosis can occur when ulcers in the distal stomach or duodenum cause fibrosis or scarring, sometimes resulting in gastric outlet obstruction. A, B and E are complications of gastric ulcers but present with different features; B is particularly rare. D is not a complication of gastric ulcers, because they do not become malignant, but gastric cancers can have ulceration by the time of diagnosis.

5. C

The combination of multiple peptic ulcers with no obvious cause together with diarrhoea and weight loss should prompt further tests to exclude Zollinger–Ellison syndrome. (The diarrhoea and weight loss are consequences of malabsorption because of the very acid environment in the small bowel.) Zollinger–Ellison syndrome is caused by a gastrinoma. Measurement of the fasting gastrin level, while not receiving PPIs, is indicated. B is a test for neuroendocrine tumours.

6. D

Up to 5% of gastric ulcers are malignant. Therefore it is essential that repeat OGD with biopsy is carried out after completion of treatment. This is not the case for duodenal ulcers, which are almost always benign. If the gastric ulcer has healed and the patient does not need to continue on non-steroidal anti-inflammatory drugs (NSAIDs), then the PPI can be stopped. Retesting for *H. pylori* is not routinely done for uncomplicated peptic ulcers unless the patient later becomes symptomatic, in which case a carbon urea breath test or faecal antigen is appropriate.

7. D

Options B, C and D are all indicated for *H. pylori* eradication (other PPIs can be used instead of omeprazole). However, B and C are contraindicated because of the history of penicillin allergy. For all patients, it is essential to ask about allergies when taking a history or issuing a prescription. A may relieve this patient's dyspepsia but will not treat the infection. E is a recognised second- or third-line treatment for *H. pylori* infection but is associated with a lower rate of adherence because of its adverse effects and poor palatability.

8. D

NSAIDs are common causes of dyspepsia as well as gastritis, erosions and ulcers. Remember that they can be purchased over the counter in supermarkets and pharmacies, so they need to be asked about specifically. A and other bisphosphonates can cause oesophageal ulceration and so should be taken with plenty of water while sitting upright. B, C and E can lead to dyspepsia and other abdominal symptoms but not visible inflammation.

9. D

These symptoms are most suggestive of functional dyspepsia. Some patients with functional dyspepsia will have symptomatic benefit from *H. pylori* eradication. It is reasonable to check D rather than B in someone who has not previously been treated for *H. pylori* infection. A minority of young patients with symptoms suggestive of functional dyspepsia require investigation with A or E, but both investigations are almost always normal. C is a test for younger patients with diarrhoea to determine if they have conditions such as inflammatory bowel disease.

10. A

This is a difficult scenario and requires careful discussion with the next of kin if the patient lacks capacity. The prognosis in a patient with reduced oral intake and advanced dementia is poor. Nastrogastric tubes and IV fluid cannulae are often pulled out in this scenario and are not a long-term solution. Percutaneous endoscopic gastrostomy (PEG) does not improve long-term survival and is associated with a significant 30-day mortality after insertion in dementia. A pragmatic approach is to allow the patient to eat and drink at risk, after appropriate speech and language assessment to guide the safest consistencies.

Small intestine

1. D

The symptoms and family history raise the possibility of coeliac disease. A and B are advised in cases of a weakly positive tissue transglutaminase antibody level or IgA deficiency only. C is used in the diagnosis of primary biliary cholangitis. E is reserved for use in specialist centres for patients who choose not to introduce gluten into their diet for diagnosis or who have had some gluten ingestion. The IgA level should be tested with anti-TTG antibodies, because IgA deficiency can lead to a false negative result and is more common in people with coeliac disease.

2. E

The source of bleeding is probably the small intestine in view of the normal OGD and colonoscopy. A, B and D are radiological investigations that would assess for only structural abnormalities. E is a non-invasive test that shows the mucosal lining of the intestine and is most likely to identify the site and cause of any bleeding points. C may also be used, but it is an invasive test and does not enable examination of the entire length of the small intestine in one go.

3. E

Current smokers have an increased risk of Crohn's disease. Smoking also has an adverse effect on its clinical course, with a poorer prognosis. Smoking cessation reduces the risk of disease relapse and recurrence after surgery. In contrast, smoking has a protective effect in ulcerative colitis. A, C and D may help the patient's general well-being but have no effect on the symptoms. B is likely to exacerbate the symptoms if a stricture is present.

4. B

Crohn's disease can affect any part of the GI tract, but it is most commonly identified in the distal ileum. Small bowel radiology may show evidence of ulceration and complications of Crohn's disease such as stricturing.

5. C

These blood test results show a macrocytic anaemia. This most commonly occurs as a result of vitamin B_9 (folic acid) or vitamin B12 deficiency. Vitamin B_9 (B) is absorbed in the proximal small intestine. Vitamin B_{12} (C) is bound by intrinsic factor to form a complex absorbed in the terminal ileum. Deficiencies of vitamins A, C and D do not result in a macrocytic anaemia.

6. B

All the answers are potential causes of diarrhoea. However, the main clue is that the symptoms started following a cholecystectomy. The gallbladder stores bile before it is released into the small intestine. Removal of the gallbladder can interfere with the recycling of bile salts, resulting in diarrhoea. Therefore answer B is most likely.

7. D

Adenocarcinoma and carcinoid tumours are the most common primary cancers affecting the small intestine. The combined symptoms of flushing diarrhoea and abdominal pain suggest carcinoid syndrome, which occurs because of the release into the circulation of serotonin and tachykinins from carcinoid tumours.

8. A

The increased faecal calprotectin level suggests ongoing gut inflammation. Prednisolone is not used as a long-term treatment, because it does not effectively maintain remission and due to its potential adverse effects, which include osteoporosis. C has a limited role in the treatment of Crohn's disease. D is best avoided in women of childbearing age because of the risk of congenital deformities and miscarriage. A step-up approach to treatment is usually used, first with azathioprine or mercaptopurine before progressing to biologic agents (e.g. infliximab).

9. B

Coeliac disease results in inflammation and damage to the endothelial villi, particularly affecting the duodenum and jejunum. During upper GI endoscopy, the endoscope is routinely inserted as far as the second part of the duodenum. Coeliac disease is diagnosed when biopsy samples taken from the second and first part of the duodenum shows increased intraepithelial lymphocytes and flattening of the villi. A, C and E are incorrect, because these are parts of the stomach, which is not affected by coeliac disease.

10. E

All the pathogens listed can cause malabsorption. The presence of periodic acid–Schiff–positive macrophages containing non–acid-fast Gram-positive bacilli is diagnostic of Whipple's disease. This condition is also much more common in men. Villous atrophy is usually present in B and C.

Large intestine

1. B

Antibiotic use increases the risk of *C. difficile* diarrhoea. It is also associated with PPI treatment. A, C, D and E usually occur after eating contaminated or undercooked foods.

2. B

In view of the presenting symptoms and family history, investigation of the entire large intestine is required. Therefore E is inappropriate as a single test, because it examines only the left side of the colon. A and D are suboptimal tests and should be used only to exclude significant colorectal pathology. Colonoscopy has advantages over CT pneumocolon: it allows polyps to be removed and samples of any abnormalities to be obtained for biopsy, without radiation exposure.

3. D

A and B are associated with the presence of hundreds to thousands of colorectal polyps. Hereditary intestinal polyposis syndrome (Peutz–Jeghers syndrome) causes benign hamartomatous polyps. The family history meets all of the Amsterdam criteria for hereditary non-polyposis colorectal cancer (Lynch's syndrome). The right-sided location of the cancer also supports this diagnosis. *MUTYH* polyposis is an autosomal recessive condition.

4. E

All the answers are potential complications of diverticular disease. However, the presence of gas under the diaphragm (subphrenic gas) indicates a perforation. A and D usually causes abdominal pain with or without pyrexia. A fistula may form between the bowel and bladder, vagina or other adjacent organ, presenting with passage of stool through

that structure. No symptoms of bleeding are reported; when it occurs it is usually fresh, red and mixed in with the stools, because the most common site over diverticulae are in the sigmoid colon.

5. D

A, C and E are forms of gastroenteritis but are not usually responsible for hospital outbreaks. Norovirus, which can be aerosolised and is highly infectious, is responsible for hospital outbreaks. B is unlikely in patients without risk factors, for example antibiotic use, and usually results only in diarrhoeal symptoms.

6. D

Because of the history of iron deficiency anaemia, an investigation is required to examine all the large intestine, so E would not be suitable. A, B and C require a full laxative bowel preparation and the ability to roll, so they would be difficult for this patient. In view of the patient's age and comorbidity, a minimal preparation CT would be most appropriate to exclude any significant colonic pathology.

7. C

The symptoms and positive stool test results indicate *C. difficile* diarrhoea. There are no features of severe infection, for example pyrexia, increased white cell count, evidence of severe colitis or an increasing creatinine level. A and B may increase the risk of *C. difficile* infection but are not used in its treatment. There is no strong evidence for D. Metronidazole is normally used for mild to moderate infection, because it is cheaper than vancomycin. However, vancomycin is preferred in severe disease because the clinical response is faster and the failure rate lower than with metronidazole.

8. B

The normal mucosal appearance at colonoscopy and thickened collagen plate on biopsy are consistent with collagenous colitis, a type of microscopic colitis. Budesonide is the treatment of choice in symptomatic patients. Mesalazine and immunomodulator drugs are occasionally used in the treatment of microscopic colitis but are more commonly used for inflammatory bowel disease.

9. B

The only abnormality detected at colonoscopy is in the rectum. The aims of surgery are to preserve the anal sphincter muscles, to prevent problems with faecal incontinence, and as much of the large intestine as possible. C and E do not include resection of the rectum. A includes removal of the anus and sigmoid colon, which is unnecessary in this case. D includes removal of the entire large intestine, which is not required.

10. B

The patient is showing features of acute severe colitis, with a stool frequency of more than six times daily, pyrexia and tachycardia. IV hydrocortisone is the initial treatment. This is escalated to ciclosporin or infliximab if there is failure to respond to hydrocortisone. E is used in the treatment of less severe presentations of ulcerative colitis and in patients who have responded to hydrocortisone. D is not used as an initial treatment in severe disease.

11. D

The overall risk of perforation during a diagnostic colonoscopy is quoted as about 1 in 1000 procedures. It may be lower for more experienced endoscopists. The risk of perforation is increased when therapeutic procedures such as polypectomy are carried out.

12. A

The review and adjustment of diet is generally the most helpful initial step in the management of abdominal bloating in a patient who is otherwise well and when other causes, for example ascites, have been excluded. The 'FODMAP' diet, in which the intake of fermentable sugars is reduced, is particularly helpful. Limiting consumption of carbonated drinks and excess fibre may also be beneficial. B is unlikely to help this patient. C is used for dyspepsia. E, for example domperidone, can be used in the short term as an antiemetic. The duration of symptoms makes pregnancy an unlikely cause, so D is unnecessary.

Liver disease

1. A

Non-selective beta-blockers, such as carvedilol or propranolol, are effective in both primary and secondary prevention of variceal bleeding. They decrease portal pressure by reducing cardiac output and causing vasoconstriction of the splanchnic arteries. B is used to treat alcohol misuse. C is used in the treatment of peptic ulcers but had no role in the secondary prevention of variceal bleeds. D is a diuretic used to treat ascites. E is a mucosal protector that can be used in the treatment of banding-induced oesophageal ulceration, although it has uncertain efficacy.

2. C

The prodromal symptoms and recent travel history are in keeping with hepatitis A. It is the most common form of hepatitis worldwide, with epidemics associated with poor hygiene and sanitation. The patient has no reported risk factors for hepatitis B or C, such as intravenous drug misuse. Hepatitis D can survive only in the presence of hepatitis B.

3. E

All these options may present with confusion in patients with known excessive consumption of alcohol or alcohol-related liver disease, but this patient has the classic triad of confusion, ataxia and ophthalmoplegia consistent with Wernicke's encephalopathy. Urgent treatment with IV thiamine is required to prevent progression to Korsakoff's psychosis, which is irreversible. Hypoglycaemia can occur because of the depletion of glycogen stores within the liver, and is easily overlooked.

4. C

The patient's bronzed skin, diabetes and family history of liver disease would be in keeping with a diagnosis of haemochromatosis. His heart problems may indicate a cardiomyopathy, which is another feature of the disease. Iron studies typically show a markedly increased serum ferritin, increased transferrin saturation and low total iron binding capacity. Diagnosis is confirmed with genetic testing for haemochromatosis. A and B are markers of autoimmune liver disease. D is a marker of glycaemic control in patients with diabetes. There are no risk factors to suggest hepatitis C (option E).

5. C

This is a cholestatic picture of abnormal LFT results, which is most likely related to her recent course of flucloxacillin. Medications such as antibiotics are frequent causes of abnormal LFT results in otherwise well individuals. No further investigation is needed, and liver function typically returns to normal within 2–3 months. Although this patient's obesity is a risk factor for non-alcoholic fatty liver disease (option E), this would typically cause a hepatocellular picture of abnormal LFT results. B would also cause a hepatocellular picture.

6. E

The results of the blood tests and genetic studies fit with a diagnosis of hereditary haemochromatosis. The aim of treatment is to reduce the body's iron stores. Therefore C and D would be inappropriate. A is an iron-chelating agent used as a second-line treatment if venesection is not tolerated, for example if the patient is anaemic or IV access is poor. One unit of blood contains about 250 mg of iron. Venesection is usually needed every 1–2 weeks for the first 6 months to remove the excess iron, and 2 or 3 units per year thereafter to maintain the level of ferritin within normal limits.

7. D

The cholestatic LFT results, increased IgM concentration and non-specific symptoms of tiredness and itching are typical of primary biliary cholangitis. The anti-mitochondrial antibody test result is usually positive. E can cause a similar pattern but is normally present in patients with inflammatory bowel disease and at a younger age. B causes a hepatitis (increased levels of transaminases rather than ALP) and increased IgG. There are no reported risk factors for A or C.

8. B

Positive surface antigen and e antigen results are in keeping with hepatitis B infection. The positive IgM indicates that this is an acute infection. IgM is replaced by IgG in chronic infection or carrier states. People who are vaccinated against hepatitis B are surface antibody–positive. A hepatitis A IgG–positive result indicates previous infection.

9. E

The cholestatic picture from the LFT results and the positive ANCA result are in keeping with primary sclerosing cholangitis (PSC). About 80% of patients with PSC have ulcerative colitis. A, C and E can all have a role in the investigation of abnormal liver function, but MRCP would be most useful. A characteristic bead-like pattern is produced by the multiple strictures throughout the bile ducts. D is used as a therapeutic rather than diagnostic tool, for example for dilating strictures or inserting stents. B provides no diagnostic information about the liver.

10. E

These findings are in keeping with a hepatocellular carcinoma. CT typically shows an enhancing lesion within the arterial phase, with washout in the portal phase. An α-fetoprotein concentration of > 400 kU/L is also highly suggestive. Liver metastases and other liver lesions are usually hypoattenuating (lower density).

11. D

An increased IgG concentration and positive smooth muscle antibody result would be in keeping with autoimmune hepatitis as the cause of this patient's abnormal LFT results. Immunosuppressants and steroids such as prednisolone are usually the first-line treatment. Azathioprine is often added as a steroid-sparing agent. A, B and C can be used but are not first line. B should be avoided in women of childbearing age, because of its teratogenicity. E is used in the treatment of primary biliary cholangitis.

12. B

The normal GGT level makes it unlikely that the excess ALP originates from the biliary tree. Increased ALP commonly has a bony cause, for example osteomalacia or Paget's disease. ALP can also be increased in the third trimester of pregnancy, but the patient's age makes this unlikely. Transaminases, i.e. ALT and AST, are present in skeletal and cardiac muscle.

13. B

If a patient with liver disease becomes acutely confused, encephalopathic or unwell with fevers, it is essential to determine the precipitant. The commonest causes are sepsis, electrolyte disturbance (e.g. uraemia or hyponatraemia), GI bleeding and medications (e.g. opiates). Spontaneous bacterial peritonitis is particularly common in this setting, so a diagnostic tap should always be carried out for white cell count and culture.

Pancreatic disease

1. E

B and D are used to investigate causes of diarrhoea; however, the description in this scenario is more suggestive of steatorrhoea (excess fat in the stool). The history of alcohol excess points towards chronic pancreatitis as the underlying cause. A, C and E can all be used to investigate the pancreas, but E is the most appropriate test; it is carried out to diagnose exocrine pancreatic insufficiency.

2. E

All the options listed potentially cause jaundice. The obstructive symptoms, i.e. the dark urine and pale stool, suggest a post-hepatic cause. E is the most common cause of painless obstructive jaundice. The patient's age and significant weight loss are further clues to suggest a more serious underlying pathology. A may present with similar LFT abnormalities but usually presents with pain.

3. A

This woman has acute pancreatitis. This is most commonly caused by gallstones, and if found, is an indication for cholecystectomy. Gallstones can be diagnosed by using A, C or E (and sometimes B if they are radiopaque). US is the most appropriate imaging modality for diagnosing gallstones, because it is readily available and does not use ionising radiation. C is used to look for complications, such as peripancreatic collections or pseudocysts. D is a crucial investigation in all those presenting with acute abdominal pain, to look for serious pathology such as a perforated viscus.

4. B

All the options listed can cause abdominal pain, but the acute symptoms and markedly increased serum amylase concentration point to B as the diagnosis. The LDH and corrected calcium concentrations are indicators of severity. E is unlikely to be a cause of the increased temperature and abnormal blood test results. D is the potential underlying cause for the acute pancreatitis.

5. C

All the options listed can result in acute pancreatitis. Gallstones are the most common cause, and the patient's age, sex, BMI and multiparity are all risk factors. There is nothing in the history to suggest other causes.

6. B

The clinical features and radiological findings support a diagnosis of pancreatic cancer. Treatment is palliative. The aim is to relieve the patient's jaundice; this can be achieved by ERCP and stent insertion. The presence of liver metastases, and the patient's age, means that E would be inappropriate. D is usually reserved for patients for whom ERCP has failed or is unsuitable. C would be unsuitable as a single treatment and because of the widespread nature of the cancer.

7. E

Each of these options has a role in the management of chronic pancreatitis, as suggested by the scenario. However, pancreatic enzyme supplements are likely to have the greatest effect in treating this patient's pancreatic exocrine insufficiency and thereby relieving his steatorrhoea. A is crucial in preventing further pancreatic damage and repeated attacks. About 50% of patients with pancreatic endocrine insufficiency will go on to develop diabetes.

Biliary disease

1. C

Pain, fever and jaundice, also termed Charcot's triad, are the clinical features of ascending cholangitis. This is usually caused by blockage of the biliary tree by gallstones, but it can also occur secondary to strictures. This patient has signs of sepsis and needs prompt treatment with IV antibiotics and ERCP to allow removal of the common bile duct stone and drainage of the biliary tree. No further imaging is necessary. A cholecystectomy is indicated in future to prevent repeated attacks.

2. A

These symptoms suggest cholangitis. Gallstones can cause obstruction at any level within the biliary tree. However, the features in this case are most commonly associated with a stone within the common bile duct. Stones within the gallbladder are usually asymptomatic. They can cause pain because of biliary colic or cholecystitis, but not jaundice. Rarely, jaundice can occur because of a stone impacted in the cystic duct, causing extrinsic compression and obstruction of the common bile duct; this is called Mirizzi's syndrome. E is normally a cause of chronic pancreatitis.

3. B

The clinical features suggest gallstones. The recurrent self-limiting nature of the attacks indicate biliary colic. This occurs as a result of intermittent obstruction of the cystic duct by a gallstone. A and D are caused by more prolonged blockage of the cystic duct. The pain is usually more persistent and may be accompanied by a fever and localised tenderness. Pain from E is usually epigastric and does not radiate to the shoulder.

4. D

Courvoisier's law states that in the presence of jaundice, a palpable non-tender gallbladder is unlikely to be caused by gallstones. It is usually an indicator of a pancreatic or gallbladder cancer. In this case, the signs of sepsis (fever, tachycardia and hypotension) make A and C less likely, and the absence of jaundice makes B less likely. An empyema is an uncommon complication of cholecystitis, in which the gallbladder becomes distended and filled with pus, usually causing a swinging fever and pain. A tender palpable gallbladder can occasionally be felt. E will often result in tender hepatomegaly.

5. **C**

The pain and cholestatic picture from the LFT results point towards biliary obstruction. This is probably secondary to a common bile duct stone. The patient is not jaundiced or haemodynamically unstable, so further imaging should be performed before considering any invasive intervention. MRCP is more sensitive and specific than E and avoids the use of ionising radiation. D is used as a therapeutic tool rather than as a diagnostic test. There is no indication for A or B at present.

6. **A**

With the exception of C, all the options listed can cause jaundice. The LFT results show an obstructive pattern, suggesting cholestasis. B typically presents with pain and fever. The significant weight loss points towards a more worrying aetiology, and the radiological findings are consistent with a cholangiocarcinoma with liver metastases. E also causes strictures, but these tend to be multiple and located throughout both the intrahepatic and extrahepatic biliary tree. It usually presents at a younger age (25–40 years) and is strongly associated with IBD.

Emergencies

1. **D**

When varices are the suspected cause of GI bleeding, IV terlipressin should be given soon after presentation; it lowers portal pressure which can stop the bleeding. It is also continued for 72 h after endoscopy. Broad-spectrum antibiotics, for example cefotaxime, should also be given in this scenario, because there is a high incidence of sepsis. IV omeprazole has a role in patients who have received endotherapy for bleeding peptic ulcers, for example by adrenaline (epinephrine) injection and other modalities. The value of tranexamic acid in upper GI bleeding is uncertain.

2. **B**

This scenario can occur in clinical practice, and it is not always possible to achieve haemostasis with adrenaline (epinephrine), clips, cautery or haemostatic spray at endoscopy. Interventional radiology with embolisation should be the next step, before surgery. The gastroduodenal artery supplies this region of the duodenum.

3. **D**

Prothrombin time is the most sensitive indicator of liver function. Both clotting factors and albumin are made in the liver and are indicators of liver synthesis; however, albumin has a much longer half-life, so it takes longer to reduce in cases of acute damage. AST and bilirubin will both be increased, indicating liver damage.

4. **D**

The increased prothrombin time indicates liver damage. *N*-acetyl cysteine should be administered: it is beneficial even 24 hours after a large paracetamol overdose. Charcoal will not be beneficial. Fresh frozen plasma is not given unless there is bleeding, because its use means that measurements of prothrombin time cannot be interpreted.

5. **A**

All these features may be present in cases of intestinal obstruction. Absolute constipation is usually associated with large bowel obstruction. Vomiting is the predominant symptom with proximal small bowel obstruction. It can be difficult to differentiate between large and small bowel obstruction on the basis of the history alone, so abdominal radiographs may be required.

6. **E**

This scenario strongly suggests acute intestinal ischaemia. This can occur as a result of thromboembolic events and is characteristically associated with an increased lactate level. Colonic ischaemia predominantly affects the 'watershed' areas. These have fewer vascular collaterals and occur at the borders of the territories supplied between major arteries, for example close to the splenic flexure between the superior and inferior mesenteric arteries.

Integrated care

1. **A**

In a premenopausal woman with iron deficiency anaemia, the most likely cause is menstrual blood loss. Coeliac serology should be checked. Unless there are any concurrent GI symptoms or a strong family history of bowel cancer, endoscopic investigations are not required in this setting. Dipstick urinalysis for microscopic haematuria is suggested if the cause remains unknown after GI investigations.

2. **D**

After appropriate dietary advice, including the recommendation to drink plenty of fluids, a stool softener or osmotic laxative is indicated. A polyethylene glycol–based product is often used. Stimulant laxatives are recommended for occasional use. Prucalopride can be used if trials of laxatives fail to help. Transanal irrigation is an option in significant ongoing constipation that has not responded to the above measures, as well as in defecatory disorders, in which biofeedback may also help.

3. C

A change of bowel function that is sustained, i.e. has lasted for > 6 weeks or so, is an alarm feature and therefore merits prompt investigation to exclude a structural cause, for example obstructing colorectal cancer. A colonoscopy would be the most appropriate investigation. A is a suboptimal test and can miss colorectal pathology. B and E should be carried out to look for causes of change in bowel habit; however, significant underlying pathology should always be excluded.

4. B

This scenario suggests 'non-alcoholic' fatty liver disease. This is more common in patients with type 2 diabetes, central obesity and hyper-cholesterolaemia. The other diagnoses should be considered and a liver screen carried out, together with an abdominal US. Treatment is to address risk factors and advocating weight loss, increased exercise.

5. B

Gilbert's syndrome is the commonest cause of an isolated hyperbilirubinaemia (it is predominantly unconjugated in nature). A similar pattern occurs with haemolysis, which is less likely. Abnormal LFT results would be expected alongside the increased bilirubin for all the other options. Mirizzi's syndrome is a rare condition where a stone in the cystic duct compresses the common bile or hepatic duct, thereby leading to jaundice.

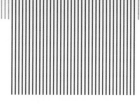

Index

Note: Page numbers in **bold** or *italic* refer to tables or figures, respectively.

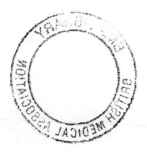